Fighting
CANCER

A Nontoxic Approach
to Treatment

ROBERT GORTER, MD, PHD,
and ERIK PEPER, PHD

for Noel with best luck
for disease-free biography

Robert 29.8.11

North Atlantic Books
Berkeley, California

Published by
North Atlantic Books
P.O. Box 12327
Berkeley, California 94712

Cover design by Suzanne Albertson
Book design by Brad Greene

Printed in the United States of America

Fighting Cancer: A Nontoxic Approach to Treatment is sponsored by the Society for the Study of Native Arts and Sciences, a nonprofit educational corporation whose goals are to develop an educational and cross-cultural perspective linking various scientific, social, and artistic fields; to nurture a holistic view of arts, sciences, humanities, and healing; and to publish and distribute literature on the relationship of mind, body, and nature.

North Atlantic Books' publications are available through most bookstores. For further information, visit our Web site at www.northatlanticbooks.com or call 800-733-3000.

Library of Congress Cataloging-in-Publication Data

Gorter, Robert, 1946-
    Fighting cancer : a nontoxic approach to treatment / Robert Gorter and Erik Peper.
      p. cm.
    Includes index.
    "Emphasizing the need for a new model of cancer treatment that nurtures the body's intrinsic cancer fighting mechanisms, Fighting Cancer presents an innovative, non-toxic approach to healing this rampant disease"—Provided by Publisher
    ISBN 978-1-58394-248-2
    1. Cancer—Immunotherapy. I. Peper, Erik. II. Title.
    RC271.I45G67 2011
    616.99'4061—dc22

                                                                2010039986

1 2 3 4 5 6 7 8 9 SHERIDAN 15 14 13 12 11

Table of Contents

Acknowledgments

This book has provided the opportunity to review thousands of the research studies and clinical trials that validate the therapies used in the Gorter Model. Developing the book has also involved a review of current theory on the human body's inherent anticancer mechanisms. In this context, the Gorter Model is designed to work synergistically with these immune defenses.

We both appreciate the contribution of our cross-cultural experiences. Being born in the Netherlands and training in the sciences in the United States and Europe, we feel that our international work has given us a more neutral point of view that extends beyond cultural belief and practice patterns. This viewpoint is reflected in a healthy skepticism toward traditional scientific beliefs and an openness to other perspectives that enhance health and quality and meaning of life. This book reflects our commitment to that exploration over the past three decades. It is also proof of our longtime collaboration and mutual trust—and our ethic to serve people who are in need.

We thank Jana Asenbrennerova for superb photography of our patients and the clinic. We thank Gary Palmer for his photography and support. We thank Dianne Shumay, who provided honest and critical feedback that made the book so much better. Finally, we thank our editor, Nancy Faass, whose in-depth review of the research literature contributed significantly to the manuscript.

—Robert Gorter, MD, PhD, and Erik Peper, PhD
  Cologne, Germany, and Berkeley, California

I wish to express gratitude for the opportunity to provide care over the past three decades for my patients, who have been highly conscientious in their use of the therapies and in working toward their own healing and personal development. Secondly, I want to express my great appreciation to the city of Cologne, which has selected our clinical center as a model program, from among more than a hundred medical facilities, as a destination health care program. And thirdly, I want to thank Erik Peper for his lifelong friendship and active support in documenting the protocol that has been the focus of much of my professional life's work.

Finally, I want to express my gratitude to Rudolf Steiner (the founder of anthroposophy), as without his spiritual science I would not have found the insight, strength, and inspiration to pursue as I did. I also thank all my colleagues and friends who through the many years have given support, knowingly and unknowingly, that has lead to the development of the Gorter Model.

—Robert Gorter, MD, PhD

My perspective about cancer evolved from researching in 1971 references documenting spontaneous remission of cancer to when my mother's identical twin sister developed breast cancer in 1995 and died the next year. My mother never developed breast cancer and died thirteen years later at the age of ninety-five. How could this be?

As I continue to read more and more about healing and treatment, I still cannot comprehend why nontoxic treatments are so often denied even if they act only as a placebo (which can have a significant success rate). Yet today extremely toxic substances and destructive procedures are commonly promoted as the only choice in cancer therapy. This also raises questions of efficacy and of malpractice. So often the medical culture implies that if a patient dies after surgery, chemotherapy, radiation, or hormone treatment, the health professional can state, "We did all we could have done." However, if the same patient died after treatment with unconventional medicine and without the extreme suffering, the practitioner would be called a quack and possibly be sued for malpractice because he or she did not follow standard care.

Acknowledgments

I thank my many students and clients who gave me the opportunity to collaboratively explore strategies to optimize health. I thank Rick Harvey for his ongoing support and for always being there to answer any question. The writing would not be possible without unconditional support and caring from my wife, Karen.

Most important, my twenty-year friendship with Dr. Robert Gorter resulted in my appreciation of his nontoxic immune-enhancing therapy to treat cancer. To create, develop, and implement the Gorter Model is a testament to his dedication and courage. I am sure that a hundred years from now, nontoxic immune therapy will be provided to patients at every stage of cancer. In the future, people will wonder what let our society continue toxic treatments without actively supporting immune therapy such as the programs developed by Dr. Robert Gorter.

—Erik Peper, PhD

Prologue

The path I am on now is so incredibly beautiful. I feel I have a free life surrounded with love and lovely things. I have learned to get rid of unimportant things in my life and have banished the things that once caused obstacles in my life. I have learned to forgive myself and have also forgiven others.... In coming to terms with moments and issues in my life, I have received bonus time. Every day is good and every moment is good.

Your life is not a rehearsal: Live Now. Enjoy. Now.

Carolien van Leusden, a forty-five-year-old mother who survived Stage IV metastatic breast cancer

You bought this book because you or someone you love has cancer. The dreaded word that stopped you in your tracks: Yes, deep inside you knew there was something wrong, and yet you hoped it was something else. Cancer can be a life-threatening illness, a chronic disease to live with, or a disease to be cured. It is a crisis, yet a crisis that is also an opportunity—an opportunity to live fully in whatever time is remaining. It is the opportunity to mobilize and support your own self-healing processes and optimize the medical treatments and integrative/holistic approaches to support your own healing.

This book describes the Gorter Model, an integrative approach to cancer treatment that mobilizes the immune system and that is currently offered at the Medical Center Cologne in Germany and elsewhere in Europe and the Middle East. The majority of patients receiving this treatment have experienced stabilization of their disease and improved quality of life. A number of Stage III and IV patients have had complete and sustained remission, documented by scans and other conventional testing. Some of these patients have been interviewed on video, and these documentaries are available at www.medical-center-cologne.com.

The following account is from Heinz Hagemeyer, a five-year survivor in total remission of Stage IIIb metastatic prostate cancer. This quote reflects his initial reactions to his diagnosis:

I was shocked when the doctor told me that my PSA level was too high.... I sensed that it was probably cancer. Of course I was devastated. I went to bed for three days. I couldn't get up, but couldn't stay there either.... I was just upset because of that stupid diagnosis, but why should I become depressed now? I decided to live a smarter life. At that moment I quickly jumped out of bed. I had just overcome the first obstacle on my path.

The first impulse is often to ask why, why me, why now? This question can be transformed to, "How can I listen to *myself* as well as to my health care providers and take action on my own behalf so that the time I have left has quality and not just quantity?"

The choices of treatments are daunting, and it is very difficult to assess whether treatment in any form will significantly prolong our lives or improve our quality of life. This is true whether it's a traditional medical approach, a holistic one, or no treatment at all. Despite all expert opinions, the evidence for healing strategies is often clouded, and the actual data tend to be ambiguous and unclear. Regardless of the seriousness of the prognosis, the specific type of cancer, or the probability of survival, there are numerous documented cases of remission and a total return to health for patients with all types of Stage IV cancers. Remission sometimes occurs even when the cancer has spread to other body organs and there is overwhelming metastasis and consequently a poor prognosis. There are always outliers, patients who receive a fatal prognosis and who somehow become completely better with treatment, without treatment, or despite treatment.

For the patient who has just received a cancer diagnosis, the future is unknown and unwritten. It is not clear when we receive the diagnosis whether we will live or succumb to the disease or the treatment's side effects. In some cases the surgical operation is a success, but the patient may not survive. In other cases, patients live with cancer as a chronic disease or have a partial remission. They may survive five years and thus be labeled cured even though they may later be diagnosed with a totally new cancer or a recurrence of the previous cancer—or they become cured and healthy. There is no guarantee of the future.

You can use the mental shock of the cancer diagnosis as an opportunity to make the present more meaningful. Consider it a chance to grow and focus those aspects of your life that give meaning and value whether you live one month, one year, or fifty years. Your illness is a time to ask, to give, to receive, and to experience love, self-respect, and support. The support and love of family and friends help protect you in the ongoing battle against cancer.

The healing journey is a challenging battle in which you want to listen to yourself, become attuned to your intuition and your inner voice, and act upon it. If it does not feel right, stop. Apply this equally to the opinions of your family, friends, and health care providers. Gather people around you who give you energy. If you feel drained by someone's presence, reduce contact with that person. Surround yourself with people and resources that nurture your spirit and increase your energy.

Do not follow either conventional medical or holistic health recommendations unless you feel that it is the right decision for *you*. As a patient, you will be flooded with suggestions and choices to make, and they may become overwhelming. The medical experts, integrative providers, and your friends and family members will all offer suggestions—for example, go to see the radiologist at Stanford, take 10 grams of vitamin C, or get acupuncture after you have chemo? Be open to exploring the options within and outside the traditional medical framework. Before acting on any of them, *stop* and listen to yourself. Make choices that are congruent with your values, not those of the people around you. Once we receive a cancer diagnosis, most of us become overwhelmed, and it's tempting to feel powerless. In some situations, we may feel infantilized. We wish to have someone else make it all right. Again *stop* and ask yourself, "Is this what I truly want to do?" Remember, your immune response will be more powerful if you make the choices than if you acquiesce to the demands of others. Whatever choice you make, do it fully and make it your own. Take your life into your own hands!

In many cases, the desire to recover from the illness implies returning to how you were before the illness occurred. You *cannot*, however, go backward and be as you were before the illness began. Healing is a dynamic, forward-moving process. You are your past, and the healing process is an opportunity to move forward and grow beyond the illness and the conditions that caused it. Make every day count. None of us know how much time we have. Regardless of how much time, aim toward becoming whole by embracing love, hope, and faith.

We recommend developing an openness to options that include medical as well as complementary and lifestyle treatment choices. There are many things you can do to support your own immune system and self-healing processes. Do the things that make you feel better, more grounded, and more energized! Many of the holistic health approaches to self-care are a helpful complement to treatment, and there is a surprising amount of research on integrative cancer treatment.

As Elizabeth Simpson wrote in the Canadian newspaper *The Globe and Mail*,[1] "Traditional cancer treatment says I have an 80% chance to die, holistic approaches say I have a 20% chance to live. I want to go for the 20%."

This book describes a comprehensive approach to cancer based on enhancing the immune system in the fight for health. It includes an overview, a description of the Gorter Model of treatment and the research behind the method, and strategies to support your own immune system. As you read the book and begin the self-care practices, you may find it helpful to view some of the video documentaries of patients who have gone through the Gorter Model treatment approach and have experienced total remission despite Stage IV cancer. Visit www.medical-center-cologne.com.

We encourage you to explore the additional books below to help you make lifestyle changes that support your health and your immune system. Each of these books offers an approach that will help you on this journey. At every step of your healing, you want to feel as supported, safe, and empowered as possible. Nurture yourself with healing foods, consciously manage stress, share and experience love, and live your dreams *now*.

We recommend the following resources:

Useful Sources
Documentaries about the Gorter Model

These videos include interviews with patients who have overcome cancer: www.medical-center-cologne.com/Documentaries.php

These documentaries were made by an independent nonprofit, patient-based foundation (www.kanker-actueel.nl) that, over time, followed cancer patients receiving the Gorter Model treatment. Their personal stories describe the treatment and the changes they made in their lives that resulted in complete and sustained remission of end-stage cancer.

General Perspectives

Servan-Schreiber, D. *Anticancer: A New Way of Life*. New York: Viking, 2009.
A superb description of how patients can contribute to their own care.

Nutritional Support

Beliveau, R., and D. Gingras. *Foods to Fight Cancer: Essential Foods to Help Prevent Cancer*. New York: DK Publishing, 2007.
Excellent overview and description of foods and herbs that help fight cancer and promote the immune system.

Regeneration and Stress Reduction

Peper, E., K. H. Gibney, and C. Holt. *Make Health Happen: Training Yourself to Create Wellness.* Dubuque, IA: Kendall-Hunt, 2002.

A sixteen-week structured stress-management and healing approach with detailed guided instructions that help us live with our bodies—a path that offers emotional, physical, and spiritual strength through changing our internal language, images, and somatic responses.

Kabat-Zinn, J. *Full Catastrophe Living.* New York: Delacorte Press, 1990.

Describes the basis of mindfulness mediation that is used with many patients. A very helpful manual that offers background information and practical exercises.

Singing Your Own Song and Finding Your Path

LeShan, L. *Cancer as a Turning Point.* New York: Plume, 1999.

Written by a master clinician using case studies to show how listening to yourself and doing what you truly want improves your quality of life and sometimes lead to remission of cancer. This outstanding book provides numerous useful practices.

Being Open to Possibilities and Listening to Yourself

Van Leusden, C. *My Path.* 2008. Available at www.carolienvanleusden.com.

This book is the inspiring emotional account of the journey of a patient using conventional medicine backed by complementary therapies and spiritual guidance. The book describes how she chose a path through the cancer nightmare of metastatic breast cancer and is still here to enjoy the Now.

Part I
ASKING QUESTIONS

●

Chapter 1

CHALLENGES IN THE WAR ON CANCER

Getting a second chance, getting the opportunity to live again, is something your mind can't handle. It really takes a while before you realize it's actually true. I am grateful to God. But there really are no words to express my gratitude.

HARMEN WAGENMAKER,[2] PATIENT WHO HAD END-STAGE CHOLANGIOCARCINOMA BUT HAS BEEN IN COMPLETE REMISSION FOR MORE THAN SIX YEARS SINCE BEING TREATED WITH THE GORTER MODEL

To tell patients that they have only a 10-percent chance of survival is to play God—no one actually knows or understands all the factors that contribute to recovery and healing. For the individual patient it is never a question of 10 percent. The patient recovers (complete remission), continues to live with the disease (partial remission or stability of the disease), or dies from the cancer or from complications of the treatment (described as progression).

Second-Guessing Cancer

In reality, our knowledge is relatively limited. We can almost never predict the exact outcome when cancer is diagnosed early, although the accuracy of the prediction does increase with the severity of the disease. There are patients who have recovered from every known cancer despite the gloomy statistics and are alive today, even when their condition appeared to be fatal.[3]

In 2005 Harmen Wagenmaker was diagnosed with inoperable end-stage bile-duct cancer (cholangiocarcinoma), with liver and pancreatic metastases, and with severe jaundice (icterus). He was given less than three months to live. The only intervention Harmen underwent at the university hospital of Utrecht in the Netherlands was the insertion of a stent to improve bile flow to the duodenum.

After eight months of nontoxic treatment with the Gorter Model at the Medical Center Cologne (MCC) to mobilize his immune system, Harmen returned to the hospital for a computed tomography (CT) scan. The scan documented a complete remission. Now, six years later, he is still in complete remission and continues to live a full and active life (see the video documentary available at www.medical-center-cologne.com):

At the end of August 2005, while I was on holiday, I was hospitalized and diagnosed with Stage IV liver cancer. There was nothing to be done. The cancer was already too far advanced for any chemotherapy or radiation.

When I heard that my life was over, I decided to go to Cologne to see Dr. Gorter. He told me, "I can't make you better. But maybe the treatments will catch on. That will extend your life for a while, and with this therapy you'll have a good quality of life."

The Approach of the Gorter Model

This book describes the Gorter Model, a clinical approach to immune therapy that has been used to successfully treat cancer in thousands of patients, most of whom have had end-stage (Stage IV) disease. In numerous cases, this treatment has not only induced remission (i.e., stopped the progression of the cancer) but has also brought about complete remission for as long as nine years. In practically all of these cases, once complete remission was achieved, the cancer never returned.

The treatment consists of pro-healing therapies that support immune response and enhance other self-healing functions in the body. There is a growing body of research on this type of approach to cancer treatment. Thousands of studies have documented the safety and efficacy of the therapies used in the Gorter Model.

There are many unknown factors that contribute to recovery and survival from a cancer diagnosis. The Gorter Model was developed by Robert Gorter, MD, PhD, who himself recovered from Stage IV testicular cancer (poorly differentiated germ-cell carcinoma) in 1976 by using nontoxic treatment—that is, without the use of chemotherapy or radiation. Thus, this model is based on self-experience, extensive research, and decades of clinical experience.

The Gorter Model includes a number of medical interventions to enhance immune function, primarily therapeutic fever (fever-range, total-body hyperthermia), localized hyperthermia, a form of inoculation using immune cells (dendritic cell vaccination) to "restart" or improve immune activity, and other immunity-enhancing approaches such as nutrient infusions and trace elements. In this chapter, descriptions of the treatment are drawn from interviews with Harmen Wagenmaker. Accounts from other patients are also included throughout the book. As Harmen describes,

> *For the first six months I received fever therapy every month, then twice every three months, and then every six months, always in combination with vaccination with injections of dendritic cells. Fever is induced, and your heart is monitored carefully. This treatment lasts three to four hours. I also received an IV each time with vitamin C and selenium. I was only given nontoxic natural substances—nothing that would tax my body.*

The model can be used alone, as is usually the case, or in combination with conventional cancer treatment. Ideally, in the future this form of nontoxic therapy will be offered as the first-line treatment approach when patients are initially diagnosed, rather than as the last resort when traditional cancer treatments have been unsuccessful.

Expanding the Continuum of Care

We believe that there is value in expanding the conventional model of cancer treatment, which focuses primarily on destroying cancer cells that are already present. We recommend that the treatment model be broadened to nurture the body's intrinsic cancer-fighting mechanisms. This means providing additional support for the immune system, reducing stress (physical and emotion patterns that suppress the immune system), and minimizing toxic exposures (such as cigarette smoke, occupational hazards, environmental toxins, and some forms of estrogen and other endocrine disregulating substances). The protocol also emphasizes a healthy lifestyle and psychological healing. As Harmen notes,

I never paid any attention to my health, and I'd been neglecting myself. I used to eat everything in sight—I love great food. Now I've willingly started to limit what I eat to healthier foods. I also make it a point to live as positively as possible—that's part of my recovery.

Approximately 96 percent of the 3,500 patients treated at the MCC come to the center with a diagnosis of Stage IV (terminal) cancer. To date, fewer than 4 percent of all patients have entered treatment with a Stage III diagnosis. Because the therapies used in the Gorter Model have only about thirty-five years of research behind them, we initially limited our caseload to patients who had no further treatment options and no hope of survival.

The Gorter Model involves at least two fundamental processes: (1) medical procedures to treat cancer and (2) therapies to mobilize and improve immune function. In terms of mind-body factors, of the patients we see, the most successful are very conscious of their decision-making processes and actively embrace their illness as a motivation to create healthier, more meaningful lives. Patients make the most of the treatment and also follow a healthier lifestyle. At the same time, they tend to accept and embrace their illness as an opportunity to live a more meaningful, purposeful life.

Patient Outcomes

As just mentioned, nearly all of the patients who have sought care at the MCC have come to the center with an initial diagnosis of terminal disease with no remaining therapeutic options. They thus considered the MCC to be their last hope. Nevertheless, 380 patients have achieved complete remission. Depending on the type of cancer, the remission rates have averaged 18 percent for malignant melanoma, 22 percent for breast cancer, and 48 percent for brain tumors (Stage IV glioblastoma multiforme). In cases of far-advanced forms of metastatic prostate cancers with a Gleason score of 9 or 10, 14 percent of patients experience complete and sustained remission.[4]

At the MCC, partial remissions were seen in roughly 60 to 70 percent of all cancer patients with solid tumors who had received at least three vaccinations with dendritic cells. Many of these remissions lasted for five years or more. Of the hundreds of patients treated with the Gorter Model who experienced complete remission, there has not been any reoccurrence (with three exceptions, all of whom were persistent smokers).

The average complete remission rate of 48 percent for patients with primary brain tumors (such as Stage IV glioblastoma multiforme) is impressive. This outcome is remarkable because the one-year survival rate for conventional treatment (radiation in combination with Temodal) is 28 percent of patients—and only 1 percent of patients survive for three years.[5]

Currently there are hundreds of patients treated for cancer using the Gorter Method who are still alive five or more years later. Generally, these patients have lived significantly longer than their statistical prognosis, and they have experienced an improved quality of life without the debilitating side effects of toxic therapy. As mentioned previously, patients who show the best response have received at least three vaccinations with dendritic cells and are active participants in their own healing processes.

Clinical Documentation

Patients routinely receive examinations, blood work, and scans at the medical centers in their own communities or countries. This serves as a form of "third-party verification" of the efficacy of treatment with the Gorter Model. Even patients who do not go into complete remission at the MCC frequently survive three times longer than their projected life expectancy and usually experience enhanced quality of life. As Harmen notes,

> *Six months after I began the treatment, I had a scan done. There was no longer any cancer in the liver. Nothing at all! Nothing bad! In general that just doesn't happen. Another scan was done four months later. Again there was nothing on the scan. A third scan was done, and when I heard that there was nothing on the scan or in the blood, I thought,* I'm going to be OK.

The Need for New Models of Treatment

Cancer is on the rise worldwide—and it continues to be lethal. Today, about 50 percent of all people in Europe and the United States will be diagnosed with cancer, and about 70 to 80 percent of all these people will eventually die of the disease. This is true despite the fact that most will be diagnosed early on and will receive all possible forms of therapy directed at killing or eradicating the cancer cells. Surprisingly, death rates for cancer have not improved significantly in the past fifty years.[6]

There are a few rare successes, such as treatment for certain forms of testicular cancer and for specific types of chronic leukemia (myeloid leukemia). However, the war against cancer initiated by President Nixon in 1971 has not reduced the number of fatalities. Nor has it reduced the percentage of the population that contracts cancer. This implies that the fundamental treatment model merits reevaluation.

Stalemate in the War against Cancer

The general perception today is that mainstream medicine has been quite successful in treating cancer. Health professionals, the media, and the public all believe that if we spend enough money, we will be able to find the cure for cancer. Yet despite the annual expenditure of more that $100 billion by the National Cancer Institute since 1971, and at least an equal amount by pharmaceutical companies, data show that nearly the same percentage of people are dying now as in 1950, as shown in figure 1.1.[7]

Over the past fifty-six years, the death rate from cancer has decreased by only about 7 percent. In contrast, heart disease and stroke death rates have decreased by 66 and 76 percent respectively due to changes in diet, medication, and other forms of treatment. Bacterial pneumonia used to be another deadly disease. However, with the advent of improved diagnostic procedures and appropriate antibiotics, this is now a highly treatable condition.

Figure 1.1. Leading cause of death of all ages. Note that there has been almost no change in cancer death rates over the last fifty-five years, unlike heart disease and stroke. Data adapted from the National Vital Statistics System, CDC/NCHS, Health, United States, 2009, Figure 18.

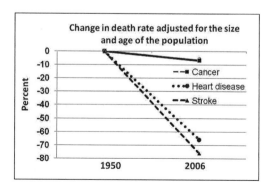

The 7-percent decrease in cancer in the last fifty-six years suggests that the fundamental model of treatment may be an incomplete approach. Most likely this decrease in the cancer death rate is due to changes in lifestyle such as the reduction in smoking. The drop in the number of cigarette smokers has had a greater impact in reducing lung cancer and other forms of cancer than has any known treatment strategy.

Although we are taught that mammogram screening reduces the death rate due to breast cancer, the research data are much more ambiguous.[8] Despite early diagnosis, the outcome of metastatic breast cancer has not improved, even with aggressive and destructive treatment approaches. As with other forms of cancer, the primary treatment strategies are to cut it out with surgery, burn it out with radiation, destroy it with chemotherapy, or block it with hormone treatment.

Today, the five-year survival rate of metastatic breast cancer is about 20 percent. This means that of every five women with metastatic breast cancer, only one will survive five years.[9] It may even be possible that the aggressive treatments increase the cancer death rates because general anesthesia, chemotherapy, and radiation all act as carcinogenic agents, suppress immune function, and disturb the body's inherent and natural cancer defenses. This also means that the immune system becomes less able to cope with new cancer cells that spontaneously develop once treatment is completed. Research has shown that patients who receive chemotherapy and radiation (or radiation exposure via multiple CT scans) are much more likely to develop another cancer in their lifetime, often within the next few years.

Innovation Rather than Incremental Change

Recent improvements in conventional cancer therapies reflect incremental changes in surgical techniques, diagnostic procedures, radiation, chemotherapy, new patented pharmaceuticals, and treatment protocols. These are all procedures embedded within an incomplete paradigm.

What is needed is a new and broader perspective that will offer a significant decrease in death rates.

Generally, clinical improvements, like cultural changes, do not occur incrementally—they occur as large, tectonic shifts. For example, in the early nineteenth century nearly 25 percent of women who delivered their babies in hospitals died from childbed fever due to sepsis caused by strep bacteria *(Streptococcus pyogenes)*. In the 1840s, the Viennese physician Ignazius Semmelweis observed that women in the maternity wards who were treated by medical students had death rates that were three times higher than women in wards staffed by midwives. He hypothesized that the medical students were carrying infection directly from the autopsy room to the women in labor. He then ordered the students and physicians to wash their hands with chlorinated solution before and between examining patients. This resulted in a major drop in the death rate to less than 1 percent for the women in labor, a twenty-five-fold decrease in mortality.

Many other innovations were essentially unrecognized at the time yet have radically changed the world in which we live. Think of the impact of water purification, lasers, the computer, the air conditioner, the electric light bulb, and the internet. Each went unrecognized as a significant change and yet totally transformed human capacity. These unexpected events are labeled "black swans" by Nassim Nicholas Taleb in his remarkable book *The Black Swan: The Impact of the Highly Improbable*.[10] It is the highly improbable that is always seen as obvious in hindsight. In the example of the physicians who did not wash their hands after performing autopsies, hand washing was the unusual, highly improbable factor that had a major impact on the transfer of contagious diseases.

Another example of the effect of innovation on medicine is the accidental rediscovery of penicillin in 1928 by the British bacteriologist Alexander Fleming. This occurred with the realization that staph bacteria *(Staphylococcus aureus)* could be destroyed by the mold *Penicillium notatum*.

The same observation had been made earlier in 1896 by a French medical student, Ernest Duchesne. However, the medical applications of this discovery were not recognized until the 1940s, when Howard Florey and Ernst Chain isolated the active constituent and developed a powdered form of the medicine. In the case of antibiotics, once the initial discovery had caused a radical change in perspective, ongoing incremental changes occurred. The first antibiotics were modified, and new antibiotic drugs were developed to improve clinical outcomes.

However, it was the initial shift in perspective—the realization of the effectiveness of antibiotics in destroying bacteria—that had the greatest impact. The analogy is similar in the field of transportation. The radical shift occurred with the development of the internal combustion engine and the car. It totally changed and replaced the horse-drawn transportation system. The conceptual change was the invention of the car. A series of smaller incremental improvements made cars more usable and more comfortable. However, the initial invention at the beginning of the twentieth century was the ground-shifting event, which was underappreciated at the time.

As with the discovery of penicillin, we propose that the discovery of a more comprehensive nontoxic approach to the treatment of cancer has probably already been discovered and rediscovered multiple times. The research bears this out.

The therapeutic application of induced fever (hyperthermia) was used successfully at Memorial Sloan-Kettering Hospital in the 1870s by William Coley.[11] Hyperthermia was further explored by Charles Kettering (cofounder of the Sloan-Kettering Cancer Center and vice president of General Motors), who designed the first hyperthermia chamber. Today, more than 1,700 research papers have been published on clinical trials of induced hyperthermia (both total-body and localized hyperthermia). Hyperthermia has been studied by American researchers from the Mayo Clinic to the University of Texas, as well as throughout Europe, in Japan, and worldwide.[12] This is a nontoxic cancer treatment approach that has the potential to create a paradigm shift in the fields of medicine.

The Origin of Aggressive Cancer Treatment

The current approach to cancer treatment is based on research published in *Cell Pathology* in 1859 by Rudolf Virchow, a professor of pathology at the Charité Hospital of the University of Berlin in Germany (see figure 1.2). Virchow had studied cancer extensively under the microscope. He observed that cancer cells are abnormal and have the capacity to grow quickly and massively, destroying healthy tissue and leading to the death of the patient. He then postulated that the most logical treatment for cancer would be to rid the body of these destructive cells. All current *anti*cancer therapies originate from this concept—to kill the cancer cells by all means possible.

The same concept underlies much of current medical treatment: *anti*biotics, *anti*hypertensive medication, *anti*depressants, and *anti*-inflammatory medications all describe the common framework for fighting disease. The treatment is viewed from a single perspective: to oppose the process. Antibiotics, for example, are prescribed worldwide, with prescription levels in the billions over the course of a decade. These medications are given without usually asking how the body's own immune system could have been mobilized to fight the disease apparently caused by bacteria.

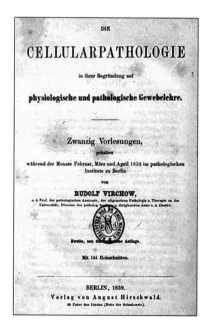

Figure 1.2. Rudolf Virchow, *Cell Pathology*, 2nd ed., 1859 (in German)

13

The current approach to cancer treatment is to aggressively destroy the cancer in the hope that after this assault, the body will be able to regenerate and reestablish a vibrant new state of being. However, in many cases what remains is a crumbling infrastructure in a dysfunctional state whose survival is uncertain.

To draw an analogy from military experience, we know that to win a war, you have to nurture and support the civilian infrastructure and not just destroy the enemy. The remarkable recovery of Germany and Europe and the establishment of democracy after World War II were not the result of the destruction during the war, but of the massive financial investment of the Marshall Plan by the United States. In the process of rebuilding nations from the ruins of war and embracing the previous enemies (Germany and Japan), everyone benefited. A similar approach is needed for the treatment of cancer—not just the destruction of harmful cells, but also a fundamental support for the healing infrastructure of the body. The same paradigm—a focus on the body's own healing forces—can be applied to the prevention of cancer as well.

Engaging the body's own healing mechanisms and protective functions expands the capacity for healing tremendously. A combative approach is only part of the solution. Again, the analogy can be made with warfare. Most wars are lost if you only fight *against* something. To win you have to have the population on your side and fight for a positive good. Guerilla warfare can be successful against overwhelming military odds if the guerillas are fighting for a highly positive goal such as independence.

Killing cancer cells may be only part of the solution. The current focus on fighting, killing, removing, or inhibiting cancer cells usually means opposing the biological systems of the body. Almost all cancer treatments are designed to oppose or destroy the "bad cancer cells," but doing so also damages many normal cells in the body. This is true of chemotherapy, radiation, surgery, and antihormonal medications that block estrogen or testosterone.

Even if there were a magic chemotherapy that would kill all cancer cells on a given day, in the real world thousands of new cancer cells would emerge within a few days. It is a known scientific fact that cancer cells appear by the thousands every day in every animal and human being on the planet, in response to our environment. Thus, it is a half-truth, an illusion that the cure of cancer lies in the killing of cancer cells.

Introducing Immune Therapy

Although most people don't realize it, cancer cells are being formed in all inner organs all the time, even in health-conscious people who eat organic food and take daily antioxidants and fish-oil supplements. However, when we're healthy, there is an ongoing balance between the spontaneous development of new cancer cells and our bodies' immune activity to identify and eliminate the newly formed cancerous cells as rapidly as possible.

What is being overlooked in this war against cancer are the inherent prohealth processes within our bodies. These processes are present in all of us, and they are active all the time in any healthy individual—our immune defenses protect most of us from cancer, most of the time. The body recognizes deviant cells that have become cancerous, and an empowered immune system effectively destroys these deviant cells.

A paradigm shift always requires patience. Today, the primary approach to treatment is through the use of pharmaceuticals, radiation, and surgery. It will take time before a new paradigm is implemented because of the belief system firmly implanted in the minds of health care providers and the public alike. In addition, changes are often resisted because of economic interests of medical equipment manufacturers and the pharmaceutical industry—what would happen to all the mammography clinics or radiation equipment if the current approach were superseded by immune-supportive approaches?

This inflexibility has been shown in the treatment for heart disease. Insurance companies reimburse customers for bypass surgery to treat coronary heart disease but often do not pay for Dean Ornish's lifestyle programs, which have demonstrated actual reversal of coronary heart disease at significantly lower cost.[13] In another example, doctors prescribe antihypertensive medication because they often do not have the time to teach patients the lifestyle changes that would reduce their hypertension without medication.

Our perspective focuses on a continuum of therapeutic approaches. This means not only aggressive cancer treatments that reduce the growth of malignant cancer cells but also supportive treatments that maximize the self-healing potential of the body. The goal is to engage regenerative processes, strengthen the patient's own immune system, and restore the ability to continuously eliminate abnormal cells.

A Note to the Reader

If you have cancer, want to prevent cancer, or want to restore your immune system, this book describes the philosophy and treatment approach of a very successful nontoxic therapy for cancer. It consists of supporting the immune system through therapeutic fever and inoculation with immune cells, as well as the use of botanicals and supportive nutrients. The model also encourages patients to mobilize their own self-healing potential through a healthy lifestyle.

This approach strengthens the body's natural immune processes to support a better quality of life, increased physical energy, and greater well-being, with none of the negative side effects of more toxic forms of treatment. Almost all patients using the Gorter Model outlive their prognosis and experience tangible increase in quality of life. In numerous cases, Stage IV patients have experienced complete and sustained remissions of their disease and have achieved ten-year survival. These success stories are presented in video documentaries in which patients tell their own survival and remission stories. These video documentaries, which can be viewed at www.medical-center-cologne.com, have been made by a Dutch patient-based nonprofit foundation (www.kanker-actueel.nl). We look forward to the day when this treatment is available to every cancer patient and provides the foundation for public health cancer prevention and education. In the words of Harmen Wagenmaker,

I've been cancer-free for more than five years. My energy is back. I'm living my normal life, I'm making music, I'm painting. I do have to take better care of myself now. I have to rest more, but I feel great. I look healthy, and I can do everything I could before. I have my life back. What more could anyone want?

Chapter 2

QUESTIONS I WISH
I HAD ASKED

When I had melanoma, I wish someone had stopped me right after my first surgery and asked, "What are the data on the risks and benefits of a second surgery? Is this second surgery really necessary? What can you do to mobilize your immune system and your health?"

ERIK PEPER

Both authors have been through the experience of cancer and its aftermath. Years later, we still remember the tremendous impact of that initial diagnosis.

In Dr. Robert Gorter's case, he developed germ-cell carcinoma (called poorly differentiated "teratocarcinoma" in those days) at age twenty-six. At the time of diagnosis, the carcinoma had spread throughout his body, and he was diagnosed as having Stage IV. As he notes,

At that time, I decided not to reveal my end-stage cancer diagnosis to prevent being stigmatized as having a fatal disease, and thus being shunned by others. Instead of focusing on the disease, I put all my energy into building a professional career.

As a practicing physician, knowing that chemotherapy and radiation would inflict massive toxic side effects without much hope of a prolonged life expectancy, I decided to decline these options. Instead, I initiated immune therapy to restore the anti-cancer defense mechanisms in my body. I decided to administer mistletoe (Viscum album) *injections, a widely respected plant-derived medication used in Europe for over eighty years, and therapeutic fever (fever-range, total-body hyperthermia). It took me about one year to achieve complete remission. It has now been thirty-seven years ago since I was given that end-stage cancer diagnosis, and I continue to live all these years to the fullest without any signs or symptoms of cancer.*

In Erik Peper's case, he developed melanoma thirty years ago and had two surgeries, which were successful. He explains,

When I developed melanoma, I had surgery to remove the skin cancer. The surgery successfully removed all the cancer. The edges of the incision (the "margins") were totally clear and cancer-free. However, because it was melanoma, the doctor indicated that a second surgery was necessary: "We should remove another two inches around the edge."

Knowing what I do today, I would have asked about the absolute benefits of a second surgery. Of every hundred patients who get melanoma, how many develop a recurrence after the first surgery? How many melanoma patients benefit from a second surgery? Based on the data, today I would probably decline that second procedure.

Another question I wished I'd asked is, "How can I boost my own immune system?" But that question never came up. The timeline and the procedures seemed like a foregone conclusion, automatic. The surgeon simply said, "Come back in two weeks, and we'll do it again."

Drawing both on our clinical experiences as working health professionals and on our own life experiences, we would like to offer some perspectives on the options available to cancer patients, which include coping with a cancer diagnosis, dealing with stress, asking for a second opinion, and getting the best information possible. Rather than viewing your initial diagnosis as a firm prognosis, consider it the first step.

Even if you have Stage IV cancer, the essential question is "What can be done about it?" This is important. Cancer is challenging to predict—sometimes chemotherapy or radiation seems to reduce the cancer load, and the patient appears healthy again. However, for many patients the cancer soon comes roaring back with a vengeance. It is possible that, in some cases, the patient may have lived longer and with a better quality of life had there been no treatment at all. In other cases, despite all interventions, the person dies.

It is vital to carefully review all the treatment options available and explore which therapies are right for you. Before you begin any treatment, discuss the following with your health care provider:

- If I do this treatment, how will my quality of life be different compared with no treatment?
- How would treatment affect my condition compared with only palliative treatment for pain?
- How much longer will I live if I received the treatment versus opting not to have the treatment?

The goal of the book is not to offer false hope, but to expand perspectives and offer scientifically legitimate resources and approaches to medical treatment that can be explored. This information is provided to stimulate intelligent, respectful dialogue.

Coping with a Cancer Diagnosis

When we get a cancer diagnosis or have a heart attack, even the strongest among us are terrified. Yet how we respond at a time like this—and the decisions we make—may affect the rest of our lives. It's tempting to lapse into panic or pure fear, like a deer caught in the headlights. Often patients go into a kind of emotional shock. We may begin to "disassociate"—going numb or lapsing into denial. It's understandable that we may feel a little helpless at times, and that we fear death.

However, it's important to resist that train of thought. If we accept the first diagnosis as final and consider cancer a death sentence, we are less likely to explore other options. Even if one is near the end of life, a negative mind-set could result in decisions that sacrifice quality of life to buy a little bit of time. Whatever the case, you want to gently work with your thoughts so you can bring yourself back to a more centered state of mind. Make time in the midst of the furor to think what *you* really want.

It can be difficult to stay objective at a time like this—difficult for the patient, the family, and even for the health care provider. We all slip into our own mental comfort zones, back to our core beliefs, for better and for worse. Patients may feel as if they're in the eye of a tornado—everyone around them is telling them what to do, which makes it hard to sit back, stop for a moment, and ask, "What are the actual facts here? What are the data? What is the reality?"

Cancer Is a Twenty-Year Disease

By the time cancer becomes diagnosed, it has usually been present (undetected) for at least five to ten years. Cancers are usually diagnosed when they are growing rapidly and have become so large they can be felt by touch (what doctors call palpation). Yet patients are often encouraged to make quick decisions about their treatment, even when the cancer is not life-threatening—despite the fact that the tumor has been growing in their body for years and years.

Giving Yourself Time for Decision Making

Although your condition may be treated as an emergency, in most cases you have time to make a careful, considered decision. Often the cancer is discovered by accident. Under other circumstances, it might not have been discovered for months or even years. This means that when you are diagnosed, unless you have a condition that is immediately life threatening, you have more time to make decisions than you realize. Clearly, there are always exceptions, but this gradual progression is true in the majority of cases. The following chart (table 2.1) shows the rate of doubling for cancer cells.

Cancer is a Slow-Growing Disease

9 days – 2 cells

1 year – 16 cells

2 years – 235 cells

3 years – 4,096 cells

4 years – 65,536 cells

5 years – 1,048,576 cells

6 years – 16,777,216 cells

7 years – 268,435,456 cells

8 years – 4,294,967,296 cells

Table 2.1. Progressive growth of cancer

In cases of breast cancer, for example, there must be four to ten billion cancer cells present before they can be detected with mammography. So, although a cancer diagnosis seems like a crisis situation, you usually still have time for a careful decision. Give yourself that time.

The Fast Track to Treatment

When we're diagnosed with a serious illness, often we feel as if we're on a speeding train. It's difficult to process everything that is happening to us. In many cases we're moved into a high-speed treatment path that begins with a brief discussion and then a series of appointments, diagnostic procedures, and interventions that may not be clearly explained or more often not clearly understood.

In the process, we receive a series of unspoken messages. The rapid move from discussion to the appointment calendar implies that there is only one approach to treatment. The doctor's recommendation for treatment also conveys the unspoken message, "If you do this treatment, you have a chance of surviving." The other part of the unspoken message is, "If you don't do it immediately, you'll die sooner."

Throughout the decision-making process, we each have to deal with our own mortality. We're trying to cope with issues that are almost too much to grasp, and too overwhelming. The fact that our doctor, a well-trained Western physician, is having us scheduled for a series of immediate treatments gives the impression that this is the most effective approach to treatment, without question.

Yet the actual research and long-term follow-up data on treatment are often not as clean and clear as we would wish. At times the only benefit is for the short-term, rather than the long-term. Many patients endure intensive treatment and gain just a few weeks or months of life expectancy. In some cases, the drugs kill the patient before the disease does. For those Stage III or IV patients who survive the complete chemotherapy cycle, 70 to 90 percent experience a recurrence of their cancer, often within three to nine months. If you think about everyone you've ever known with cancer, you may find examples of this in your own experience.

When I was diagnosed with intestinal cancer, the tumor was surgically removed, and the report indicated that it had not spread. But six months later, secondary tumors were found in my liver, and they were not operable. We got a second opinion from a large hospital in a nearby city— they indicated that chemotherapy was necessary, but we later learned that there were other treatments that they had not told us about.

By autumn, the prognosis was bad. I tolerated the chemotherapy well but was told that the liver cancer was not responding and was not curable. So we made an appointment for a consultation in Cologne. We found that Dr. Gorter's treatment could be done in combination with chemotherapy, so we decided to do that. We also discussed this treatment with our oncologist. He said, "If I were in your shoes, I wouldn't know what to do." He understood that we were looking for more options.

TRUUS KLEIJ-SWAN, FIVE-YEAR SURVIVOR OF COLON CANCER
WITH MULTIPLE METASTASES IN LIVER, LYMPH NODES, AND
PERITONEUM WITH IMPROVED AND STABILIZED DISEASE,
TREATED WITH THE GORTER MODEL

Dealing with Stress: What You Can Do

When we receive the diagnosis, we're tempted to move into panic—essentially the *stress response,* and stress inhibits healing. In the simplest terms, the role of "flight or fight" is to get us to safety—so we can run for dear life or stand in our defense (rather than thinking of a saber-toothed tiger, think of being pursued by an angry, rabid dog). In the process of mobilizing to run or fight, the body switches into a highly streamlined mode. Any function that isn't absolutely essential to our survival is shut down. This includes digestion and immune function. We only reactivate these functions later when we've reached a place of safety and can relax. Then the immune system kicks back in, into the *regeneration response,* so we can rest, restore, and heal. (See Part III for more information on coping with stress.)

So as long as we are in the stress response—especially chronic stress reaction—the immune system tends to be inhibited.[14] When patients receive a diagnosis such as cancer or AIDS, many go into a state of stress, and the immune system "turns off." Even those who have been doing quite well, up to this point, tend to do poorly from then on. It's vital that we not give in to that fear, but really work with it. The immune system is ultimately our first line of defense against cancer. If we want to beat the cancer and retain our day-to-day quality of life, it is essential that we stay in a calm mode and keep stress at a minimum.

Stress Blanks Out the Mind

The following brief exercise will give you the sense of how fear affects us all.

Quickly wrap your arms around your chest (hug yourself) in a protective gesture. Tighten your stomach muscles, gasp, open your eyes wide, and arch your back as if recoiling from danger. Breathe rapidly and shallowly. Stay this way for a moment without moving.

Now take a moment to think about your response—most people find that their thinking stops and that they blank out. In a state of fear and self-protection, it's almost impossible to really listen and make decisions. Yet often this happens in a more subtle form when we hear the diagnosis, "You have cancer." For our bodies, this is a signal that our survival is threatened. When that happens, we regress to our most basic reflexes: to fight, to run, to freeze, or to hide.

The instinct to hide or withdraw may be the most basic of all responses. In the face of danger, even reptiles freeze in place or retreat to safety.[15] Our human version of this primal response is to feel immobilized, stuck, and utterly numb. It's vital to step back, catch your breath, and rethink options. At that point, you can mobilize your energy and resources so you can take a proactive approach. It is helpful to have time to get some perspective on the situation, regroup mentally and emotionally, and then move outward into action.[16]

Taking a Moment for Yourself

Remind yourself that everyone produces cancer cells all the time. You often have more time than you think. Your own cancer has been growing for years, and it happened to be discovered at this point, so you now have a diagnosis. But if you had not been tested and received this diagnosis, the cancer would still be growing or stagnating without immediately threatening your life. So usually you have more time to gather information about your options.

Finding Your Center

Use your own personal style of decision making. When you're under pressure, how do you make good decisions? What has supported you when you've made your best decisions? Draw on these kinds of resources now so that you can stay as centered as possible.

Restoring Your Energy

Take time to catch your breath. Go for a long walk. If you can take a brisk walk in a natural setting, so much the better—walk on the beach, in the woods, or by a river. The most effective way to cope with major stress is to do some form of physical activity for about an hour—ideally exercise that will divert your attention. Physical activity tends to be more centering than quiet activity such as meditation. It can be very difficult to relax and become still when we're feeling highly stressed.

Working Off the Stress

Reduce your stress. In the case of a cancer diagnosis, your survival has just been threatened, so by definition you have triggered a stress response. Physical activity, even just a brisk walk, following stress completes the stress response and switches us back into the relaxation response. At that point, you'll probably feel better prepared to go back to your family and friends, talk openly about your situation, and share and reflect on what needs to be done.

Keeping Your Immune System Engaged

Feel the shock of the diagnosis, acknowledge it, and then do whatever you need to stay proactive. Seek support. Look for survivors who are positive role models. Whenever possible (and appropriate), continue to exercise to work off the stress. If you can't run, walk. When you're too tired to work out, do gentle movements such as yoga or curative eurhythmy.[17] Fit these suggestions to your own lifestyle.

Gathering Information

Stay objective and get the best data (see Appendix B for resources on the Web). You'll want to begin gathering information on your options. Take a balanced approach. You don't want to exhaust yourself with research or get overwhelmed by conflicting opinions. However, you do want to become well informed. You can begin by asking sensible questions. Your options should also include nontraditional approaches to treatment and also immune support such as good nutrition, meditation, and activities that are joyful and fulfilling and give you a sense of meaning and purpose. (For more on this perspective, see Part III.)

Remembering That You Are Unique

Accept that no one can truly predict the path of your illness or healing. Research and clinical data are useful because they help define statistical trends. Yet ultimately the data cannot predict the specific outcome for any given individual. If fifty men take part in a study, and the average of their prostate-specific antigens (PSA) scores is 60, that still does not predict the score of any single individual, who might have a PSA of 10 or 120. Nor will the research be able to predict an individual's outcome. Group averages do not predict individual responses. Consider that George Burns smoked cigars and lived to be 103. Julia Child cooked with lots of butter and lived well into her nineties.

Supporting Your Immune System

Explore programs such as the Gorter Model, Dr. Dean Ornish's program for cancer, or other integrative medicine approaches. They provide useful guidelines such as (1) better diet, (2) antioxidant supplements, (3) walking or bicycling for exercise, (4) stress reduction, and (5) group support. Consider developing your own personal lifestyle program to improve your immune function.

Asking for a Second Opinion ... and a Third

I took the information on hyperthermia to my doctor. After he read through the material, he spontaneously said, "If I had known this, it would have helped my brother. [His brother had recently died of prostate cancer.] I'd definitely give it a try." My pharmacist said the same thing.

The urologist said, "I'm not familiar with this. I cannot give you an opinion. But if you want to do this, you have my support."

HEINZ HAGEMEYER, SIX-YEAR SURVIVOR OF METASTATIC PROSTATE CANCER WITH MULTIPLE LYMPH AND BONE METAS-TASES (STAGE IIIB), TREATED WITH THE GORTER MODEL

Before making any decision, whether it involves surgery, chemotherapy, or integrative medicine, stop and ask yourself, "What is best for *me?*" You want a clear sense of your full range of options. Get more information, rather than assume that the first diagnosis or treatment option is the only option. Even for patients at Stage IV, there are options that may provide an improved quality of life and prolonged life expectancy. Getting a second opinion does not mean you are doubting your physician. You simply want to look at your condition and the treatment from more than one perspective.

It's often very challenging to know what to do. One of Dr. Peper's clients for pain management was Carole Palmer, a woman with terminal pancreatic cancer. Using breathing and imagery techniques, she became totally pain free. However, she confided that she wished she had talked to a naturopath when she was initially diagnosed instead of waiting until the disease had progressed too far. Carole notes,

I would have started eating better, cut back on sugar, and changed my lifestyle. My oncologist told me there was nothing else that I needed to do as far as diet or exercise was concerned. But now I see that there are other ways of looking at this.

Remember that when you hear that there is nothing you can do, it often induces a feeling of helplessness. This sense of powerlessness can actually suppress your immune system. Research has shown that this can lower your defenses, which allows the cancer cells to grow more rapidly.[18]

By taking control of basic aspects of your life, you will have a greater sense that you are doing something on your own behalf, whether you are improving your diet, creating a more positive state of mind through imagery, or supporting your body through deep breathing, walking, qigong, or eurhythmy. Whenever you experience empowerment, that feeling enhances your immune functions and actually inhibits cancer cell growth.

Think about the following when seeking additional advice:

Seeking a second opinion—Consider the qualities you value most when seeking a consulting physician. For many patients, medical expertise paired with compassion is highly appreciated at a time like this.

Getting another perspective on your diagnosis—Get an opinion from a physician who does not know your diagnostic label or prognosis. When physicians know the formal diagnosis, they may begin thinking in terms of a predefined approach to treatment.

Taking economics out of the equation—Make sure that there are *no* economic or social connections between the second physician you see and the physician who gave you the diagnosis. You do not want to be seen by a partner or colleague who could benefit economically from the treatment. In addition, you want to be seen by someone with no financial investment in your outcome. Every surgeon and every practitioner who will potentially treat you may have an unconscious incentive to encourage you in a certain direction. You also want to be seen by providers who are not professionally affiliated. Ideally, you want someone with a fairly different point of view who can give you a fresh perspective.

Evaluating your options—Consult with someone who uses a different approach to treatment. There is also value in advice on nutrition and exercise. One of the key questions is, "How can you change your lifestyle to mobilize your health?" We are not suggesting healthy lifestyle as a cure for cancer, but it can be an important complement to treatment.

Bringing an advocate to your appointments—Bring a close friend or advocate to your appointments. Have your advocate keep notes and ask questions. It is often difficult to ask questions when we are stressed, especially if the health care provider is a respected expert and authority.

Recording any instructions—When you're receiving detailed instructions that you must follow at home, record them as an audio file on your cell phone or other digital device (be sure to ask the health provider for permission) or write them down.

Avoiding quick decisions—Avoid making snap judgments in time of crisis. Take the time you need to think through your decision. Sleep on it and talk with those you love.

> *We examined Dr. Gorter's treatment critically (I tend to have healthy skepticism about almost everything). When we met with him, he didn't raise our expectations. The goal we set was more time, with good quality of life. And we've achieved that at every stage of treatment. It's been important to me that he never mentioned the word "cure." He never made false promises. But now, I am more than two years in complete remission from a Stage IV brain tumor.*
>
> DIRK VD BOOGAARD, SURVIVOR OF BRAIN CANCER
> (STAGE IV GLIOBLASTOMA MULTIFORME), TREATED WITH
> THE GORTER MODEL

Different Approaches to Medical Care

Often we're not aware of how much of our world is defined by our culture, our family, our friends, and our coworkers. We often see health and illness as they are defined by the medical professions and the broader society. This is as true for doctors as it is for patients.

For a brief glimpse of how different cultural perspectives affect treatment, consider American versus French approaches to women's health.

In the United States, when a middle-aged woman develops fibroids (myomas), the uterus is usually removed since she is no longer of child-bearing age. As a culture, we're practical people, everything happens fast, and we tend to be fairly aggressive in our approach to treatment.

The French, on the other hand, place a high value on beauty and the aesthetics of the body. Many of the gynecological surgeons are female physicians, trained in surgical techniques not offered in the United States. They opt to keep the uterus and perform a myectomy, which surgically separates out the fibroid tissue from the uterine wall and extracts it. In addition, they almost always retain the cervix because of its role in a woman's sexuality. The survival rates in both cultures are comparable, but since more and different quality-of-life factors are taken into consideration in the French approach, the French model leads to an overall better quality of life.[19]

Cancer Care

Cancer is also approached differently in Europe. The differences are not tremendous, but as you'll see in Part II of this book, there are other approaches included in treatment.

Often, we tend to take the current standard of care for granted. Yet new research sometimes indicates that a different approach might be more effective. For example, an extensive study in Norway of breast cancer found that women who got no screening at all had lower rates of breast cancer than did those who were screened and received mammograms. (The imaging process used in mammography involves X-rays and radiation exposure. Radiation has been linked to cancer for more than seventy-five years, since the time of Marie Curie. In fact, many of the early researchers who worked with radioactive substances died of cancer-related disorders.)

In this study, the health of more than 220,000 women was tracked over a period of six years.[20] At the end of that time, the total incidence of invasive breast cancer remained 22 percent higher in the group of women who had been screened routinely compared with those who had not received mammograms. (For every 100,000 women in the population, 1,909 women in the screening group developed breast cancer compared with 1,564 in the group that had never been screened.)

Higher incidence was observed in screened women at every age, and the longer the study progressed, the higher was the incidence observed in the group that had received mammograms. However, it is difficult to change conventionally accepted practice. Just reflect on the major controversy that erupted in 2009 when the U.S. Preventive Services Task Force (USPSTF) recommended that low-risk woman should receive fewer mammograms.[21] Many organizations with vested interests in performing mammograms initiated lobbying and protested against changing the recommended guidelines.

Lifestyle Therapy

We all have cancer cells in our bodies all the time, and cancer cells are continuously being created. The occurrence of cancer cells is increased by the exposure to cigarette smoke ("tar"), ionizing radiation, barbeque smoke, pesticides, household products, industrial chemicals, and viral infections, among many other factors.[22] The fact that we survive is a credit to the immune system (see chapters 3 and 4 for more background on exposures and immune function).

Recent research by Dr. Dean Ornish shows the immune function's tremendous power to affect the course of cancer.[23] Ninety-three men with confirmed prostate cancer took part in this study. One group simply received "watchful waiting," which means that they were periodically monitored by measuring their prostate-specific antigens (PSA). The other group followed a vegetarian diet, took supplements (antioxidants), exercised (walked thirty minutes a day, six days a week), and used stress management techniques such as yoga, breathing exercises, and relaxation.

At the end of twelve months, both groups were evaluated. Among those who had only monitoring for their condition, six grew worse and were given chemotherapy and radiation. The PSA levels in that group worsened (went up) by 6 percent on average.

Among the men in the lifestyle program, no one got sick, and the average PSA improved (decreased) by 4 percent. Both groups had their immune function evaluated through a simple blood test that measured the aggressiveness of natural killer (NK) cells—immune cells that target and destroy cancer cells. The blood tests indicated that men in the lifestyle group had NK cells that were seven times more capable of destroying cancer. This research shows that it is important to keep your immune system strong and fully engaged so that you can continue to fight the cancer and maintain a good quality of life, in addition to any form of treatment that you and your physician may choose.

Get the Best Information Available

Physicians who work with cancer patients have a challenging job, and this sometimes results in a sense of unconscious bias in favor of the treatment to which they have committed their life and their career. Without realizing it, they may not give patients the entire picture or the full range of options.

It is not unusual to learn of patients who opt for multiple rounds of chemotherapy, radiation, or surgery, yet only extend their lives by a few weeks or months at great cost to their quality of life. In the case of elderly patients, sometimes they survive only a matter of days following the treatment, with exceptional suffering.

Quality of life is as valid and important an issue as is life expectancy. For example, in recommending radiation treatment, the oncologist sometimes understates or nullifies the possibility that the patient could develop chronic, persistent bowel and bladder incontinence, or a second primary cancer in that region within a few years.

What Is the Risk?

Make it a point to ask specifically how much time the treatment will buy you.

What are the differences between doing the treatment and not doing the treatment?

Ask very specifically how the treatment will affect your quality of life.

One patient with untreatable bone cancer was given two years to live. He opted for an experimental chemotherapy treatment that resulted in debilitating and disabling side effects, including nausea and vomiting, profound exhaustion, peripheral neuropathy, and bone-marrow suppression, and he was unable to do anything for days after each treatment. His immune system became so suppressed that he developed a series of viral infections and even an extreme case of the measles even though he had had them as a child. He still died two years after the diagnosis. It may have been possible that his quality of life would have been much better without the chemo.

One of the major points of confusion in understanding actual risk is the difference between *relative risk* and *absolute risk.* Consider a hypothetical condition that kills two people in a hundred. If a new drug is introduced and one person survives, in absolute terms that is a 1-percent absolute benefit—because one additional person in a hundred has survived. However, because twice as many people survived (two rather than one), the drug company will report the medication as reducing relative risk by 50 percent. In practical terms, the absolute risk reduction was 1 percent.

The Second Cancer

Usually, after routine chemotherapy and radiation, the risk of developing a second primary tumor increases significantly. For some patients, a tumor may also be just the tip of the iceberg. They may have cancer throughout their system that will later resurface in another form and at other locations within the body.

About 80 percent of patients opt for chemotherapy, and about 60 percent of patients receive radiation. Both these treatments suppress the immune system significantly. Treatments that involve either of these cancer-causing toxins lower one's immediate risk on the one hand but increase future risks on the other. Doctors are aware of these risks and are trapped in making diabolic choices weighing possible immediate benefits against possible long-term risks.

The data on survival rates can also be confusing. Researchers think in terms of five-year survival rates. For example, if a patient is cured of one form of cancer for five years, and it recurs in another form, that patient is still considered cured of the initial cancer. Patients who survive five years and then die soon thereafter are also considered treatment successes.[24] Remember that the overall death rate for cancer has not been significantly reduced over the last fifty years. In addition to any other form of treatment you might choose, it is always a good idea to mobilize your immune system in your defense.

Questions to Ask

In sum, what is the key to realistic information that you can apply in your own life? You will want to ask about data on *absolute risk,* rather than *relative risk.* The following questions to ask your physician are adapted from *Matters of Life and Death: Risks versus Benefits of Medical Care* by Eugene D. Robin, who was professor of medicine and physiology at Stanford University Medical School.[25]

- For how long does this treatment typically prolong life?
- In absolute terms, if a hundred people get the treatment, how many will benefit?
- What is my personal benefit?
- How many more days, months, or years would the treatment extend my life?
- What are the risks of the treatment?

- What are the temporary side effects, and what are the permanent side effects?
- Do the benefits outweigh the risks?
- If I did nothing other than pain medication, what would my quality of life be, compared to the quality of life I would have during and after chemotherapy or radiation treatment?
- How much time would I spend receiving treatment and recovering from the treatment?

With some cancers, patients who opt for *no* treatment actually live longer than do those who receive treatment, according to new research. Knowing this, patients find it useful to ask,

- How much longer could I live if I have this treatment versus not having the treatment?
- If the treatment does not work, what would I do next?

Potential Risks of Diagnostic Testing

Of all the patients who are given X-rays or CT scans, one in fifty patients will receive more radiation exposure than is allowable for workers in the nuclear industry. At times the patient will receive an excessive dosage because of multiple scanning or technical or operator errors.[26] Remember that every time you get a CT scan, an X-ray, or radiation treatment, the radiation exposure can potentially suppress your immune system. This can increase the risk of developing cancer. This is also true for surgical procedures under general anesthesia.[27]

We are not suggesting that you forego necessary testing or treatment, but rather that you choose these interventions carefully, after thinking through the potential consequences.[28] For example, think twice about obtaining tests that only provide information but will not actually change treatment strategies. In terms of diagnostic workups, you might find it helpful to ask the questions such as those developed by Robin:

- What are the benefits of this test?
- What are the risks of this test?
- How accurate is the test—that is, how often are the results inaccurate (referred to as false positives and false negatives)?
- What do you expect to learn from this test, and will the information make a significant difference in my treatment plan?

If the test results will make no difference in your treatment plan, carefully consider whether you want to expose yourself to additional risks induced by this diagnostic procedure. On the other hand, the test may help confirm that the illness has stabilized and offer hope.

The fact that the cancer has stabilized is pretty remarkable. It's been almost four years since I began treatment in Cologne with Dr. Gorter, after I was diagnosed with incurable liver cancer. Every nine weeks a scan is made, and the radiologist writes a report. For more than four years now, my situation has been stable. The liver tumors are getting smaller and smaller. Periodically I speak with the oncologist in my town. Although he was skeptical of the treatment at first, he thinks I'm doing well and shows more interest in what I am doing. The blood counts are good; the scans are good. I'm in pretty good shape. So we just keep taking one day at a time.

TRUUS KLEIJ-SWAN

Chapter 3

WHY ME?

Beth and I have always been close—we're identical twins. One evening two years ago, our husbands were taking us out to dinner, and we were getting dressed. I noticed that she looked different—her left nipple was actually inverted. When I asked her about it, she said it was just "a little cyst." (Honestly, I still can't figure out why she hadn't gone to the doctor. I was terrified for her and begged her to see her doctor right away.) It turned out to be a huge cancerous mass in her breast, more than five centimeters wide. The next year passed like a blur, with one procedure after another, three rounds of chemo, a mastectomy of her left breast, radiation, then a mastectomy of her right breast (just in case), and exhausting hormone injections.

I panicked when she got the diagnosis, and within days I was sitting down with my own ob-gyn for a complete breast exam and a referral for a mammogram. No sign of cancer. How many times since then have I asked myself, "Why Beth and not me?" We have the same father, the same mother, come from the same egg, and lived in the same house for eighteen years—we are so alike, we even finish each other's sentences. Why her? Why did it have to happen to her?

JENNIFER

The question, "Why one person and not another?" cannot be answered with a simple explanation. Clearly, a model based on one isolated case almost never explains cancer. The case of Beth and Jennifer makes it clear that cancer is not just a matter of "bad genes." Cancer is hardly ever caused *just* by exposure to cigarette smoke, radiation, asbestos, polychlorinated biphenyls (PCBs), pesticides, or any of the thousands of other chemicals in our homes, gardens, offices, factories, oceans, or air.

Sorting through the Issues

In the case of the identical twins, whatever the factors, the end result was that one twin developed cancer, and the other did not. Although they come from the same genetic source, they are still not totally the same. Even in utero they experienced slightly different environments and nutrients because each placenta was attached differently to the uterine wall. Once they reached college age, they chose different schools, ate different foods, lived in different environments, and were exposed to different carcinogens (Beth had a roommate who smoked; Jennifer did not). They experienced different sexual histories and viral exposures and developed slightly different coping styles.

All these factors (and many others) affect the immune system. In the example of breast cancer, due to the tremendous influence of environment and lifestyle, on average there is only an 18 percent correlation for breast-cancer risk in identical twins. This means that environment and lifestyle account for 82 percent of the risk.[29]

Why was I the one to get lung cancer? I don't smoke. I've taken 1000 milligrams of vitamin C every day for the past fifteen years. I haven't eaten meat for more than seven years. I exercise at least five times a week, jogging, and racquetball with Raoul. Why me? My neighbor is five years older than I am, smokes (a lot), drinks (a lot), and barbecues at least once a week. Damn, this is so unfair!

MICHAEL

Although environmental exposures and lifestyle factors have been found to contribute to 70 to 80 percent of all cancers, genetic factors also play a key role sometimes. High stress at home or work, if it's intense enough, can also compromise the immune system. It's important to sort out these factors whenever we can, because we want to minimize the exposures we *can* control.

If you're dealing with cancer yourself, or that of someone you love, rest assured that almost everyone finds cancer overwhelming. Even researchers are hard pressed to offer a clear-cut model of what causes cancer. We do know for certain that many factors promote or deter cancer growth. When biological, environmental, personality, and stress-response factors augment or amplify each other, the immune system becomes less effective. In the absence of strong immune defenses, cancer may develop.

A Question of Balance

Rather than focusing on a single cause, there is value in looking at a number of factors that contribute to cancer. Taking a "systems approach" means supporting immune competence, reducing exposure to toxins, and minimizing other factors known to promote cancer.

Rebuilding the Terrain

This approach also takes into account the body's general health—our inner "terrain." Terrain includes the body's chemistry and biological rhythms such as temperature. Viewing the body as an entire ecosystem with its own unique balance suggests strategies to both treat and prevent cancer.

Cancer growth is controlled by the strength and aggressiveness of specific immune cells within the body. In many cases, when cancer develops, it's because the immune system has a reduced ability to recognize or destroy the cancer.

On the other hand, if there is a massive exposure to toxic chemicals or radiation, the immune system can be overwhelmed by the level of exposure or the aggressiveness of the cancer cells.

There are many factors that can increase or decrease immune competence and immune burdens. If the immune system is less competent, it is less able to cope with the burden, and the cancer increases. Health can be enhanced by reducing the toxic burden or by supporting the immune response.

System Overwhelm—Increasing the Immune Burden

The development of cancer cells can overwhelm our immune defenses if the exposure to carcinogens is frequent, intense, or long-lasting. An example of frequent exposure would be seen in a heavy smoker. Intense exposures may occur as industrial accidents or disasters such as the meltdown at Chernobyl. Long-lasting exposures might occur, for example, in a house that leaks radon on an ongoing basis.[30]

In terms of cancer, the balance of health reflects the relationship between immune competence and the cancer load. A poorly functioning immune system may be able to cope with day-to-day exposures (and the random cancer cells that result). Balance is maintained as long as the system is not challenged by metabolic stress due to an aggressive virus, chemical exposure, or other factors as shown in table 3.1.

Immune Burdens	Immune Strengths
Radiation exposure weakens immune cells and healthy tissue	Radiation treatment to destroy cancer cells
Chemotherapy weakens immune cells	Chemotherapy destroys cancer tissue
General anesthesia tends to suppress immune function	Reducing the cancer burden through surgery
Stress in almost all forms, including psychological stress such as fear or grief, suppresses immune function	Increasing immune competence through immune therapy

Exposures to Minimize	Positive Lifestyle Factors
Persistent viruses: Epstein Barr, hepatitis B and C, human papillomavirus	Minimizing viral exposures; nipping infections in the bud
Common chemicals in our homes, gardens, workplace, air, and water, which are eventually stored in fat tissues of the body	Minimizing chemical exposures
Sedentary lifestyle and weight gain; "Bad" estrogens produced by fat tissues of the body	Walking 30 minutes, 6 times a week reduces cancer risk significantly
Common foods: refined sugar, transfats, charred meat	Eating fruits and vegetables every day including a range of phytonutrients reduces cancer risk significantly
Chronic physical, mental, or emotional stress	Effective stress management through meditation, yoga, sports, counseling, or other means
Irregular sleep patterns	Adequate sleep, in rhythm with light and (complete) darkness

Table 3.1. Examples of factors that increase or decrease immune competence

Chemotherapy and radiation produce a fairly rapid response since the chemo toxins and radiation destroy the cancer cells. Once the cancer burden is lower, the immune system may be able to restore balance. However, both chemotherapy and radiation can damage many other cells in the body and also tend to decrease immune competence at the same time. Thus although these therapies can reduce and destroy the targeted cancer, they increase the risk for future cancers if the immune system is impaired by the treatment procedures.

The Tipping Point for Cancer

As immune capacity drops, vulnerability to cancer increases. Once the number of immune cells falls below a certain level or the immune system is less competent at recognizing and destroying cancer cells (or the number of cancer cells increases and reaches critical mass), the system cannot cope adequately with the cancer load. When immune capacity is overwhelmed by toxic exposures and health burdens, the immune system can no longer prevent cancer.

For example, radiation exposure compromises immune competence, which lowers immune function and increases the risk of future cancers. In addition, exposure to high-energy radiation treatment increases damage to genetic DNA and RNA. At the same time, once immune function falls below the threshold level, cancer emerges. The interactions are highly complex and are schematically illustrated in figure 3.1.

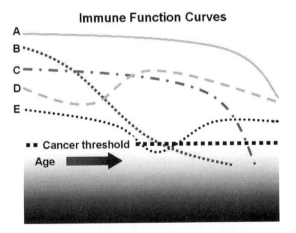

Figure 3.1. Illustration of different life patterns of immune function

Immune Function Curves

This graph illustrates five life stories (chosen from an infinite number of patterns of disease progression or recovery). Each pattern can be seen in terms of a threshold model that represents a tipping point for the development of cancer. Those who had low exposures and strong immune function were able to avoid cancer. These are theoretical patterns based on a view of immune function and disease.

A. **Healthy aging immune system.** Tom was born with strong immune function. By the time he retired at seventy, his immune system was no longer as vital, but he was still able to fight off the minor infections and died cancer free at eighty-five.

B. **Compromise due to viral infection.** Bill was also born with a healthy immune system. However, his immune function never fully developed because he was vaccinated early and given aspirin or Tylenol (acetaminophen) at the first sign of a fever. When he got hepatitis C from a transfusion while traveling oversees, his immune system possibly couldn't handle the infection, and he eventually developed liver cancer.

C. **Weakened immune function.** Ann seemed to catch every cold that came along (the story of her life). The house she purchased as a newlywed was in an upscale community, but located near a huge refinery. By the time she reached her forties, she was diagnosed with breast cancer that metastasized within a matter of months.

D. **Immune function strengthened through lifestyle.** Sarah had terrible allergies as a kid. In college, she started doing yoga, began eating lots of fruits and vegetables, and minimized her allergy exposure. From then on, her health seemed to get a little better over time, and she was able to live a relatively long, healthy life.

E. **Weak immune system strengthened after surviving cancer.** Paul was the guy in the back of the class that you never noticed. He enjoyed gardening but didn't bother with sunscreen. After beating skin cancer, he turned over a new leaf, became a racquetball fanatic, and got healthy.

The information here is not intended as a cookbook approach to cancer. This disease is so complex that it requires a comprehensive model. If you got cancer even after working hard through your lifetime with a healthy diet and exercise, it is important not to think that your efforts were for naught. If there were a single cause, we would have beaten cancer long ago. Every individual case reflects unique elements, and ultimately each patient, working closely with health care providers, will need to find his or her own dynamic balance to achieve a good quality of life and work toward healing.

Treating Cancer

Both cancer prevention and treatment are multidimensional. The major goals are to reduce the cancer burden while simultaneously enhancing immune competence. Until recently, the major focus of cancer treatment has been on reducing the cancer burden through toxic treatments such as radiation and chemotherapy. However, these forms of treatment also reduce immune competence and increase the burden on the immune system. They also cause a number of debilitating side effects.

In integrative oncology, cancer can be treated with "anticancer" therapies while providing immune support with "proimmune" therapies. In this approach, the immune system is enhanced to mobilize the body's self-healing potential. New cancer treatments such as the Gorter Model provide nontoxic therapies that enhance immune competence with only minor side effects.

An initial cancer diagnosis naturally prompts a response such as, "Why me?" This diagnosis prompts us to reexamine our values and ultimately requires a change in how we look at our life. So the question "Why me?" could be reframed as, "How can I use this experience for personal growth?" or "What can I learn from this experience?" Once the question is reframed, a shift in perspective occurs—from helplessness and powerlessness to hope and empowerment. Research data have shown that depression is often associated with a decreased cancer survival. Thus the experience of being proactive, of taking action on your own behalf, literally turns on the immune system and enhances our immune competence.[31]

Chapter 4

NEW PERSPECTIVES ON CANCER

One day, I was brushing my hair, and I noticed that one of my breasts looked unusual. I had it checked, and it turned out to be a malignant tumor. The surgeon removed the tumor and a lymph node that had been affected. I was also given radiation treatments. From then on, I went back to the hospital for checkups every few months. That was in 2003.

In 2006, I had a relapse. They did a scan and found that the cancer had metastasized to my bones, across the spinal column, the pelvis, a shoulder blade, my breast bone, both collar bones, and the crown of my skull. I was started on hormone injections.

The tumor markers went down a little, but I was in a bad state. I had four collapsed vertebrae. I lost a lot of weight and had trouble walking. My husband had to help me out of bed in the morning. I couldn't sit up by myself.

When we read an article about the Medical Center Cologne, the approach seemed sensible to us. Dr. Gorter explained the research on these therapies and their experience with patients. Neither my husband nor I have any patience with vague, flaky ideas, but we understood the methodology and the biochemical background. This made sense to us, and we decided to do it.

MRS. HENNY HOEVE, SURVIVOR OF STAGE IV METASTATIC
BREAST CANCER, TREATED WITH THE GORTER MODEL AND NOW
IN REMISSION FOR OVER FIVE YEARS

How Cancer Develops: We All Have Cancer All the Time

If you select any healthy individual at random and draw a sample of blood at any given moment in time, in just a few millimeters of blood (about a tablespoon) it is possible to detect thousands of cancer cells. In cancer patients, the number of cancer cells is a hundred times greater.

In our bodies, cancer cells occur at random almost every day in response to many factors:

- chemicals in our food, such as dyes, pesticides, and preservatives, and foods such as sugar, trans fats, and charred meat[32]
- exposure to environmental toxins (there are nineteen known cancer-causing chemicals in cigarette smoke alone)
- chemicals found in many homes, including aerosol sprays, air fresheners, dry-cleaned clothing, certain cleaners and disinfectants, some hobby supplies, paints, paint strippers, solvents, and wood preservatives
- carcinogenic environmental chemicals such as chlorine, gasoline, and PCBs
- viral infections such as Epstein-Barr, viral hepatitis, human immunodeficiency virus (HIV), and human papillomavirus (HPV)
- mutations both inherited and acquired during life time

This continuous battle against toxins and infection is waged daily. The damaging effects from fighting infections or mopping up toxins increase oxidative stress. This unbalanced chemistry in the body may trigger or promote the development of malignant cells.

Cancer under the Radar

We generate cancer cells in our bodies all the time. However, the immune system can usually destroy the malignant cells as they develop, thus preventing the growth of cancerous masses, or tumors. As long as the immune system is able to identify and effectively eliminate these malignant cells early in their development, we do not develop clinical cancer.

The immune system is a highly complex organ that is located throughout the body. Interestingly, only about 2 percent of all immune competent cells are present in the peripheral blood stream flowing to all organs and the limbs. Fully 98 percent of all immune cells are found in the inner organs—strategically located to destroy emerging cancerous cells.

In the normal course of events, with this protection in place, the number of cancer cells never reaches critical mass. With a vigilant immune system, the level of malignant cells remains below a threshold level or tipping point that our immune response can handle. When the immune system is effective, it has the capacity to detect and destroy cancerous cells as soon as they develop.

The immune system needs to be competent enough to identify and destroy these cells. If cancer appears as a life-threatening disease, it is a sign that one arm of the immune system—our cellular immunity—is compromised. When the body's efforts at destroying cancer fail, a tumor can form and then begin to develop and spread.

It is important to understand that *the development of cancer always reflects a deficiency in immune function—a major shutdown of the body's immune defenses.*

Basic Immunity

Research has provided comparable examples of how immune function maintains control throughout the body. We know, for instance, that the majority of people carry strep bacteria at one time or another, without ever developing a streptococcus infection. Similarly, staph bacteria are carried by about 40 percent of the population at any given time without causing staphylococcus infection.

These pathogenic bacteria can remain in the body for decades without manifesting as disease. Then, seemingly "out of the blue," a respiratory infection or even a life-threatening pneumonia develops, with the same bacteria as the causal agent. How is it possible that after thirty years an acute infection can suddenly occur? What about the patient is different this month from last month? And how is this patient different from another who does not develop a clinical disease?

All healing originates with our bodies' immune capacity. Even when we use antibiotics, the bacteria are not completely wiped out. The drugs work to lower the bacterial load so that our own system can knock them out more quickly and restore our usual balance. The answer is usually found in the immune system.

Fighting Cancer: What Goes Wrong?

When evaluating cancer patients for the status of their immune response, without exception, we see some type of immune system failure or shutdown.

Immune therapy is designed to restart these functions and target the cancer. The Gorter Model is an innovative approach to mobilize and restore a patient's own immune function and enable the body to reverse the cancer. By enhancing the body's own defense mechanisms against cancer, healing is maximized. The same process is important in preventing and fighting cancer, and it can even bring cancer patients into complete and long-lasting remission.

There is a state of equilibrium that enables our bodies to cope with the development of infection or cancer cells. When we're healthy, the immune system destroys malignant cells as they develop. When cancer occurs, what has gone wrong?

No Fever, No Fight. One of our primary protections against cancer turns out to be fever. As the body mounts a fever, an entire army of immune defenses is put on active duty. Even a mild fever doubles the number of immune cells actively circulating in the body, and also enhances their functions. A number of these cells play a major role in keeping cancer in check.

One Arm of the Immune System Shuts Down. When the immune system gets out of balance, it puts us at greater risk for cancer. If the system is tied up fighting allergies or chronic (viral, bacterial, or parasitic) infections, this may occur at the expense of our cancer-fighting cells.

No Recognition of the Cancer. Many standard immune defenses appear to be inactive in cancer patients. The cells that would identify cancer cells and the natural killer (NK) cells that would destroy the cancer are dysfunctional. If the body does not recognize malignant cells, no defense can be mobilized.

Fewer Immune Defenses. When cancer cells are not identified and no defense is mounted, the cancer can gain a foothold and begin growing unchecked. Once the number of cancer cells reaches a threshold level—critical mass—they will manifest as "clinical cancer," usually within a particular organ of the body such as the breasts, prostate, pancreas, or liver.

Loss of Immune Balance

These factors each play an important role in the loss of balanced immune function.

Fever Launches Our Immune Defenses

Most of us are accustomed to thinking of fever as inconvenient or potentially dangerous. But fever is one of the keys to an immune system that is working effectively.

On average, a newborn has seven viral infections in the first year of life and other illnesses throughout childhood that cause fever. These bouts of fever prime and activate the development of the immune system. Frequently, we find that patients who develop cancer are unable to mount a fever, their core body temperature is significantly lower than the norm, and they did not experience fevers as a child.

A number of researchers and clinicians have documented in large scientific studies that if a significant fever does not occur in childhood at least four to five times before age six (time of changing teeth), the immune system may not develop and mature fully. Data suggest that this increases the risk of developing both allergies in puberty and cancer in adulthood.[33]

Suppression of fever in the first year of life with nonsteroidal anti-inflammatory drugs (NSAIDs) such as aspirin or Tylenol (acetaminophen) is associated with a significant increase in food allergies, hay fever, asthma, dermatitis, and eczema as compared with children who did not have the fever-suppressing medication.[34] This is possibly an early indicator of a dysfunctional immune system. In addition, if a vaccination is given to children and the child receives NSAIDs, the child will be less likely to show a competent immune response to the agent of the inoculation. By blocking the fever, the immune system may be inhibited from producing the appropriate responses.

The Efficient Immune System

Your immune system functions somewhat like an exterminator that keeps your body clear of invasive cells. Immunity functions in two major approaches: to trap invaders and to kill them.

Trapping Invaders

The arm of the immune system that traps invaders is targeted at bacteria, viruses, yeast, and parasites—as well as anything likely to cause an allergic reaction (i.e., allergen). This is described as the *humoral immune system* because it is present in the body's fluids (once referred to as "humors").

The key players in this system are the antibodies—protein fragments that stick to the surface of a microbe like Velcro and then trap it in mucus and dispel it. (This is what happens when you breathe in germs or pollen and then sneeze. Your immune system has just "trapped" the allergen and disposed of it.)

Antibodies by themselves are unable to trap cancerous cells. Since antibodies are not generally effective in dislodging cancer, they are generally insufficient in preventing cancer or fighting it once a malignancy develops.

Because the cancer cells occur within the cells and tissue of the body, they are regarded by the immune system as the body's own *(autologous)*. Thus, the humoral immune system does not target cancer cells. Malignant cells are not identified as invaders, and therefore they are not treated as if they were dangerous.

Fighting Cancer

The task of identifying and destroying harmful cells lodged within our bodies' cells or produced by the body itself is relegated to the *cellular immune system.* When this cellular immunity is compromised or shut down, the body becomes vulnerable to cancer.

Cellular immunity includes white blood cells, such as T cells, and other infection fighters. Only humans and mammals have this sophisticated form of immunity. Lower animals such as birds and reptiles do not have this aspect of immune function. This system includes cells that detect cancer, others that destroy it, and some that clean up the debris after these skirmishes are over. When cancer develops, it often means that cellular immunity is compromised.

Detecting Malignant Cells

Cancer cells develop all kinds of hiding (escape) mechanisms inside the organs of the body and thus make detection by the immune system more difficult. *Dendritic cells* are the immune defenses that identify the cancer. Cancer can gain a foothold if these dendritic cells are impaired or fail to detect the malignant cells early on. When dendritic cells are effective, they work superbly to indentify cancerous cells and to alert thousands of immune cells to the specific identity and location of the cancer.

Destroying the Malignancy

Cancer cells are always harmful and represent a huge threat to the body as a whole. Once a cancer cell has been identified, our bodies call up one of the premier fighting forces of the immune system, such as the NK cells. These powerful cells are the "exterminators" that destroy tumor cells and other precancerous cells such as cells chronically infected with viruses like hepatitis C.

These NK cells and cytotoxic cells launch their attack by puncturing a hole in the cell wall of the cancer cell. The NK and other cytotoxic cells then inject certain enzymes that dissolve the cancer cell within a few hours *(lysis)*.

Mop-up Operations

Other cells of the immune system, the so-called *granulocytes*, provide "mop-up" operations by eating up the debris of dead cancer cells and digesting them completely. This process, known as *phagocytosis*, clears the body of dangerous oxidants and toxic cancer-specific proteins that are left behind after the NK cells have done their job.

The *antioxidants* that we get in fresh fruits and vegetables contain the raw materials our bodies use in the mop-up operations that clear away the debris from these tiny inner battles. When full-blown cancer develops, it is usually because the cellular component of the immune system is no longer active or has been severely compromised.

At the Medical Center Cologne, when I meet with new patients living with cancer, we do a two-hour interview and history. I explain to them what I think we can realistically do. At that point, I give them background on cellular immunity and immune therapy—how it works, what it does, and what the research literature says. I also describe our experiences with therapeutic fever. Depending on the needs of the patient, at that point we discuss different treatment options.

ROBERT GORTER

Once we met with Dr. Gorter, we had a good feeling about the information we received, and the results have been very positive. In fact, the treatment has really worked out far better than we'd dared hope for.

MRS. HOEVE

When Immune Balance Is Lost

Under normal conditions, both the humoral and the cellular immune system collaborate by supporting each other's functions. However, if the immune system is tied up fighting allergies or chronic infections with viruses, bacteria, or parasites, the humoral immunity will predominate at the expense of cellular immunity. When that happens, there are fewer active cells from the cellular immune system to identify cancer and fewer to destroy it.

At first, we came for dendritic cell injections and fever therapy six or seven times a month, and twice a week for localized hyperthermia. The cancer had spread everywhere, and the metastases are in my bones, so I also took medication to help rebuild bone tissue. I have very few side effects, except that I get a fever the day after the dendritic cell therapy. Sometimes it's like a heavy flu, but I know that means the treatment is catching on. My tumor markers have dropped, and there's even some healthy bone growth.

MRS. HOEVE

When a patient is receiving hyperthermia, all kinds of metabolic and immune processes are accelerated. Fever improves circulation, and improved blood flow facilitates the absorption of medication and nutrients. With breast or prostate cancer, a hormone blockade therapy is usually initiated, which usually works more intensively during and

55

after fever treatments. We see this enhanced activity with essentially all medications.

Robert Gorter

New Options for Treatment

Immune therapy is designed to restart the immune system and restore cellular immunity. This new paradigm, described in Part II, is based on more than thirty-eight years of modern scientific research and thousands of studies conducted worldwide. These therapies are now being incorporated in clinical practice in a number of medical centers around the world. Immune therapy is provided as a specific protocol, and it is also used in combination with treatments such as surgery, radiation, chemotherapy, hormone injections, and other forms of immune treatment.

The Gorter Model offers new and effective options in cancer therapy and a range of nontoxic approaches to treatment. Patients using this protocol often report that within two days of treatment, they have more energy, feel more alive, and have none of the negative side effects usually associated with chemotherapy, radiation, or hormone treatment therapy. The Gorter Model offers documented potential for the partial or complete remission of Stage III and Stage IV cancers.

At least 60 percent of patients with end-stage cancer show partial remission and live many years longer than their previous prognosis, without the debilitating side effects often associated with conventional treatment.

I didn't dare dream of ever living a normal life again. If I wanted to get into the car, Jan had to open the door, and then help me get in, one leg at a time. I just couldn't do anything anymore. I could hardly climb the stairs.

But after three years of the treatment, I can do almost everything I used to do before my illness. Yesterday I went to Amsterdam on my own, by train and trolley. When I got to my daughter's, I walked up the stairs with no trouble. (She lives on the fourth floor.) I'm very happy about it. It's a totally different life. And I have been stable in this tremendously improved condition for three years now.

MRS. HOEVE

Part II
IMMUNE THERAPY

●

Chapter 5

THE GORTER MODEL

When I took the job as a receptionist nine months ago, I really expected that the cancer patients would be depressed and fearful. To my surprise they are relaxed and smiling when they come in, and often well enough after the treatment to go out and enjoy Cologne with their families. What makes this surprising is that all these patients have Stage III or IV cancer.

RECEPTIONIST AT THE MEDICAL CENTER COLOGNE

The Medical Center Cologne is located in a spacious community hospital in Cologne, Germany. Although this is a large teaching hospital with modern equipment in the hallways, there are plenty of windows to the outside, and the halls are filled with light to create a healing environment. The space is supportive and nurtures healing.

We know from the research that healing is supported when the environment feels safe—a quality so often underestimated in modern clinics. Yet research data show overwhelmingly that when the physical environment feels safe and inviting, healing is promoted.[35]

The healing environment is also embodied in the approach of the clinic. Treatment never causes debilitating side effects, and approximately 80 percent of the patients experience either remission or extended longevity. Many find that they are actually energized by the treatment and better able to enjoy their daily lives.

Each patient is treated with courtesy and respect. There is time for every patient, which is so different from the stress that sometimes occurs in many oncological treatment centers. At the Medical Center Cologne, patients are not queued up, waiting for hours to see their physician or

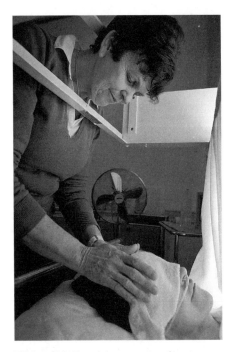

Figure 5.1. Receiving compassionate care during fever-range, total-body hyperthermia (photo by Jana Asenbrennerova)

to receive treatment. They are addressed by name when they come in, and the medical staff is ready for them, so that they are not made to wait.

The waiting room is comfortable and relaxing, with thoughtful touches such as a cappuccino machine and lots of licorice (for the patients from Scandinavia and Holland!), home baked cookies and pies, organic bananas, grapes, and apples, and organic juices. Just being in the space feels normalizing. Patients can also go downstairs to the hospital cafeteria, where they can dine outside on the terrace. The hospital food is not mass-produced—there are tasty local dishes and even the same desserts that one would buy in neighborhood pastry shops. Special diets are accommodated and vegetarian, halal, and kosher foods are always available.

Everything that can be done for the comfort of the patient is done. There is a real sense of caring and compassion.

The Gorter Model Protocol

This chapter provides an overview of cancer treatment using the Gorter Model. It begins with a description of the training and background of Dr. Robert Gorter, who developed the model, and then outlines the various components of the program. The specific treatment strategies are explained in the chapters that follow: chapter 6 describes the role of fever and fever therapy (hyperthermia); chapter 7 explains dendritic cell vaccinations, which serve to restart the immune system; and chapter 8 gives an overview of the use of the botanical mistletoe *(Viscum album)*, antioxidant infusions, and other immune-enhancing approaches.

The Medical Center Cologne was founded by Robert Gorter, MD, PhD, and has been under his direction for the past twelve years. The center is dedicated to the treatment of cancer using immune-supportive therapies. Dr. Gorter developed this program after more than thirty-five years of clinical experience, after surviving cancer himself, and after having been a program director in the field of AIDS treatment and research for four years.

Dr. Gorter earned his medical degree at the University of Amsterdam Medical School in the Netherlands, where he graduated as a family practitioner in 1973. He completed his second postdoctoral training at the University of California–San Francisco (UCSF) Medical School in 1986. Dr. Gorter served as a full UCSF faculty member from 1986 to 2008. Additional education includes a doctorate from the University of Witten/Herdecke in Germany in 1993, where he continues to serve as a faculty member. His training is foremost in conventional Western medicine with postdoctoral work in the United States, Germany, and the Netherlands. He also completed specialty training in anthroposophical medicine in 1973 in Arlesheim, Switzerland, with an emphasis on oncology.

Dr. Gorter opened his private practice and health center in the heart of Amsterdam in 1974. Only a few weeks after opening his practice, he was diagnosed with far-advanced, Stage IV testicular cancer—at that time described as "teratocarcinoma," which is a type of cancer currently defined as germ-cell carcinoma. He was able to recover successfully through nontoxic treatment—that is, without the use of chemotherapy or radiation. His treatment consisted solely of therapeutic fever (hyperthermia) and injections of a known oncologic botanical, the European mistletoe. This experience motivated him to further explore new, nontoxic approaches to cancer therapy.

In the 1980s Dr. Gorter served as physician and researcher on AIDS at San Francisco General Hospital in the world-renowned Ward 86. He continued his involvement in research within the emerging field of immune therapy when Ward 86 became part of the UCSF AIDS Program. Subsequently, for four years Dr. Gorter was medical director of the Department of AIDS Epidemiology and Biostatistics at UCSF. He was also highly active in program development in the initiation of the AIDS Health Project, the Coming Home Hospice movement, and the Visiting Nurses' Association home care services for HIV/AIDS and cancer patients.

Almost all that is known about the progression of HIV infection into AIDS comes from the seminal research on this initial cohort of patients living with HIV infection, whose progress was tracked in long-term follow-up studies by the Department of AIDS Epidemiology and Biostatistics. Dr. Gorter was intrigued by the fact that a few people with HIV infection never progressed to AIDS or AIDS-related complex (ARC). These patients were called "long-term nonprogressors." The research on HIV/AIDS and the immune system helped Dr. Gorter better understand immune function.

This work, conducted at the very beginning of the AIDS epidemic in the United States and Europe, provided Dr. Gorter the opportunity to be involved in the research and clinical care that first defined the complex elements of the human immune system. These studies from UCSF Medical Center have resulted in the most extensive knowledge base on immunity in HIV infection in our time.

When Dr. Gorter moved the focus of his work to cancer treatment a decade later, he integrated what he had learned in clinical practice and program development. He applied clinically relevant research on immune therapy to develop nontoxic, immune-based therapies for the treatment of cancer. Drawing on what he learned as an AIDS researcher and on his clinical experiences, he began developing a cancer treatment program based on the principles of intensive and targeted immune restoration.

Dr. Gorter has also participated in research on botanicals that address cancer, as well as other forms of immune suppression. In Berlin he founded the European Institute for Oncological and Immunological Research, which he directed until 2001. This Institute was affiliated with the Free University (Freie Universität), and Dr. Gorter was also asked to lecture regularly to medical students and young doctors in this field. The main focus of his research was to document possible efficacy of *Viscum album* (mistletoe) in both oncological patients and patients with chronic viral infections, like HIV and hepatitis C virus (HCV). For one clinical study with *Viscum album* in HIV/AIDS, he received a personal Investigational New Drug (IND) approval from the Food and Drug Administration to conduct phase II and phase III clinical trials. When applied correctly, mistletoe has been shown to promote major improvement in quality of life and also to significantly prolong life expectancy in cancer patients with solid tumors.

Currently, almost 70 percent of all cancer patients in Germany, Switzerland, Austria, and Central Europe receive mistletoe *(Viscum album)* by prescription, making it the single most commonly prescribed anti-cancer medication in these countries of all forms of pharmaceuticals and botanicals combined. Dr. Gorter is convinced he owes his own complete recovery in part to mistletoe, and thus he has been committed to clinical research on this botanical.

Dr. Gorter has spent more than two decades establishing and refining effective methodology for immune therapy. He has pioneered the integrated use of therapeutic fever (fever-range, total-body hyperthermia). He has also worked extensively with an approach that essentially vaccinates the immune system to restore latent immune function. This therapy, described as dendritic cell vaccination, is used in combination with mistletoe botanicals, antioxidant treatment, and other immune-restorative agents. Components of these approaches to treatment have also been independently studied in thousands of clinical trials conducted at research centers in the United States, across Europe, and in Australia,

New Zealand, and Japan. Summaries of the most relevant research are included in the chapters that follow.

The Program at the Medical Center Cologne

The Gorter Model is designed to restore and enhance immune function, enabling the immune system to aggressively and effectively combat cancer cells throughout the body. The treatment protocol is also enhanced by self-care approaches such as diet, meditation, imagery, and physical activity. This comprehensive program can also be used in combination with conventional cancer therapy, such as chemotherapy, radiation, hormone blockage, or other treatments. Therapeutic fever is also used in combination with immune therapies that include interleukin, interferon, and various other treatments. These various approaches have been evaluated in hundreds of clinical trials worldwide.

Conditions that have been successfully treated with the Gorter Model include almost all metastasized solid tumors, such as breast and prostate cancer; lung, brain, liver, and colon cancer; and bone cancer.

At the Medical Center Cologne, when I meet with new patients, I always begin with a two-hour interview and history taking. I explain to them what I think we can realistically do.

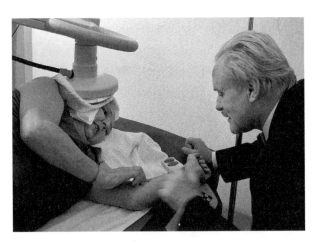

Figure 5.2. Robert Gorter explaining to a patient how her brain cancer is being treated with local hyperthermia (photo by Jana Asenbrennerova)

At that point, I give them background information on immune ther-apy and cellular immunity—how it works, what it does, and what the research literature says. I also describe our experiences with therapeutic fever and local hyperthermia. Depending on the needs of the patient, at that point, we discuss different treatment options.

ROBERT GORTER

Immune Therapy in Cancer Treatment

The Gorter Model is designed to improve immune function through comprehensive treatment that restores the normal activity of the immune system. Some patients have *impaired immune function,* which occurs when the patient is unable to mount a fever. This means that the immune system has no way to launch a major response to combat cancer cells that begin amassing. Fever therapy is provided using a safe, carefully monitored protocol.

Some other patients have *impaired immune signaling:* the cells that normally identify cancer and trigger an immune response are inactive. These vital cells are reintroduced into the body to activate cancer sur-veillance functions of the immune system. This makes it possible for the body once again to destroy cancer cells from within.

The ultimate goal for each patient is to restore and empower the immune system and all its primary functions. The basic elements of the Gorter Model are the integration of the therapies and protocol in a schedule designed specifically for each individual patient. Treatment may involve some or all of the following therapies to optimize immune function or to directly destroy the cancer cells.

Fever-range, total-body hyperthermia to restart the immune sys-tem. Practically all cancer patients have a below-average core temperature and are unable to develop a fever—thus they are unable to activate their immune system. To reactivate immune function, a controlled fever is

67

induced to artificially heat the body. This process is known as therapeutic fever (see chapter 6).

Localized hyperthermia to selectively kill cancer cells. Heat therapy can also be applied specifically to the area of the tumor, referred to as local, localized, or regional hyperthermia. At the Medical Center Cologne, almost all patients receive this form of treatment, particularly if they have entered the final stages of cancer. Local hyperthermia is exceptionally safe because it increases the temperature of cancer cells within the tumor to 42°C (107.6°F) without increasing the temperature of adjacent normal cells or cells in the rest of the body. Research has shown that cancer cells begin to die *(necrosis)* at 38.8°C (101.8°F), and at 42°C (107.6°F) almost all cancer cells are destroyed.

Vaccination with dendritic cells that enhance immune defenses. All patients receive injections with dendritic cells to restore adequate immune function. These immune cells, cultured from the patient's blood, are described as autologous, monocyte-derived dendritic cells. Dendritic cells have the job of detecting cancer and then mobilizing the immune system, particularly natural killer (NK) cells and related immune cells such as T cells that destroy cancer cells. Dendritic cell vaccinations are used in conjunction with fever-range, total-body hyperthermia, and also with local hyperthermia (chapter 7).

Intravenous (IV) therapy with vitamins, minerals, trace elements, antioxidants, and glandular extracts. Antioxidants include vitamins and minerals that quench the oxidants that are the by-product of fighting infections and destroying cancer cells. Low antioxidant levels have been clearly linked to cancer. While antioxidants can be obtained from a good diet, IV therapy provides these nutrients efficiently and at much higher levels, which have been found to be significantly more therapeutic in combating cancer. This medical application is widely used in integrative and nontoxic cancer treatment in Europe and the

United States. The infusions are generally well tolerated and are given at a dosage that is specific to the individual patient (see chapter 8).

Botanical mistletoe therapy. This approach was developed in the early 1920s by the Austrian scientist Rudolf Steiner (1861–1925), PhD, and the Dutch physician Ita Wegman (1876–1943), MD. Mistletoe *(Viscum album)* is utilized in the clinical treatment of cancer throughout Europe for a wide range of cancers. A highly refined form of the botanical is used in injectable form to enhance immune function and reestablish circadian temperature rhythm. Mistletoe is widely used in conventional European oncology and is described in more detail in chapter 8.

Treatment with oncolytic viruses that destroy cancerous cells. The Newcastle disease virus has been found to selectively kill human cancer cells without harming healthy tissue or other aspects of patient health. At this point, there is approximately forty years of research on the use of this virus in oncology, in more than twenty-five clinical trials conducted in Europe, the United States, and worldwide. Newcastle disease virus makes the cancer more visible to the immune system. Additional information on this mechanism of action and the treatment protocol is given in chapter 8.

Lifestyle and mind-set. Healthy lifestyle and mind-body medicine have become widely accepted essentials in any holistic treatment plan. Healing is promoted by maximizing support from the environment and from within. This support activates immune function, enhances basic health, and ultimately benefits the whole person. Health professionals at the Medical Center Cologne encourage patients to live a health-promoting lifestyle, and some of these self-care concepts are provided in chapters 9 through 15.

The Clinical Setting

The treatment implies hope, although not all patients improve. At the Medical Center Cologne, in cases of Stage IV glioblastoma multiforme, aside from the 48 percent of patients who experience complete remission, roughly 40 to 60 percent show partial remission. Some die in the course of treatment, which would be expected since the vast majority of patients enter the program with end-stage disease, major tumors, and extensive tissue destruction, physical depletion, and immune compromise. Many are also physically compromised from previous applications of surgery, chemotherapy, and radiation. This makes the stabilization of their disease all the more remarkable. Their improved health and quality of life are reflected in the patient interviews available at www.medical-center-cologne.com.

Treatment at the Medical Center Cologne does not debilitate patients. Even patients with Stage IV cancer often report that they feel a certain sense of vitality and are able to maintain or improve their quality of life throughout much of the course of their illness.

In 1999, I was diagnosed with breast cancer. It had already spread to eight lymph nodes. My breast was surgically removed, but after much thought, I declined radiation and chemotherapy. I opted for a nontoxic follow-up treatment, but also continued to go back to the hospital for my scheduled checkups.

During the next six years I was in remission, but eventually developed bone cancer. I was able to beat the cancer two more times. When I developed the third recurrence, I received radiation treatment. However, the pain returned, and I had to walk with a cane because it hurt a great deal just to move.

At that point I decided to go to Germany for treatment at the Medical Center Cologne. With the treatments I have received in Cologne, the pain is gone and remains gone. In fact, after six months, I can walk again. Many of the tumors are gone, although a few remain. But the pain is gone and I feel quite well, so I have a good feeling about this therapy.

IEDJE ABBENHUIS, A DUTCH WOMAN LIVING IN BELGIUM, AND A LONG-TIME SURVIVOR OF BREAST CANCER WITH MULTIPLE BONE METASTASES

Chapter 6

THERAPEUTIC FEVER

I would cure all diseases if I only could produce fever.

PARMENIDES, GREEK PHYSICIAN AND PHILOSOPHER,
510 BC

Fever and heat therapy have been recognized for their beneficial effects on health since antiquity. Ancient Greek medicine, Roman hot sulfur baths, Finnish saunas, European and American spa treatments, Japanese hot tubs, Native American Indian sweat lodges, and therapeutic hot springs worldwide are examples of how various cultures have used simple forms of heat as a way of both cleansing and healing. Traditionally there have been two forms of heat therapy: whole body and localized applications. This chapter will discuss modern innovations to both approaches, as applied in the treatment of cancer.

Fever turns out to be one of the missing links in understanding cancer. Most cancer patients have a lower core temperature and cannot mount a fever. Thus they are unable to activate their immune system. We know scientifically that fever is a protective mechanism. When body temperature reaches 101.3°F (38.5°C), the immune system shifts into a state of alarm. At this temperature, the level of immune chemicals in the bloodstream doubles, and immune defenses throughout the body increase. Within six hours, almost every major defense within the immune system doubles its efforts.[36]

This process appears to be dormant in many cancer patients, who typically report never having experienced a fever. To reactivate the immune system in these patients, the Gorter Model uses a process of controlled fever referred to in the scientific literature as *fever-range, total-body hyperthermia*—a form of treatment in which the entire body is heated to a moderate fever temperature of approximately 101.3°F (38.5°C).

As a result, the immune system is activated in the same way as a natural fever would activate immune response, such as to an infection. This approach is necessary to raise the body to a therapeutic fever range, unlike traditional methods such as sauna methods and the hot tub, which do not affect core temperature or achieve temperatures that are as high as the temperature range that occurs during a fever. In the Gorter Model, fever-range, total-body hyperthermia is provided to about 70 percent of all patients. The following quote describes the experience of Fatima Galamba, a patient with breast cancer who received fever-range, total-body hyperthermia and has been in complete remission for two years, with no sign of cancer on any of the scans taken at the hospital.

> *Nothing led me to suspect that I had breast cancer. I'm a strong woman. I've always been strong and active.... I've always done my work with energy and commitment. I've always been very healthy—one of those people who never misses a day of work.*
>
> *I was initially diagnosed with breast cancer in the summer of 2005 and had breast surgery, eight sessions of chemo, twenty-five sessions of radiation, and medication. Although I went into remission and felt better, in 2007 I learned that the cancer had metastasized to my bones, and my oncologist told me that it was incurable.*
>
> *I see cancer as a disease I have to deal with. But I want to live. If other people can survive cancer, so can I. My attitude is that I will do whatever it takes.*
>
> *In August 2008 I began treatment at MCC, despite severe bone pain. At that point I had nothing to lose and everything to gain, so I decided to do the hyperthermia and dendritic cell treatments. The treatments at MCC had no significant side effects, although the two hours of hyperthermia were tough for me. The localized was no problem at all. I*

experienced the dendritic cell vaccinations as a severe flu with headaches and nausea that lasted for about six hours. It was unpleasant, but I knew it would be over after just a few hours.

After three treatments the pain went away. It was totally gone, and I stopped taking painkillers. I have felt good ever since.

Four months after my first treatment at MCC, I went for a checkup with my original oncologist, and they did a PET scan. The bone cancer was gone. There was no trace of the cancer visible on the scans—they had disappeared. In September 2010 another PET-CT scan still showed no recurrences, and I am still in complete remission. Now I am hopeful about the future. God will decide when my time has come. But I know that I will live for many years to come.

Localized heat treatment is another approach used in the Gorter Model in which localized heat is applied to the tumor tissue. In other cases, a "region" or area of the body is selectively heated, again so that only the cancer cells increase in temperature. The local heating increases the temperature within the malignant cells to 42°C (107.6°F) so that they die, due to the increased intracellular lactic acid production. Only the cancer cells are increased in temperature, which leads directly to cell death. The localized high temperature and resulting cancer cell death also activate the immune system. The surrounding healthy cells are not affected. Localized hyperthermia is used with approximately 99 percent of patients.

Fever: Foe or Friend?

In our culture, there is a pervasive fear of fever. Many people see fever as the cause of illness, rather than the body's natural attempt at healing. While fever racks the patient, the mother, father, lover, friend, or caretaker stands by, feeling powerless. It is no wonder that at the first sign of a fever, we quickly reach for medications such as aspirin or Tylenol

(NSAIDS—nonsteroidal, anti-inflammatory drugs). The medicine represents hope and recovery. Giving medication implies a cure. (And so does the advertising.)

The message is that if you can just reduce the fever, the disease will go away. So the caretaker feels empowered by giving fever-suppressing medication. There is the belief that reducing the fever is a way of fighting the illness.

Ironically, the fear of fever is misplaced. Unless the fever is too high (40.0°C/104°F or above) for weeks at a time, no harm occurs. Fever signals the immune system to mount an increased defense and sets the process of healing in motion. In fact, fever is the natural response of all mammals to infection or illness. This is true for cats and dogs, elephants and tigers, horses and humans. Research has made it clear that fever is not the enemy; it is the friend of healing. This scientific rationale, supported by thousands of research studies, provides the basis for hyperthermia treatment at the Medical Center Cologne and other medical centers in Europe, Japan, and worldwide.[37]

The Importance of Body Rhythm in Cancer

When we are well, our core body temperature has a rhythmic pattern. It is lower in the morning and increases in temperature toward the later afternoon—the difference can be as much as 1.8°F (1.0°C) or more. The temperature difference decreases as we age.[38] The pattern is often noticeable in children, who may become flushed and rosy cheeked in the late afternoon. They may run a higher temperature as if they have a low fever. These mild fevers normally decrease as the evening progresses.

In patients with cancer, core body temperature tends to be lower than normal—for many it is more than 1°F lower. Many report that they have frequently felt chilly over the last few years and often have cold feet and hands. This is an indicator that their body has difficulty regulating temperature and suggests a disruption of the normal bio-logical rhythms.

In addition, there may be an inconsistent pattern in the rhythm of their temperature over a twenty-four-hour period. Figure 6.1 shows the different core temperatures and twenty-four-hour temperature rhythms of healthy adults, as compared with patients with cancer before and after treatment with the Gorter Model.

In clinical practice, doctors observe that many cancer patients simply don't develop fevers, and cancer patients often report that they were never ill. Their core temperature is on average 0.8°F (0.5°C) lower than in healthy people, and their natural temperature circadian rhythm is absent.

Patients often report that they may have had brief bouts of a sore throat, a cold, or a cough, but these illnesses were never accompanied by a fever. Many of these patients, like most people in industrial soci-eties, habitually use aspirin, Tylenol (acetaminophen), or antibiotics at the first sign of a fever. Antibiotics are another medication that tends to suppress fever.[39]

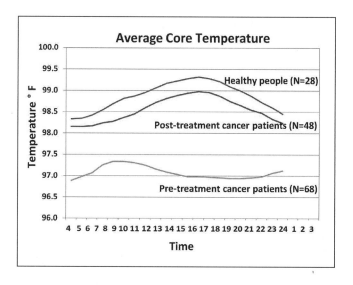

Figure 6.1. The average rectal core tempera-ture for twenty-four hours of healthy adult controls and cancer patients before and after treatment (from Gorter, unpub-lished data)

With frequent use of fever suppressants, the immune system may never mature adequately or become fully activated. Without an all-out effort by the immune function to completely wipe out an infection, many bacterial and viral infections tend to linger and become chronic. In addition, the immune system is prevented from opportunities for a "work out" and becomes less and less adept, leaving the body more vulnerable. This can set the stage for developing cancer.

Part 1. Fever-Range, Total-Body Hyperthermia

Fever-range, total-body hyperthermia is a nontoxic treatment that is often linked to improved temperature regulation in the body. The treatment is well tolerated by practically all patients and can be provided in combination with a range of other therapies. In the past twenty-five years, more than a thousand clinical trials on induced fever-range, total-body hyperthermia and localized hyperthermia have been conducted, and thousands of scientific articles have been published in the peer-reviewed medical literature. Hyperthermia has also been studied for chronic pain, asthma, and other chronic or recurrent respiratory infections, urinary tract infections, and immune deficiency.

More than seven hundred research studies have focused specifically on cancer treatment using total body hyperthermia. Research on fever therapy for cancer has been performed in medical schools and research centers since the 1980s. These studies have been conducted primarily in the United States, Germany, and Japan, but also in Australia, China, Denmark, Italy, the Netherlands, New Zealand, Norway, South Korea, and other countries. American research has been conducted in FDA-approved studies at centers such as the Mayo Clinic, University of Pennsylvania, University of Texas, and Duke University. These studies reflect a global dialogue between researchers across the world that has systematically defined effective fever therapy.

At the Medical Center Cologne, fever-range, total-body hyperthermia is given to approximately 70 percent of all patients. Because fever is a stress to the system, it is usually not given to patients with severe cardiac decompensation or to patients with brain cancer because it potentially can evoke cardiac difficulties or an epileptic seizure. For almost all other patients, fever-range, total-body hyperthermia has no negative side effects, or risks. Usually when patients complete the fever-range, total-body hyperthermia treatment, they feel cleansed and energized. In many cases, this hyperthermia treatment is provided first in the protocol to simulate the fever response of the body.

To personally understand and experience the nature of fever-range, total-body hyperthermia, one of the authors (Erik Peper) volunteered to experience a treatment:

When I arrived at the clinic for my hyperthermia treatment, the nurse checked me in and then helped me settle into the hyperthermia chamber, which is essentially a light tent/box heated by infrared lights [see figures 6.2a and 6.2b].

My head was outside the tent, comfortably supported by a pillow, which avoids any sense of claustrophobia. The doctor then began an IV infusion of electrolyte minerals to ensure that I would not get dehydrated. The infusion included antioxidants, particularly vitamin C and selenium. An electronic thermometer was provided rectally so that my core temperature could be monitored continuously. To monitor my heart rate during the treatment, the nurse also placed a few electrodes on my skin, attached with gel. (This is another step provided to ensure the safety of all patients.)

The lights inside the light chamber gradually increased my temperature. However, because the container is relatively airtight, perspiration did not cool my body, which was also covered with heavy towels to retain the heat. My temperature gradually increased. After about three hours, the lights were turned off, but my temperature continued to increase for a while because the blood just under the surface of my skin was still warmer than the rest of my body. Once my skin began to cool, the returning blood began to cool, and my core temperature very slowly began dropping naturally.

For me, the worst side effect of hyperthermia treatment was boredom and the inability to turn over while lying on my back for four and a half hours. My major concern occurred about two hours into the treatment: I had to urinate. This was solved by urinating into a special container. When the treatment session was finished, I took a shower, shampooed my hair, and felt comfortably warm, very relaxed, and ready for a meal. I went downstairs to the hospital cafeteria and ate a large salad and a delicious dessert. This is a very different experience than I imagine I would have had with chemotherapy or radiation.

ERIK PEPER

Hyperthermia can be used as the primary form of treatment or safely applied in combination with conventional therapies such as chemotherapy or radiation. Controlled studies have documented that chemotherapy or radiation in combination with total body hyperthermia becomes more effective, often with fewer side effects than chemotherapy or radiation alone. In the European Union, this combination therapy is widely available at numerous major cancer treatment centers in cities such as Amsterdam, Hamburg, Munich, Rotterdam, Stuttgart, and Utrecht.

How Fever Ramps Up the Immune Response

Fever is the signal that launches our immune defenses. Once a fever reaches 101.3°F (38.5°C), the level of immune defenses in the blood doubles within the next six hours.

Launching our defenses. Specialized proteins referred to as *heat-shock proteins* activate white blood cells and other immune defenses to increase their anticancer activities.

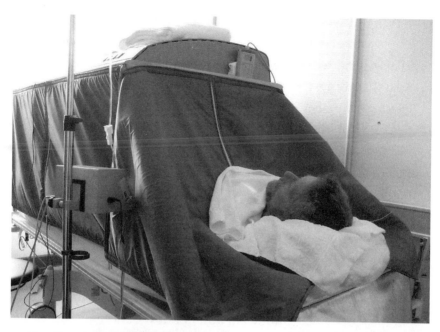

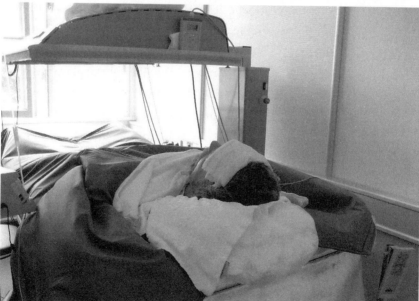

Figures 6.2a and 6.2b. Erik Peper receiving hyperthermia treatment. Note in the second picture, the nurse has placed a cool cloth on his forehead to make him more comfortable during the cooling down period.

Calling in the troops. Messenger chemicals such as interleukins and cytokines circulate throughout the bloodstream, signaling a state of alarm and recruiting immune defenses.

Search and destroy. Dendritic cells are activated to roam the body looking for malignant and virus-infected cells to identify them for destruction. When these cells are found, the dendritic cells go to the nearest lymph node and report the location of the cancer cells.

Infection fighters. Natural killer (NK) cells are the demolition crew of the immune system. They cruise the body, hunting down cancerous cells and terminating them. Other defenses, such as T cells, are targeted against specific types of infection

Ammunition. Antibodies are fragments of protein like microscopic arrows that are targeted at intruders such as bacteria, viruses, and parasites, but they also can play a role in blocking cancer cells from multiplying. This immune ammunition is produced by B cells and kills intruders and abnormal cells in the body alike. All these immune components are activated by fever.

Mop-up operations. Phagocytes, macrophages, and granulocytes are like Pac-Men or "cookie monsters" that literally swallow invaders and then digest them whole. This clears the body of dangerous oxidants and toxic cancer-specific proteins that are left behind after the NK cells have done their job. They consume dead cancer cells and also swallow up invasive bacteria and other unpleasant microbes. This process is called *phagocytosis*.

Blocking tumor formation. Tumors grow most rapidly when they are able to form new blood vessels *(angiogenesis)*. These highly primitive blood vessels are vulnerable to destruction and can actually be obstructed when immune defenses are strong.

Promoting tissue repair. Fever also enhances the body's ability to repair tissue by improving circulation. Fever promotes the release of a greater number of stem cells from the bone for repair and improves blood flow to areas where repair is needed.

The Process of Fever Therapy

The goal of hyperthermia in oncology is to induce a fever state that will activate the immune system and destroy the cancer cells. The patient lies within a hyperthermia chamber where her body is heated by specially developed infrared lamps—the safest, most natural source of warmth currently available. Infrared waves are invisible light waves close to those of visible light on the spectrum. In nature, the sun is the most effective source of infrared radiation, supporting all life processes on earth. In hyperthermia, short-wave infrared radiation penetrates the skin and warms blood vessels close to the surface of the skin. As the temperature rises in the skin and the blood flowing through the skin, the warmth spreads throughout the body, and core temperature begins to increase. Infrared light is one of the primary means used to heat the body in fever-range, total-body hyperthermia.

As the heat is gradually increased, the patient begins to perspire; but without airflow, evaporation cannot occur. Transpiration and perspiration only lead to cooling if the water can be evaporated. Perspiration is our primary means of maintaining stable body temperature. Without this process, body temperature continues to increase, raising core temperature and inducing a fever-like state. Once the fever is reached and maintained for one to two hours, the heat is very gradually reduced over the course of another hour or two.

In the Gorter Model, directly after fever-range, total-body hyperthermia treatment, patients receive an injection of dendritic cells cultured from their own blood. They usually experience mild flu-like symptoms for six to twelve hours right after the treatment. This is not the flu—it is the body's response, which indicates that the immune system is being activated. After these symptoms subside, almost all patients report less pain and a greater sense of well-being. It has been observed that patients who react with flu-like symptoms after the vaccination with dendritic cells do clearly better and show more benefit from the therapy than do those patients who cannot mount any flu-like symptoms at all. All of our patients who went in complete remission always experienced flu-like symptoms.

How Fever Activates the Immune System

The core body temperature of a human being is approximately 98.6°F (37°C), and this varies during the day, as mentioned. In total body hyperthermia, the patient's core body temperature is slowly increased to about 102.2°F (39°C), and sometimes even to 104°F (40.0°C) if it is medically appropriate.

The immune shift is triggered by an impulse from deep within the brain stem in the hypothalamus. This area of the brain contains the command center for our most basic functions, especially those our bodies carry on without our conscious awareness such as breathing, blood pressure, and core body temperature. This command center guides the autonomic nervous system, which functions "automatically." Fever is triggered from deep within the most ancient area of the brain, also present in all mammals, which demonstrates how fundamental fever is to our functioning.

Fever-range, total-body hyperthermia treatment is used to relaunch and reactivate cells of the immune system. These defenses increase targeted efforts to destroy the cancer through cytotoxicity. This selective toxicity by immune cells targets malignant cells, resulting in tumor cell death *(necrosis* and *apoptosis)*. Healing occurs as the cancer load is lowered through improved immune activity. In sum, the fever primes the immune system to destroy cancerous cells and triggers increased immune responses throughout the whole body.

I was diagnosed with colon cancer, and that spread to my liver. Although I did well on the chemotherapy, the oncologist made it clear that treatment was palliative and not a cure. So we made an appointment for a consultation in Cologne. When we learned that Dr. Gorter's treatment could be used together with chemotherapy, we decided to do that as well.

I began the fever-range, total-body hyperthermia and dendritic cell therapy in Cologne. Once you've received the treatment, you know what to expect. It's not painful, and I was hardly sick at all. I usually feel worse after the dendritic cell vaccination, but only for one day. Every nine weeks a scan is made, and they show that there are no new tumors and the liver tumors are getting smaller. The fact that my cancer has stabilized is remarkable.

TRUUS KLEIJ-SWAN

Safety and Effectiveness of Hyperthermia

The approach to fever-range, total-body hyperthermia in the Gorter Model is based on twenty-five years of clinical experience by Robert Gorter. The model differs from other treatment protocol in several ways:

- **Comprehensive therapy.** At the Medical Center Cologne, fever-range, total-body hyperthermia is usually provided in combination with local hyperthermia, injections of dendritic cells, mistletoe injections, and IV nutrients for immune restoration. This therapy enables the immune system to better identify cancer cells and targets efforts to destroy them.

- **Low intensity.** Controlled fever is maintained at a moderate temperature to safeguard the well-being of the patient. Maximum temperatures range from 101.3°F (38.5°C) to 103°F (39.5°C).

- **Carefully staged treatment.** Temperature is gradually increased for three hours and then, after a plateau of about one hour, allowed to return to normal over the course of one to two hours. The average treatment lasts four to six hours in total.

- **Optimal timing.** Hyperthermia in combination with dendritic cell vaccinations is provided six times monthly. A major difference with other hyperthermia protocols is the timing sequence. That is, the induced fever-range, total-body hyperthermia mobilizes the immune system, and then the immune system is augmented by the dendritic cell vaccinations. Thus, the body receives millions of its own activated dendritic cells, timed to work together with fever-induced immune system activation.

- **An absence of side effects.** This process involves the body's innate immune responses. Treatment is accomplished with almost no disruption or side effects—typically less than one day of mild flu-like symptoms at most.

- **Primary therapy.** This timed approach is almost always effective in restarting and enhancing immune function and competence. This method harnesses the biological healing power of fever in the treatment of cancer patients. Once the immune system is engaged, the body begins destroying cancer cells from within. This reduces the need for medication and stabilizes the body against further deterioration. These gains provide the basis for a sense of well-being, improved health, and healing, even in many patients with Stage III and IV (end-stage) cancer.

- **Complementary to conventional treatment.** Fever-range, total-body hyperthermia can be applied as part of a comprehensive immune therapy program or in combination with conventional therapy such as chemotherapy or radiation. The majority of studies have focused on this combination treatment. Research has shown that hyperthermia increases the effectiveness of conventional therapy with fewer side effects than chemotherapy or radiation treatment alone. Also, conventional therapies sustain their efficacy when given in combination with hyperthermia. In the European Union, this type of combination therapy is widely applied in most major cancer treatment centers.

Part 2. Localized Hyperthermia

Twenty years ago, Teun van Vliet was twice a world-champion indoor cyclist, and in 1988 he wore the yellow jersey in the Tour de France. In 2001 he was diagnosed with a brain tumor, and in 2006 an inoperable recurrence of the tumor was detected. Teun had another round of brain surgery (known as "debulking") and also received radiation treatment. This caused him to lose his power of speech, and to some degree he also lost memory and coordination. Within conventional oncology, nothing could be done for him. He was told that he had a year left to live at the most. Teun and his girlfriend decided to seek a second opinion, and they went to Cologne to consult with Dr. Gorter, who advised him to do localized hyperthermia in combination with immune therapy. Teun's partner soon noticed beneficial changes in his health:

> The first thing we noticed about these treatments was that they really improved his speech. He is much more lively, more active. I have my old buddy back, really. When he comes home from Cologne, his speech has improved, his motor skills have improved, he feels more energetic. Nothing but improvements. The quality of his life is definitely better. In April 2010, a new MRI scan confirmed that there is still no recurrence of the cancer, and Teun has been clinically cancer-free for more than four and a half years.[40]

To date there are more than 2,800 articles in the medical literature listed under "regional hyperthermia." Hundreds of preliminary animal studies were performed before clinical research was initiated. In conventional oncology, the majority of studies have evaluated local hyperthermia in tandem with chemotherapy or radiation. At least 230 clinical trials have been conducted in countries worldwide, including Canada, China, France, Germany, Greece, Italy, Israel, Japan, the Netherlands, and Sweden. Extensive research has been performed at the National Cancer Institute in Rome and the National Cancer Research Center in Heidelberg in Germany for more than two decades. American studies include research at the Anderson Cancer Center in Houston, at Duke University, and at Wake Forest University. Localized hyperthermia is used with all patients at the Medical Center Cologne who have solid tumors. It is an approach in which heat is initiated *only* in the tumor cell, so it leaves a healthy cell unaffected. Tumor cells have a very different cell dynamic—the membrane has an unusual surface potential, and they produce abnormal tumor-specific proteins that can also be used as tumor markers.

One of the reasons that localized hyperthermia is so effective is that cancer cells contain abnormal proteins that are coarser and thousands of times larger than normal proteins. During hyperthermia, these tumor proteins absorb the energy when exposed to an MRI-like electromagnetic field. This causes the cells to heat up to a very high temperature: 107.6°F (42°C). The heating causes the cancer cell to increase its metabolism and, therefore, its lactic acid production, which causes the cancer cells to become highly acidic (pH declines) so much that these cells die. Neighboring healthy cells are not affected at all and stay at regular body temperature.

The selective heating of the cancer cells directly causes the death of the malignant cells without affecting the adjacent healthy cells, as shown in treatment in figure 6.3.

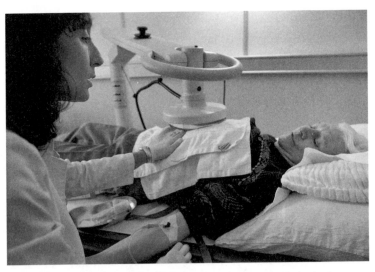

Figure 6.3. Example of a patient receiving local hyperthermia for brain cancer (photo by Jana Asenbrennerova).

In summary, cancer cells have an abnormal metabolism. Normal cells found throughout the body produce carbon dioxide as a waste product. In contrast, malignant cells produce lactic acid. When the cancer cells within a tumor are heated to 42°C (107.6°F), the production of lactic acid increases rapidly, and the cells become highly acidic (pH goes down).[41] As metabolism speeds up within the tumor cells, they essentially self-destruct and drown in the lactic acid that they produce. Healthy tissue surrounding the cancer cells is unaffected by the localized heat used in the treatment. The same biological dynamics occur to a reduced degree during normal fevers of 101.3°F (38.3°C), in which cancers become more and more stressed and produce more lactic acid.

Making Cancer Visible to the Immune System

Cancer cell are also able to hide (cloak themselves) from the immune system, thereby avoiding detection. Total-body fever therapy and localized hyperthermia both disrupt this cloaking mechanism. Whether it is local or fever-range, total-body hyperthermia, each degree of increase in temperature causes cancer cells to undergo greater stress until the lactic acid production has increased to such a degree that the cancer cell is threatened with suffocation. The cancer cells will try to fight off their impending death by putting all their energy into surviving, thus dropping their escape mechanisms. Once cancer cells drop their escape mechanisms, they are more easily detected by dendritic cells, which now can better "see" the "naked" or uncloaked cancer cells. As a result, the dendritic cells are better able to obtain an image of the cancer cells' ID—their profile or antigen.

As Robert Gorter notes,

The electro-hyperthermia equipment used for localized hyperthermia causes no risk of burns and can be focused exclusively on any area of the body. Unlike fever-range, total-body hyperthermia, with this localized technique we can selectively heat tumor cells. This enables us to provide interventions for areas of the body that would normally be difficult to treat such as the lungs, bone, and the head. The fact that hyperthermia can be efficacious in treating brain tumors was borne out by a recent Phase III study for patients with brain lesions, in which hyperthermia proved to support significantly better results in terms of illness-free time and survival when compared with radiation and/or medication.

Localized hyperthermia is a highly effective means of destroying cancer cells without causing toxicity, particularly when used in conjunction with other immune-supportive therapies such as vitamin C infusions, thymus peptides, and mistletoe extract. In addition, most patients are provided with dendritic cell injections since the heating process makes cancer cells more vulnerable for destruction by the immune system. The efficacy of dendritic cell vaccinations is enhanced by simply injecting them during or right after a fever period.

At the Medical Center Cologne, even patients with primary or secondary brain tumors or metastases of the breast or lung are successfully treated in this way without any side effects. Statistically, the research shows that about 72 percent of all patients with Stage IV glioblastoma multiforme die within the first year after diagnosis, and only 1 percent survive for three years. At the Medical Center Cologne, 48 percent of all patients with Stage IV glioblastoma multiforme go into complete and persistent remission following a protocol of at least three dendritic cell vaccinations and twenty-four sessions of local hyperthermia.[42]

Localized Hyperthermia Research and Clinical Trials

As mentioned, approximately 2,800 articles have been published to date on regional or localized hyperthermia. Among the fifty most recent studies on localized hyperthermia, the majority (thirty-two) involved the use of hyperthermia with chemotherapy. The majority of the other studies evaluated localized hyperthermia in combination with surgery and with radiation. The others involved some form of immunotherapy provided in combination with the local hyperthermia treatments (primarily tumor necrosis factor alpha—TNF-alpha). Researchers have documented that conventional treatments (e.g., chemotherapy and radiation), when used in combination with localized hyperthermia, clearly work more effectively and have fewer side effects than when used alone.

Only a handful of large clinical trials have focused on localized hyperthermia as a stand-alone treatment, perhaps due to the lack of economic incentives. We predict that in the future, patients who desire a nontoxic approach to cancer will be treated with localized hyperthermia, paired with some form of immunotherapy such as those offered at the Medical Center Cologne.

Total Body Hyperthermia Research and Clinical Trials

Induced total-body hyperthermia was first studied in animal models twenty-five years ago, and then in humans over the past twenty years, both in cancer patients and in healthy volunteers.[43] Initial studies explored the most effective ways to administer the therapy, defining the length of treatment,[44] heat sources,[45] optimal temperatures,[46] and the effects produced. Treatment has been applied as a freestanding therapy, in combination with immune therapies such as dendritic cell injections,[47] and with conventional therapies such as radiation,[48] chemotherapy,[49] or hormones.[50] Decades of research have shown that hyperthermia is a safe procedure for the greater majority of patients and many types of cancer.[51]

Effectiveness. Natural killer (NK) cells play an important in destroying the cancer cells. Hyperthermia is effective in recruiting NK cells into action.[52] When dendritic cells are also provided through inoculation, they activate toxic (cytotoxic) T cells, alerting them to the cancer tissue in the body. Working in combination, these immune cells have inhibiting effects on tumor growth.[53]

Safety and duration. Studies conducted in the 1980s and 1990s established hyperthermia as a safe form of treatment.[54] Studies in Germany have also confirmed the safety of infrared radiation as an optimal heat source.[55] This is the form of heat used at the Medical Center Cologne in fever-range, total-body hyperthermia. In terms of the length of the therapy, early studies provided hyperthermia for a duration of thirty to sixty minutes, but most treatment provided today is typically two to four hours, depending on the patient's response, plus a cooling-down period of one to two hours. The Gorter Model utilizes a protocol of at least three to four hours in which the temperature is gradually increased over the course of two hours or longer, followed by a sixty-minute interval when the temperature is maintained at a steady level (plateau) before cooling to restore normal temperature.

Modulating core temperature. Research has confirmed that traditional forms of heat therapy such as mineral baths and Jacuzzis have a very limited effect on core temperature. A study at the Medical University of Hannover, Germany, showed that when body temperature was raised via warm baths that were gradually heated to 42°C (approx 107°F), core temperature actually increased less than 1°F (or 0.4°C) above normal.[56]

Activating the immune system. It is well recognized that the immune system ramps up and doubles the level of immune activity in the blood at 101.3°F (38.5°C). Therefore, the maximum temperature used with patients at the Medical Center Cologne is 102.2°F (39°C). This moderate approach to hyperthermia increases the safety factor while effectively promoting an immune response. Research from the University of Vienna has shown in a test tube evaluation that when blood was heated to 102.2°F (39°C), the level of protective monocytes multiplied by ten times.[57] These researchers also confirmed that one of the mechanisms that promotes this increase is heat-shock proteins, a factor in the blood that plays a role in calling up the immune response.[58]

Tapping the body's intelligence. A study in Hamburg, Germany, found that an increase in body temperature alone does not automatically induce the immune response. In this research, the temperatures of cancer patients were increased with hyperthermia and compared with those of healthy volunteers who took part in strenuous physical exercise to raise their temperatures. Although participants in both groups experienced elevated temperatures, immune function increased in the cancer patients but not in the healthy volunteers. Elevated immune factors in the cancer patients included human growth hormone and the induction of NK cells and T cells.[59]

Moderating temperature. In contrast to the Gorter Model, many of the research studies use temperatures in the range of 107.5°F (41.8°C to 42°C), and in some of the studies patients were anesthetized so they could tolerate these high temperatures. We believe that unnecessary anesthesia is always to be avoided, since it can induce senility in older patients in a phenomenon known as Sundowner Syndrome, and general anesthesia is often immune suppressing.

Treatment without side effects. A German study of hyperthermia for pain in patients with fibromyalgia tracked safety and effectiveness and noted, "Side effects were observed in 14 of 69 participants (20%) but all disappeared in less than 30 minutes."[60] The study showed that hyperthermia combined with standard multimodal rehabilitation was significantly more effective than was standard therapy alone in terms of reducing pain intensity while improving quality of life.

Minimizing distress. Researchers at the Roswell Park Cancer Institute in Buffalo, New York, report that fever-range, total-body hyperthermia treatments are "well tolerated, with no significant adverse events related to cardiac, hepatic, renal, or pulmonary systems."[61] However, patients with a history of heart disease or brain tumors must be carefully screened. At the Medical Center Cologne, only 70 percent of patients are considered eligible for hyperthermia. Additional safety measures used at the center include an electrolyte IV solution to avoid dehydration and monitoring of the heart rate at all times.

Therapeutic fever in combination with conventional therapies. Hyperthermia has also been found to increase the successful use of radiation[62] and chemotherapy[63] and improves the efficacy of medications.[64] A study conducted at a medical center in the Netherlands tracked the progress of 378 cancer patients receiving both hyperthermia and radiation treatments. Over an eight-year period, a positive response was achieved in 77 percent of patients. At five years, the disease-specific survival rate was 47 percent, which is exceptional in cancer treatment. Toxicity was an issue for 12 percent of patients. Researchers concluded that in addition to diagnosis, "the number of hyperthermia treatments emerged as a predictor of positive outcome."[65]

In the majority of studies, a stabilizing therapeutic response was experienced by more than 50 percent of patients—typically 56 to 80 percent of those treated. Hyperthermia is becoming accepted throughout Europe and has been researched in the United States at university medical centers such as the University of Pennsylvania[66] and the University of Texas.[67] We predict that the next phase of this research will focus on hyperthermia as a freestanding cancer therapy for patients with inoperable tumors and for those who require or desire a protocol low in toxicity.

For more on the use of hyperthermia in cancer treatment, download the U.S. Department of Health and Human Services' Fact Sheet at www.cancer.gov/images/Documents/c5006d69-7257-47b4-a416-519ad402a243/Fs7_3.pdf.

The Role of Fever in Immunity

The research makes it clear that fever is a protective mechanism that plays an important role in fighting infection, healing wounds, and destroying malignancies.

Fever is the necessary signal that ramps up the immune response.

Fever is a basic, protective response to infection in almost all animals.[68] The U.S. National Library of Medicine affirms this, defining fever as "an abnormal elevation of body temperature, usually as a result of a pathologic process [i.e., infection]."[69] However, laypeople have assumed that fever was the *cause* of illness—not realizing that fever is the body's primary response in fighting infection.

NIH Report on Fever

One of the most insightful looks at the role of fever has come from a research team from the National Institutes of Health. The researchers performed an in-depth review of the medical literature on cancer risk. They reported that risk appears to be increased in individuals who have not experienced fewer infections. They noted "an inverse correlation between the incidence of infectious diseases and cancer risk." In other words, people who have not experienced common childhood illness and fever seem to have a greater risk of cancer.

Averting fever by the frequent use of aspirin or antibiotics may actually impair immune function. The NIH team concluded that "the occurrence of fever in childhood or adulthood may protect against the later onset of malignant disease."[70] They also pointed out that "spontaneous remissions are often preceded by feverish infections." Their final report includes hundreds of references from the medical and research literature.

A Century of Research on Fever

A number of researchers have tracked this issue in large clinical trials over the past hundred and fifty years, starting with published reports in 1854 that many cancer patients have a "remarkable disease-free history."[71] Several later studies confirmed this, reporting that people who developed cancer were rarely ill before their disease.

If it seems surprising that this premise would have gone unrecognized for a hundred and fifty years, consider the fact that scurvy among seaman caused by lack of vitamin C was not acknowledged for more than a century after it was first confirmed by a ship's physician. The doctor's recommendations were adopted 105 years later when another naval physician reported a similar finding.

In a similar pattern, studies on the importance of fever in a strong immune defense against cancer were published in the medical literature in 1854, 1910, 1934, and 1936, each study involving hundreds of patients. Researchers consistently found increased cancer risk for patients who had no history of infectious illness or fever.[72] The majority of more recent studies have corroborated these findings.

- German research published in 1983 found that cancer risk more than doubled in patients who had not experienced major infectious diseases (2.6 times greater risk). Cancer risk was more than five times higher in patients who had never experienced the common cold (5.7 odds ratio), and there was a fifteen-fold increase for those who had never experienced fever (15.1 odds ratio).[73]

- A study of skin cancer patients published in *Melanoma Research* in 1992 reviewed the medical histories of five hundred comparable patients with and without cancer. Researchers found that the patients who had experienced infections accompanied by fever had a much lower incidence of malignant melanoma.[74]

- Research published in the journal *Cancer* in 1992 evaluated the medical histories of more than two hundred patients with brain tumors, who were compared with more than four hundred similar but non-cancerous patients. Those who had experienced infections and colds had a 70 percent lower risk of cancer.[75]

How Fever Activates Immune Function

As described in detail earlier in this chapter, fever is actually the signal that mounts immune activity in response to infection, illness, injury, or malignancy. At 101.3°F (38.5°C) the immune system doubles its functions, in response to impulses from deep within the brain stem.

This increase in body temperature has been shown to call up various aspects of the immune function, including chemical messengers such as interleukin that call the immune system into action,[76] dendritic cells that identify the infection or malignancy, heat-shock proteins that activate white cells,[77] and T cells to destroy viruses and cancer cells.[78]

The Role of Fever in Immune Development

In a newborn the immune system is immature and underdeveloped. For example, protective antibodies are not made by the infant's body, and the baby relies on those transmitted before birth by the mother to her infant through the placenta. These maternal antibodies become depleted by the time the baby is about six months old. At this point, the immune system of the child must learn how to respond to invasive infections such as bacteria, viruses, and parasites and to threats from within the body such as abnormal and cancerous cells. Like any other organ system, the immune system must develop and mature if the child is to remain healthy.

On average, each newborn develops about seven viral infections in its first year of life. Researchers now view fever as a "necessary attempt by nature" to support immune system development and have confirmed that it is the process that activates the immune response.[79] Cohort studies have also shown that a child needs at least four to five episodes of high fever before age six to develop an adept immune system.

The development of immunity can be compared with the maturation of the muscles and skeleton, which only develop correctly if they are used all the time and experience periodic exertion from activity and play. That is why we encourage children to participate in sports. A child who is bed-bound or wheelchair-bound does not have the opportunity to develop a proper skeleton and musculature as a result of disuse.

The immune system can only develop fully if it is put under "stress" by defending the child against invading microbes such as viruses and bacteria. When a child experiences any type of infection, the immune system must augment its defense mechanisms and step up its activities and metabolism. In childhood, fever is important because it plays a role in immune development and maturation so the system can function properly lifelong.

A number of researchers have suggested that averting childhood infections and fever through inoculations for benign illnesses such as chicken pox and rubella may be a factor in increased vulnerability to cancer in adulthood.

- A British study published in 1977 of three hundred women with ovarian cancer found lower incidence of measles, mumps, and rubella compared to noncancerous patients.[80]
- A study published in *The Lancet* in 1985 of five hundred patients reported that approximately 6 percent of cancer patients had not developed measles in childhood compared with fewer than 1 percent of noncancerous participants in the study.[81]
- A 1986 study in the *American Journal of Epidemiology* reported that children with leukemia had experienced fewer infections in their first year of infancy, suggesting the importance of stimulating the immune system early in life.[82]

Effects of Fever Suppression

Blocking fever with medication such as aspirin, Tylenol, or antibiotics appears to compromise long-term health by impairing immune development.[83]

Absence of fever in cancer patients. In clinical cases evaluated at the Medical Center Cologne, the vast majority of cancer patients report that they are never sick and they never missed a day at work. Typically, they may have had a few days when they experienced a sore throat, a cold, or a cough, but it was never accompanied by fever. When fever did develop, it was suppressed with aspirin, Tylenol, or antibiotics.[84]

Most cancer patients also have a reduced core body temperature and lack of circadian temperature rhythm.[85] These are indications of the inability to raise temperature to a level necessary to activate the immune system.

It is possible that we have unknowingly conditioned the immune system not to respond, through our use of fever suppressants with our children.

Interrupting the fever mechanism. Surprisingly, the immune system can be trained to turn on or off in response to repeated cues, for example in response to certain medications. This trained or "conditioned" response was demonstrated in the work of Dr. Robert Ader and colleagues, published over a period of twenty-five years.[86] Researchers found that the immune system could actually be deactivated through "classical conditioning."

Applying this finding to the use of fever-suppressing medications with children, the implication is that over time the fever response can be permanently inactivated by the frequent use of medication. Childhood fevers are also prevented when vaccines are used to avoid common childhood infections. From that point on, whenever the child develops a fever, the fever process is aborted.

Suppressing the immune response. In time, the body becomes conditioned to suppress fever at the slightest hint of a fever. Since fever is the cue that activates many of the key defenses of the immune system, this also means that the immune response is cut short and never activated.

Loss of defenses against cancer. We now know that our bodies develop cancer cells every day of our lives.[87] When we have periodic bouts of cold or flu and allow our bodies to experience a fever, that provides an additional opportunity for clearing malignancies and lingering infections. If the immune system is never activated, we have lost these opportunities to destroy cancer cells while their number is still small.

Increased risk of chronic infection. Suppressing fever may also enable bacterial and viral infections to become chronic. Without fever, some of the infectious cells escape destruction, linger, and start increasing in number. Note that although we think of antibiotics as our primary protection, it is actually the immune system that protects us. The antibiotics simply lower the infectious load so the immune system can handle it more easily.

Infections linked to cancer. Specific types of chronic infection have been linked to the localized development of cancer, including human papillomavirus, viral hepatitis, and *H. pylori* bacteria. In the peer-reviewed literature, more than twenty thousand articles address the link between cancer and these three infectious agents.

- Chronic human papillomavirus infection is implicated in about 40 to 80 percent of all cervical cancers.[88]
- Various forms of hepatitis viral infections are associated with the development of liver cancer.[89]
- *H. pylori* bacterial infections have been identified as a causal factor in an estimated 40 to 80 percent of gastric cancers.[90]

Allergies, asthma, and cancer. Among children who never developed a high fever, about 30 percent develop food allergies, hay fever, and contact dermatitis (atopic dermatitis). In children who experienced episodes of childhood fever, only 5 percent develop these allergic reactions. Overuse of fever-suppressing medications has been found to increase the risk of allergies and autoimmune conditions.[91]

Increased incidence of asthma. A recent study on the effects of Tylenol exposure in childhood published in the British journal *Lancet* in 2008 reported on the health of 205,487 children ages six to seven years old from thirty-one countries.[92]

The study found that exposure to Tylenol (acetaminophen) during intrauterine fetal development or during the first year of infancy was associated with an increased risk of asthma symptoms. The risk was "dose-dependant"—the more frequent the Tylenol use, the greater the likelihood of asthma. Tylenol use, both in the first year of life and in children aged six to seven years is also associated with an increased risk of symptoms of rhinoconjunctivitis and eczema. These data suggest that by suppressing fever, the immune system becomes compromised and less functional.[93]

The Effect of Vaccines

The use of vaccines averts fevers that would normally have occurred if the child had been exposed to chicken pox, rubella, or measles instead of being vaccinated. Thus later in life when spontaneous cancer cell production in the body increases or the immune system ages and becomes less competent, cancer can progress instead of being recognized and destroyed by the immune system.

Although our society tends to the belief that vaccinations have made a significant impact in illness and death rates, for a number of vaccines the data do not bear this out. For common illnesses such as measles and whooping cough, U.S. and British data suggest that the death rate already had fallen significantly by the time the vaccine was introduced. In fact, the rates were so low at that point that vaccination apparently had little or no impact (see figures 6.4a and 6.4b).[94]

The absolute impact of vaccination is extremely small if the death rate is plotted from 1900 to the present. Thomas McKeown, PhD, a noted epidemiologist, carefully reviewed the historical medical data on immunization. He states in *The Role of Medicine,* "I conclude that the

Figures 6.4a and 6.4b. The absolute impact of measles and whooping cough (pertussis) vaccinations is extremely small if the death rate is plotted from 1900 to the present. The largest decrease in the death rate occurred before the vaccines were introduced. Used with permission from www.healthsentinel.com.

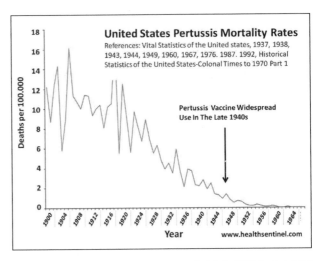

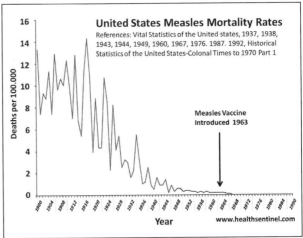

contribution of immunization on the reduction of notifications [deaths] in the last decade cannot be decided on this evidence."[95]

More pediatricians worldwide now recommend that children be allowed to experience most normal childhood illnesses and viral infections that induce fever, unless the child belongs to a high-risk group or is immune compromised.

Public policy and clinical practice. Leading pediatricians and immunologists now recommend that children not be vaccinated for benign childhood diseases such as chicken pox or rubella. It is not clear whether vaccination for these illnesses in healthy, non-immune-compromised children offers any benefit.

Polio vaccine. We strongly recommend *continuing* oral vaccination for polio because the long-term effects of this disease can be exceptionally harmful.

Conservative Use of Medication

The use of medication is an area of discretionary control within the family. The question is when to use over-the-counter drugs such as aspirin or acetaminophen (Tylenol), and when to request antibiotics. This is an issue about which parents can become informed. The goal is to open tactful dialogue with one's physician. This kind of thoughtful discussion can have a positive influence on public awareness and health policy. Although policy change may seem beyond our influence, consider the fact that twenty-five years ago, no one would have guessed that conventional medicine would someday recommend a conservative policy on the use of antibiotics or that cigarette smoking would be limited in public places.

Another key piece of this is to become more informed about the protective role of fever in health. Currently, fever in childhood is seen not only as inconvenient but also as dangerous. And this is almost never true. Although fever can be a sign of serious illness (such as bacterial meningitis), this is surprisingly rare.

The current approach to common nonthreatening childhood illnesses is to monitor the fever when the child is sick. The fever is brought down only if it goes too high—greater than 102°F (38.9°C). At that temperature, the fever can be attenuated by cooling the body with a lemon wash or giving medication.

We encourage an open discussion of these questions among both health care practitioners and parents alike, so fever can be appreciated as a healthy physiological effort by the body to support and activate immune function. The key fact that emerges from the data is that fever is the mechanism by which every major immune response is mounted against infection—and also one of our primary protections against cancer. A large body of research is testament to this.[96]

Chapter 7

RESTORING IMMUNE FUNCTION

Dendritic cell therapy has no side effects for me, except for a touch of flu, which means that the treatment is catching on. It does cause a temporary fever, which usually starts about an hour after the injection. Over the course of eight hours, the fever rises a little, in my case up to about 38.9°C (102°F).

Somehow it feels fine—I feel as though something positive is happening—I don't feel ill. Although it's a real fever, somehow my body knows that I need this. And the results are fantastic. My MRI scans over the past five years have confirmed that the treatment has been successful.

HARMEN WAGENMAKER

All healthy individuals continuously produce cancer cells throughout their lives. These cells occur on an ongoing basis, and because they develop from within the body, they are referred to as autologous. Malignant cells result from the effects of mutations and viruses and from exposure to carcinogens ranging from radiation and tobacco smoke to pesticides, food colorings, and preservatives, just to mention a few.

Combating Cancer

It is the primary task of the cellular immune system to detect these cancer cells early and destroy them. It should be understood that in any human being, cancer cells develop by the thousands every day. As long as the immune system can detect and contain the flow of newly emerging cancer cells early on, one can go through life without ever developing clinical cancer. Systemic immunodeficiency is observed in patients with advanced malignant disease.[97]

When cancer occurs, by definition the immune response is suppressed, or there has been an excessive exposure to a carcinogen. Impaired immune function often involves a drop in the number and/or the function of immune cells available to effectively detect or kill cancer cells.

Dendritic cells are one of the keys to an effective immune response to cancerous cells. The dendritic cells migrate throughout the tissues of the body, checking for abnormal cells. Dendritic cells also target cells with the potential to become malignant, due to chronic infection by a virus (e.g., a chronic viral infection in the cervix such as human papillomavirus, or HPV, which can develop into a malignancy). When an abnormal cell, such as a cancer cell, has been detected, the dendritic cell travels to a nearby lymph node and presents the "ID" (the specific antigen profile) of the cancer cell to be destroyed.

If the immune system is no longer able to recognize cancer cells, it cannot destroy malignant cells as they develop day to day. When that occurs, cancer can gain a foothold and grow unchecked. Tumor cells, which may remain undetected for years, are referred to as subclinical cancer. Over time, tumors can continue to develop without detection and amass.

Dendritic Cell Vaccination

Researchers have shown that fresh and vital dendritic cells can be introduced into the body in the form of a vaccine. If cancer is present, inoculation with new dendritic cells alerts the immune system to the presence of cancer and restarts proper immune function. This serves to mobilize the exceptional power of the immune system to identify cancer and combat it.

These dendritic cells are cultured from the patient's own white blood cells (so they are described as "autologous"). Initially, after a simple blood draw, the blood is sent to a high-tech medical laboratory where specially trained cell biologists and technicians separate out certain white blood cells (monocytes) from the blood. These cells are then cultured and transformed in seven days into a new generation of dendritic cells. This new generation of vital, activated dendritic cells is reintroduced into the patient's body through simple intracutaneous injections as shown in figure 7.1. The results are remarkable by any standard, increasing immune response, patient survival, and quality of life.

During the transformation of monocytes into dendritic cells in the laboratory, it is possible to specifically sensitize those cells to the patient's cancer if tumor tissue has been preserved during the patient's surgery.

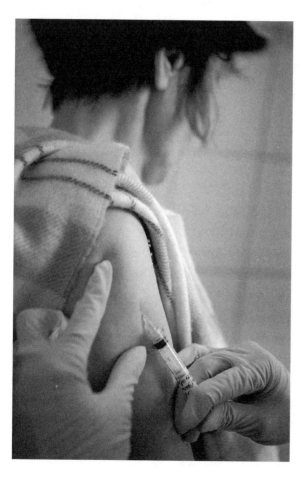

Figure 7.1. Patient receiving a dendritic cell injection (photo by Jana Asenbrennerova)

If the tumor tissue is transported to the Medical Center Cologne following surgery, it is possible to isolate the specific tumor antigens (the cancer's ID) directly from the tumor tissue. When the dendritic cells are exposed to these tumor-specific antigens, they "memorize" this particular ID. When they are reintroduced back into the body, the dendritic cells are "imprinted" specifically with the ID of the cancer cells to be destroyed. This process of educating the dendritic cells is described as "loading" the dendritic cells. However, only about 1 percent of all cancer patients seeking treatment at the Medical Center Cologne have suitable tumor tissue available. Yet the current success rate with dendritic inoculations is exceptional by any standard.

At the Medical Center Cologne, we like to use fresh tumor tissue whenever possible. The task of the dendritic cells is to recognize cells that look different. When they identify a deviant cell, the dendritic cells signal the immune system to destroy the cancer. By focusing the immune system specifically on the actual cancer cells of the patient, we are able to achieve an even stronger, targeted immune response. In case we have suitable tumor tissue available, we then load about 50 percent of all dendritic cells and leave the other 50 percent "naive" so that these dendritic cells can also recognize other tumor-specific antigens than are present in the tumor tissue sample. In this way, it is very likely that all possible tumor cells can be recognized by these dendritic cells.

ROBERT GORTER

Treatment History

Over the past ten years, the Medical Center Cologne has treated roughly 3,500 patients with dendritic cell therapy. Conditions successfully treated with dendritic cell therapy at the center have included primary and secondary brain tumors, primary bone cancer and bone metastasis, breast cancer, pancreatic cancer, colon cancer, liver metastasis of all kinds, cholangiocarcinoma, lung cancer, melanoma, and prostate cancer.

Using the Gorter Model, patients with end-stage cancer frequently experience partial remission and stabilize for several years with a very positive quality of life. Some also experience sustained and complete remission.

These outcomes reflect the positive survival rates frequently seen in the patients at the Medical Center Cologne. Dendritic cell therapy has been an integral aspect of Dr. Gorter's treatment for more than ten years. This work has pioneered a very moderate approach to hyperthermia and immunotherapy, developing safe, effective protocols that are now being validated in the peer-reviewed medical literature. Today, research centers worldwide are studying dendritic cell therapy, which continues to emerge "as a potentially powerful, nontoxic and broadly useful vaccination strategy for cancer patients."[98] Experts expect that within a few years, dendritic cells will become part of the standard treatment of various (and maybe all) forms of cancer.

Safety and Effectiveness

Dendritic cell therapy is now widely recognized as safe[99] and nontoxic[100] with minimal toxicity, at the lowest level—Grade 1.[101] This nontoxic treatment is appropriate for probably all cancer patients and all immune-compromised patients.

The injections are generally well tolerated[102] with almost no side effects except for a fever that typically starts the day of the injection and lasts four to twenty-four hours. Temporary side effects documented by Japanese researchers "were low grade fever (78%), chills (83%), fatigue (23%), and some nausea (17%) experienced on the day of the cell [injections]."[103]

Researchers have also pointed out that dendritic cell therapy offers a safe, effective, nontoxic treatment option for children.[104] Preliminary studies show that the vaccines are even more effective in younger patients[105] and in early-stage cancers.[106]

In my case, the dendritic cell therapy's symptoms were minimal and lasted no more than two days. The hyperthermia was uncomfortable for me personally, but it only took three hours. There were no side effects from the treatment. After that I felt better and could do what I wanted. So the treatment did not exhaust me and because I was not exhausted, it was much easier to stay optimistic.

HARMEN WAGENMAKER

Training the Immune System

When we vaccinate for diseases such as tetanus or measles, the injection must be repeated five to six times at defined intervals, in order to establish lifelong immunity. Vaccination improves specific immune function, but the immune system must be "trained" through repeated exposures.

To improve immune function using dendritic cells, these new cells must be injected at least six times. Patients with all forms of cancer and also patients with chronic viral infections, such as hepatitis B and C or HIV, are initially vaccinated with dendritic cells six times at monthly intervals. Thereafter, the injections are repeated once every six months for the duration of three years as "booster shots" and then at usually yearly intervals.

This ongoing dendritic cell vaccination is another aspect of treatment. Providing the vaccine on a schedule comparable to other vaccine protocols has resulted in an encouraging success rate of effective treatment. The importance of frequent vaccination in the initial stage of treatment has now been validated in scores of recent research studies.

The Gorter Model

In the Gorter Model, the first step is to induce fever—either by fever-range, total-body hyperthermia or by localized hyperthermia—provided in conjunction with the dendritic cell vaccine.

Normally, fever is initiated and controlled by certain centers in the brain stem that are also responsible for maintaining core body temperature. The location of the body's temperature regulation deep within the brain stem shows how fundamentally important core temperature is in the systems of the body and how involved the brain is in maintaining a constant temperature (independent from the temperature of our external environment).

Fever is the necessary condition that ramps up the entire immune defense system, which is essential in eliminating diseases. Fever also serves to initiate tissue repair. This is well documented in situations such as an accident or other types of events causing organ damage.

As described earlier, fever induces the immune response at 101.3°F (38.5°C). The immune system then shifts from "automatic pilot" to a highly activated state, increasing dramatically in preparation for a system-wide attack on *any* deviant cells found. Broadly focused immune defenses such as natural killer (NK) cells are also called up. In short, fever primes the body for full-force immune response and repair mechanisms.

The second step in the protocol is the dendritic cell vaccination, which provides immune defenses with the means to identify and target the cancer cells to be destroyed. Dendritic cells are white blood cells that serve as the "detectives" or the "long arm" of the immune system. They migrate throughout all the body's organs and tissues looking for the "bad guys"—abnormal or malignant cells that could be damaging to the body. When these deviant cells are detected, a complex identification mechanism is triggered in the dendritic cell. It then travels to the nearest lymph node. This is like a "military base" where hundreds of thousands of armed and hopefully well-trained soldiers, the NK cells, are waiting to serve in the body's defense. The dendritic cell presents the ID or specific antigen of the malignant cell, which launches the NK cells on a seek-and-destroy mission to eliminate the cancer.

After I had lung surgery to remove some additional tumors, we brought the material from the second lung to Cologne, because it contained active tumor cells. That tissue was used to make the dendritic cells.

<small>WIM KOOSTERBOER, FIVE-YEAR SURVIVOR OF HEPATITIS B
AND HBV-ASSOCIATED PRIMARY LIVER CANCER (HCC)
WITH LYMPH, LIVER, AND LUNG METASTASES, STILL IN
COMPLETE REMISSION</small>

Dendritic Cell Research

More than 250 research studies have confirmed the effectiveness of this approach to immunotherapy in cancer treatment. Study after study has shown that dendritic cell therapy provides "a significant prolongation in survival."[107] American studies of dendritic cell therapy have been conducted at major universities including Harvard Medical School, Stanford, UCSF Medical School, University of Maryland, University of Michigan, and University of Texas. As mentioned, in May 2010 the FDA approved dendritic cell therapy in patients with metastatic prostate cancer.

There is broad agreement that dendritic cell therapy increases the number of T cells in the body, which results in a stronger immune response.[108] Italian researchers reported, "Dendritic cell targeting... has recently been shown to confer strong and protective cytotoxic T-cell-based immunity."[109]

Studies at research centers around the world have documented the benefits of dendritic cell therapy for many forms of cancer, including brain tumors,[110] leukemia,[111] lymphoma,[112] melanoma,[113] and a range of other malignancies including cancers of the breast,[114] gastrointestinal tract,[115] liver,[116] lungs,[117] pancreas,[118] kidneys,[119] and thyroid.[120] In the United States, a controlled phase II study of metastatic prostate cancer conducted in 2009 documented the effectiveness of dendritic cell vaccinations for prostate cancer.[121] In May 2010, the FDA approved dendritic cell vaccinations as an effective therapy in metastatic prostate cancer.[122]

In terms of dendritic cell therapy, I had the first six treatments in four weeks. I would receive the injection and then after an hour and a half, I would start getting a fever. Before I got home, I would have a fairly high fever. It wasn't unpleasant—it never made me feel weak, whereas normally a fever might wear me down. Once I lie down and close my eyes, I always fall asleep fairly quickly.

When I wake up the next day or night, it has already subsided a bit. I always develop a mild headache, but I don't take anything for it because the headaches are bearable. I take it easy that day, go for a walk, and get some fresh air—and in the evening it's gone. That's it. Those are the only side effects I've ever experienced from this therapy.

HEINZ HAGEMEYER

Long-Term Survival

Dendritic cell therapy improves the outcome of cancer treatment and frequently extends life for cancer patients by several years, with improved quality of life.

- In an Austrian study of 10 patients with metastatic thyroid cancer, 30 percent had stable conditions at one year.[123]
- German cancer research on metastatic thyroid conditions found that five of ten patients survived more than three years with dendritic cell therapy—50 percent of patients.[124]
- A Polish study of leukemia patients found that eight of twelve (66 percent) patients stabilized or improved.[125]
- Research conducted in Korea with nine renal cancer patients found that six of nine (66 percent) benefited from the dendritic cell vaccine, with an average survival of two and a half years.[126]
- An Italian study followed the progress of relapsed lymphoma patients who were then treated with dendritic cell therapy and reported that almost 80 percent were stable after four years.[127]

- Japanese research documented the health of twenty-eight lung cancer patients who received dendritic cell therapy and found a two-year survival rate of 90 percent and five-year survival greater than 50 percent.[128]

Current Research

The most recent studies have found that dendritic cell injections significantly prolong patient survival. For example, a recent French study involving fifty-six cancer patients reported patient survival averaging almost four years.[129]

In a Chilean study of fifty patients, those with Stage III cancer survived an average of four years. Among those with Stage IV cancer, 60 percent responded positively to the therapy and lived almost three years.[130] This is an exceptionally positive result, since life expectancy of Stage IV patients is usually measured in weeks or months. Each of these studies involved some form of dendritic cell vaccine.

A Danish study found that dendritic cell inoculation can double the number of T cells and NK cells in the body in as little as four weeks following the injection.[131] According to British researchers at the UK Institute for Cancer Studies, "Dendritic cells are the most potent of all antigen-presenting cells, with the capacity to take up, process, and present tumor antigens to T cells and stimulate an immune response, thus providing a rational platform for vaccine development."[132] Japanese researchers conclude, "Dendritic cells loaded with tumor antigens have been emerging as a new strategy in cancer treatment."[133]

At the Medical Center Cologne, of patients with glioblastoma multiforme, 48 percent experience complete, long-lasting remission, and another 24 percent experience a prolonged period of partial remission or stable disease. This is remarkable in the context of the 5 percent one-year survival rate reported in the medical literature, for the average patient diagnosed with Stage IV brain tumors dies within the first year of diagnosis, although some patients who undergo chemotherapy

(Temodal) and radiation experience an additional six months life expectancy.[134]

In patients with Stage IV breast cancer, approximately 26 to 28 percent still go into complete and sustained remission, and approximately 48 percent experience partial remission with improved quality of life and significantly prolonged life expectancy.

This nontoxic immune therapy offers an important option in cancer treatment. Dendritic cell vaccines provide another form of treatment for conditions that cannot be addressed with standard chemotherapy or radiation, such as metastatic renal cancer[135] or melanoma.[136] The vaccine can be a life-prolonging therapy for Stage III and IV patients, and for the vast majority of patients it enhances quality of life significantly.

After I received the dendritic therapy, I recovered quickly, and the next scans confirmed that all the cancer was gone. All the scans since then have been good news. The radiologist said, "We don't believe in miracles, but this sure looks like one."

WIM KOOSTERBOER

Chapter 8

EXTENDED IMMUNE THERAPIES

When I began treatment at the Medical Center Cologne, Dr. Gorter evaluated my condition and suggested a two-week course of vaccination with the Newcastle disease virus. Before we began treatment, they took blood samples. The vaccine was given every day, skipping one day on the weekend. The first week it was administered intravenously. After that it was given by injection and also provided in a little spray, which I inhaled. We went to Cologne every other day, and took the vaccine home for the second day, where it was administered by a nurse in our city.

I was given the dendritic cells once a month. The first dendritic vaccination was eight days after a series of eight vaccinations with the Newcastle disease virus. The virus hardly produced any side effects—I'd get a little shivery and feverish, but it wasn't as intense as the cell therapy, which would send me to bed after only half an hour. The treatment worked, and a scan nine months later showed that my liver cancer was in remission and that the lung tumors were stable. Physically I felt great.

The doctors in Rotterdam were amazed, and they felt I was now well enough to have surgery to remove the lung tumors. They found that the cancer cells in the first lung had completely died (necrotized). On the X-rays, you couldn't see that there had ever been a tumor. We were so happy. In the second lung, there were still active tumor cells, although a large part of the tumor had necrotized as well. But the margins around the surgery were clean, and so were the lymph nodes— and there was no longer active cancer in the other lung or in my liver.

WIM KOOSTERBOER

In the Gorter Model, a full range of immune therapies is used to treat cancer patients. Although fever therapy and dendritic cell vaccinations are the primary forms of treatment, there are also several other complementary therapies that are incorporated, depending on the needs of the individual. The main goals of these innovative therapies are to restore and maximize immune function. The other goal is to destroy cancer cells without introducing toxic agents that can have a negative impact on immune function, and on patient's quality of life. The three major immunotherapies used are (1) botanical mistletoe to activate and balance the immune system, (2) infusions of nutrients and trace elements to support immune function and (3) Newcastle disease virus (an oncolytic virus) to kill cancer cells. These procedures support immune function without toxicity and can destroy cancer tissue directly.

The Botanical Mistletoe

I had no concerns about toxicity, because there is already broad agreement in the research literature on the safety of mistletoe. Given the findings on immune support, I felt it could actually be beneficial to me, because as we age, the immune system tends to decrease in competence. The pinprick of the needle was barely painful—it felt similar to an acupuncture needle. I noticed no response with the first series of injections—eight little shots, given every other day. It was only at the second series of injections that my body showed a reaction—a reddish welt that would take a few days to disappear. The welt told me that my immune system was responding and being activated.

ERIK PEPER

For thousands of years, European mistletoe has been used as a medicinal plant in many healing traditions. Extracts from botanical mistletoe have been used in Europe for decades to support immune function in cancer just as in Asia many Chinese herbs are used to balance energy flow in the body. Extracts of mistletoe are well studied in Western science, and hundreds of scientific articles have been published on practically all aspects of its clinical use. The clinical protocols for using mistletoe in cancer treatment were initially developed by Rudolf Steiner (1861–1925). Since that time, pharmacological research and clinical studies have shown that it provides a broad spectrum of antitumor activities and restoration of the cellular immune system.

European mistletoe *(Viscum album)* grows on various species of trees found in northern and central Europe as shown in figure 8.1. Unlike almost all other plants, it blooms during winter when there is frost and snow, and the white berries ripen a year later under the same conditions. The mistletoe's form, color, shape, and content of the plant and berries depend upon on the type of tree on which it grows. As a result, the ratio of various constituents in the plant can differ significantly, reflected in the different composition of glycoproteins, viscotoxins, and other components in the host tree. For example, mistletoe grown on species of trees such as the apple tree *(Malus)* is indicated for use in uterine, colon, and breast cancer in women. Extracts from mistletoe grown in oak trees

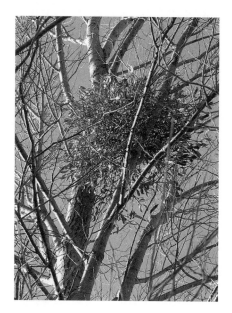

(Quercus) are used for prostate cancer and tumors of the gastrointestinal tract in men. Extracts from mistletoe grown in maple trees *(Acer)* are used for cancers of the lungs and respiratory tract, and extracts of pine tree *(Pinus)* mistletoe are used in treating brain tumors.

Figure 8.1. Mistletoe growing in winter on a deciduous tree

119

There is also seasonal variation in the level of glycoproteins and viscotoxins produced by the plant in the summer compared with those harvested in the winter. Based on the research findings of Steiner, extracts of summer and winter harvests are mixed in a centrifuge, resulting in a unique medication that includes all the possible components of the plant.

Mistletoe is currently the most commonly prescribed anticancer medication used in northern and central Europe. Fully 70 percent of all cancer patients receive mistletoe preparations, and it is usually paid for by the national health care systems, making mistletoe a more frequently prescribed anticancer medication than any other type of medication, including immunotherapies such as interleukin-2, all forms of chemotherapy, and angiogenesis inhibitors.

Mistletoe is provided as a simple subcutaneous injection twice a week, preferably in the early morning. Like dendritic vaccinations, the mistletoe extract needs to be injected in a series to evoke and maintain a significant immune response. At the Medical Center Cologne, approximately 85 percent of patients receive mistletoe. Usually, after some instruction, they find it easy to give themselves these injections, which are applied just beneath the surface of the skin using a small insulin syringe and a very fine needle.

Initially, the injection is repeated every three days. In most protocols, mistletoe is injected subcutaneously twice a week in the morning, for a period of several months to several years. Injections are typically applied in the morning when core temperature is lower. Based on each patient's progress, the injections may then be prescribed periodically at six-week intervals.

Benefits of Mistletoe

Mistletoe has been found to both prolong life and improve quality of life. Researchers studying uterine cancer reported, "mistletoe preparations such as Iscador and Abnoba Viscum have the effect of prolonging overall survival of corpus uteri cancer patients."[137] Another study, which tracked patients over five years, found "significantly improved quality of life and significantly reduced persistent signs/symptoms."[138] Numerous studies have affirmed these benefits.[139] Studies have also shown a range of other clinical benefits:

- Typically well tolerated[140]
- Low toxicity[141]
- No more than Grade I flu-like symptoms[142]
- Decreased pain due to higher serum endorphins[143]
- Prolonged survival of patients with breast cancer[144] as well as ovarian,[145] uterine,[146] and cervical cancers[147]

Enhanced Immune Function

Recent research has confirmed enhanced immune function and healing with the use of mistletoe in patients with various types of cancer, including a broad range of cancers of the digestive tract and the genital system. Studies of immune support and restoration have also involved healthy individuals and report:

- Higher levels of cellular immunity, our primary defense against cancer (eosinophils)[148]
- Greater numbers of natural killer cells *and* increased activity[149]
- Increased levels of cancer-fighting T cells and T helper cells[150]
- Increases in immune signaling chemicals (cytokines)[151]
- Higher levels of protective immune antibodies and the B cells that make them[152]
- DNA repair following chemotherapy and radiation in patients with almost all types of cancers[153]

Normalized Body Temperature

Therapeutic use of mistletoe helps to reestablish the body's natural temperature rhythm and increases core temperature by about 1°F (0.6°C).

This increase in temperature counters the poor circulation and slower metabolic rate experienced by many cancer patients, reflected in chronically cold hands and feet. Improvement in core body temperature and restoration of circadian rhythm seems to be an important marker of immune restoration. Normalized body temperature also correlates with improved outcome and survival.

Nutrient Infusions

At the Medical Center Cologne, essentially all patients receive antioxidants, nutrients, trace elements, and minerals via IV (intravenously). In addition, electrolyte minerals are given to avoid dehydration during fever-range, total-body hyperthermia. Patients also receive nutrient infusions during localized hyperthermia, to increase the efficacy of the treatment. Vitamins and trace minerals support immune function and repair mechanisms.

Research has shown that providing antioxidant vitamins and minerals by infusion restores deficiencies much more quickly than would be possible with oral supplements alone.

Regardless of how depleted patients are initially when they first arrive at the center, typically within a few days they begin to feel the beneficial effects of the infusions. Often patients leave the clinic after a week to ten days, refreshed and energized. Those who were experiencing pain initially when they entered the program almost always find that they have much less or no pain at all.

ROBERT GORTER

Sources of Oxidative Stress

Antioxidants are essential nutrients that the immune system uses to protect us against cancer. Whenever cancer cells thrive, the body combats them with "oxygen products" such as ozone and nitric oxide (NO).

These by-products of our own immune system are a necessary evil of this inner warfare, causing "oxidative stress."

Oxidative stress is a well-recognized cause of cancer that can result from exposure to a wide range of well-known carcinogens, including cigarette smoke, industrial and environmental toxins, pesticides and food additives, and thousands of other chemicals.

Researchers have found that cancer patients are often low in antioxidants and other nutrients essential in preventing and combating cancer.[154] Causes of this depletion include the following:

- Inflammation and infection[155]
- Radiation and chemotherapy
- The process of aging, which impairs digestion, reducing nutrient levels
- Diets deficient in micronutrients due to overfarmed soil, transport of food, and other commercial agricultural practices
- The body's attempts to destroy cancer cells

A study at the University of Dresden in Germany confirmed the link between oxidative stress and disease in cases of lymphatic edema. Researchers found that when markers of oxidative stress increased, the severity of patients' conditions typically worsened.

Countering Oxidants with Antioxidants

Antioxidants are nutrients found in fresh fruit and vegetables. They counter the harmful body chemistry of oxidative stress. Without *antioxidants*, oxidants persist and ricochet through cells and tissues in a destructive chain reaction. (Also, aging in general is accelerated by oxidative stress.) One of the therapies used to reduce oxidative stress is IV nutrient therapy, which has become widely recognized as an important strategy in cancer treatment.

Antioxidant Deficiencies in Cancer

A number of clinical trials have measured levels of antioxidant nutrients in cancer patients. One study of terminally ill patients reported that "the majority of patients were vitamin C deficient prior to treatment."[156] A study of patients with brain cancer found that on admission, 70 percent had subnormal blood levels of selenium.[157] This finding was also reported in a study of head and neck cancers, which reported, "patients entering the study had significantly lower plasma selenium levels than healthy individuals."[158] Studies on trace minerals involving patients with oral cancers indicated that "serum iron levels were decreased significantly in the cancer group."[159]

This research also showed that the longer patients were ill, the more depleted they became. "Patients in Stage I or II of the disease had significantly higher plasma selenium levels than patients in Stage III or IV disease."[160] The goal of nutrient therapy is to restore nutrient levels, thus normalizing function within the body.

Vitamin C Therapy

Research has shown that vitamin C has both antioxidant and antitumor properties. In the past five years, intravenous vitamin C (ascorbic acid) has been studied at research centers that include the National Cancer Institute (NCI),[161] McGill University in Canada,[162] and the National Cancer Center of Japan.[163] An NIH study published in the Proceedings of the National Academy of Science (2008) reported, "These data suggest that ascorbate as a pro-drug may have benefits in cancers with poor prognosis and limited therapeutic options."[164]

Antitumor activity. Researchers at the NIH National Cancer Institute have reported that "vitamin C at high concentrations is toxic to cancer cells in vitro [in the lab]."[165]

- **Dosage.** Japanese researchers have indicated, "Higher concentrations of vitamin C induced apoptotic cell death in various tumor cell lines including oral squamous cell carcinoma and salivary gland tumor[s]."[166]
- **Response time.** A research institute in Wichita found that when vitamin C was applied to cancer cells in the lab (with vitamin C levels comparable to an IV), the number of tumor cells began to drop within two days.[167]
- **Human studies.** Research conducted at McGill University in Canada reported that vitamin C "is selectively [cytotoxic] to many cancer cell lines and has in vivo anticancer activities [confirmed in patients] when administered alone or together with other agents."[168] This selective toxicity means that intravenous vitamin C is toxic to cancer cells, but not to healthy human cells.

Oral supplements or IV infusions? The choice of oral supplements or IV therapy is determined by the goal of therapy—whether the purpose is to prevent cancer in healthy individuals, to enhance the well-being of a patient with cancer, or to support antitumor activity.

Studies that provided terminal cancer patients with *oral* megadoses of vitamin C found no benefit when a 10-gram dosage was given once a day.[169] To examine this question further, NIH researchers compared vitamin C levels provided orally or by IV. They found that IV infusions produced blood levels of vitamin C that were "140-fold higher than those from maximum oral doses."[170] The conclusion of this NIH team was that "only intravenous administration of vitamin C [and not oral vitamin C] produces high plasma and urine concentrations that might have antitumor activity."

Types of cancers studied. The safety of vitamin C therapy was confirmed in a study evaluating patients with cancer of the kidneys,[171] and also in clinical experience with non-Hodgkin's lymphoma, colorectal, and pancreatic cancers.[172] The effectiveness of vitamin C has been evaluated for a number of other types of cancer as well:

- Lab cultures of breast cancer tissue: laboratory research found that ascorbic acid and copper sulfate inhibited cell growth.[173]
- Animal studies of ovarian, pancreatic, and brain cancers: significant decreases in cancer growth rates were noted in studies by the National Cancer Institute.[174]
- Human studies of oral squamous cell carcinoma and salivary gland tumor cells: these cancers were found to respond to IV vitamin C therapy in clinical studies.[175]
- Acute leukemia: A beneficial response to nutrient therapy was observed in 43 percent of patients with advanced disease in a Korean study.[176]

The absence of side effects. McGill researchers reported that in intravenous vitamin C therapy, "Adverse events and toxicity were minimal at all dose levels."[177] The most common adverse events reported for IV therapy with high-dose vitamin C were nausea, edema, and dry mouth or skin; and these were generally minor.[178] Of twenty-four patients receiving high doses of vitamin C in one study, one developed a kidney stone after thirteen days of treatment, and another experienced low potassium levels. Given the severity of the patients' initial conditions, researchers concluded that "intravenous vitamin C therapy for cancer is relatively safe."[179]

Findings at the Medical Center Cologne. The Gorter Model includes moderate doses of vitamin C given intravenously during hyperthermia sessions. Clinical experience at the Medical Center Cologne documents the exceptional safety of these infusions. For an average adult patient, 12.5 grams of vitamin C are given by IV in combination with electrolytes. These infusions have been found to increase the efficacy of the hyperthermia and have never lead to complications such as kidney stones or diarrhea.[180]

Selenium Infusions

Selenium (sodium selenite) is a trace mineral with major antioxidant properties that has been found "well tolerated and easy to administer."[181] Cancer patients are frequently depleted in this important nutrient. The research has shown that restoring selenium levels activates detoxification pathways, which are essential in helping the body break down and metabolize medications and clear away toxins.[182]

In the past decade, studies on selenium have been conducted in the United States, across Germany, and in Austria, China, Egypt, and India. This trace mineral is surprisingly important in supporting good immune function:

- Improved red blood cells counts[183]
- Reduced destruction of white blood cells[184]
- Increased levels of T cells[185]
- Much lower rate of infections and side effects following chemotherapy[186]
- Reduced complications and edema following radiation therapy[187]
- Inflammation brought under control quickly
- Longer survival[188]

The studies also reported the outcome of treatment for various types of cancer:

- Non-Hodgkin's lymphoma: a 20 percent improvement was found when selenium was provided in combination with chemotherapy.[189]
- Head and neck cancers: in a study involving late stage cancer, 60 percent of patients experienced reduced edema (twelve of the twenty patients).[190]
- Brain tumors: over 75 percent of patients experienced definite improvement, with fewer symptoms of nausea, vomiting, headache, vertigo, unsteady gait, speech disorders, and seizures.[191]

- Lymphedema: all patients receiving selenium infusions remained free of skin infection, whereas 50 percent of patients who did not receive this mineral developed these infections[192]

Oral Nutritional Supplements

The research shows greater benefit from IV antioxidants than from oral supplements. However, immune function can also be improved to some degree by providing nutrients in oral form. Daily oral intake of multi-vitamins, minerals, glandulars, and botanicals can help to supply essential nutrients lacking in the diet. A number of studies have found benefit from oral supplements, although reviews are mixed, and there currently are no clear predictors of what works and what doesn't.

Rejuvenation. Nutrients and other metabolic factors found in supplements can be beneficial in supporting healing:

- Antioxidants tend to slow the destructive oxidation process.
- Trace minerals serve as antioxidants and catalysts (catalysators) in the body's chemistry.
- Supplements derived from thymus and spleen tissue function as immune modulators (the active constituents are peptides extracted from protein).
- Certain botanical extracts function as adapatogens, natural chemicals that can normalize the metabolism of various systems in the body.

Preventing cancer. Nutritional supplements taken orally have been found effective in reducing cancer incidence. A study on the prevention of liver cancer was launched with approximately two thousand people in Qidong Province, China. The goal was to reduce the incidence of liver cancer by supplementing table salt and nutritional yeast with traces of selenium. At the end of this three-year study, researchers reported a 3 percent cancer rate for people who got the selenium supplement in their food and 6 percent for those receiving no supplementation.[193]

A second study, with patients who had colon cancer, reported, "Our results confirm ... low selenium levels in patients prone to colon [tumors] and show that by [oral] selenium supplementation this can be normalized."[194]

Short-term research and low-dose studies. Findings from short-term studies have been less favorable. For example, a four-month study of men with prostate cancer found that low-dose lycopene at 30 mg had no effect in slowing the development of cancer (this nutrient is found in tomatoes and tomato products).[195] Similarly, some of the studies using low dosages find no protective effect. A large two-year study on digestive tract cancers tracked the effects of two low-dose supplements: vitamin A (20 mg beta-carotene) and vitamin E (50 mg alpha-tocopherol).[196] Although trends are emerging in the research, currently there are no clear-cut guidelines on the role of oral nutrients in cancer therapy.

Reducing oxidative stress. Japanese research has confirmed that oxidative stress can be reduced with oral supplements and highlighted the value of higher doses. In a study of oxidative stress and gastritis, 244 patients were evaluated for the effects of oral vitamin C given daily for five years. Study volunteers who took 500 mg of vitamin C daily had 125-percent reductions in oxidative stress. Minimal daily doses of 50 mg of vitamin C were found less effective—participants on this lower dosage had increases in harmful oxidative stress that were four times normal.[197] Generally, higher dosages of vitamin C appear beneficial; however, they need to be adjusted for each individual.

Slowing the growth of cancer. Recent research suggests that pharmacologic levels (megadoses) are more likely to slow the progression of cancer. An NIH animal study reported that "a regimen of daily pharmacologic ascorbate treatment significantly decreased growth rates of ovarian, pancreatic, and glioblastoma [brain] tumors established in mice."[198] In a human study, prostate cancer patients who could no longer be helped by standard therapy were provided a protocol of high-dose oral vitamin C in combination with vitamin K3. Of seventeen patients, fifteen opted to continue the therapy. There were no adverse effects, and after more than a year, fourteen of these fifteen patients had survived (despite the prognosis that their conditions had progressed too far for treatment).[199] Antioxidant nutrients have also been found effective in combination with conventional medication and chemotherapy.[200]

Newcastle Disease Virus

At the Medical Center Cologne, one of the innovative approaches provided is nontoxic treatment using the Newcastle disease virus (NDV) as a form of therapy.[201] The NDV was first recorded in England in 1926 and was subsequently identified in Indonesia and other regions of Southeast Asia. Newcastle virus is not related to the avian influenza virus.

NDV can selectively infect cancer cells, initiating cell death without toxicity to healthy human cells. NDV is therefore considered a natural oncolytic virus. As an infectious agent, this virus is highly contagious to poultry, yet it has no effect on mammals and human beings except for brief episodes of respiratory infection, periodically reported among poultry workers. Newcastle disease is defined as an "oncolytic virus," which selectively infects mammalian and human cancer cells and destroys them *(apoptosis)*, yet has no effect on healthy human cells.[202]

The possible mechanism by which NDV kills cancer cells is that many cancer cells have escape mechanisms—for example, malignant cells are able to suppress intracellular interferon production. As a result, cancerous cells are able to become less visible to the immune system. NDV evolved to infect cells that do not produce interferon, which is characteristic of birds. As a result, the NDV selectively kills those human cancer cells that have suppressed their intracellular INF production. NDV is completely nonpathogenic to healthy human tissue.

When the NDV infects cancer cells, the malignant cells quickly deteriorate and die within three to four days. As the cancer cells die, they drop their escape mechanisms, and thus their ID—their tumor-specific antigens—becomes better detectable to dendritic cells.

The Patient's Experience

At the Medical Center Cologne, the NDV is used to treat more aggressive forms of cancer, sometimes as preparative support for dendritic cell therapy. Since 2002, this vital therapy has been integrated into the protocol for solid tumors to reduce the cancer load and enable immune therapy to work more effectively.

In the Gorter Model, a few hours after the NDV is administered by inhaling through a nebulizer, the patient receives injections of newly cultured dendritic cells as shown in figure 8.2. Clinical findings indicate that the use of NDV destroys cancer cells and also leads to overall better immune response.

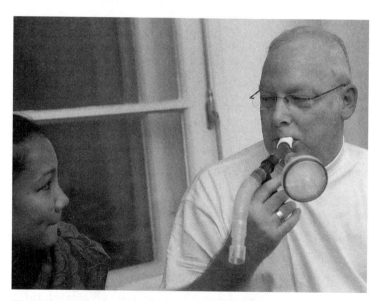

Figure 8.2. Patient inhaling Newcastle Disease virus through a nebulizer (photo by Jana Asenbrennerova)

Gorter Protocol—Newcastle Disease Virus

A three-step protocol is used to counter the ability of cancer cells to avoid detection by the immune system:

1. *Weakening the cancer cells.* On the day of treatment, an IV injection is provided in the morning containing the NDV. Many of the cancer cells immediately become infected by the virus, weaken, and eventually die in three to four days through cell death *(apoptosis).*

2. *Targeting the immune response.* Six hours later, dendritic cells are administered. Because the cancer cells have been weakened by the virus, the dendritic cells can easily recognize the sick and dying malignant cells. The dendritic cells recruit and target T cells and NK cells in an attack on the cancer.

3. *Launching a broad-based response.* Fever therapy is also provided at this time to launch a more generalized immune response, calling up not only T cells but also immune-signaling chemicals and a broader immune response.

Research on the Newcastle Disease Virus

The early literature on viral therapy was based on case reports of temporary improvement in cancer patients following viral infections or vaccinations. Initial experiments with the virus were conducted in the lab on cell cultures, and the virus's ability to destroy cancer cells was also confirmed in animal models.[203] NDV has been studied extensively in Germany, and also in Canada, China, and the United Kingdom. In the United States, the virus has been studied at Emory University Medical School, NYU School of Medicine, and several other medical centers.

Approximately thirty clinical trials have been conducted with cancer patients using this virus, with exceptionally positive survival rates. However, because the virus cannot be patented, pharmaceutical companies have had little interest in research or development. At the time of this writing, there has been a new wave of interest in oncolytic viruses, possibly based on the potential for a commercial vaccine using altered genetic material (recombinant DNA—literally genes that have been "recombined"). Currently there are almost a thousand scientific articles on the NDV, with approximately a hundred of those articles published in the past three years. This surge of scientific literature focuses on how the virus works, its physiology, and its genetics, as well as studies conducted in the lab, with animals, and in human patients.

In 1965, Cassell and Garrett were the first to use live NDV to treat human cancers.[204] Research in this area took on additional importance in 1968 when a poultry farmer who suffered from metastatic gastric cancer exhibited a spectacular recovery after exposure to the poultry virus. Following these reports, researchers began employing a strain of the NDV to treat human malignancies, and this viral strain has been found to be effective even in the treatment of advanced cancers.[205]

Researchers consistently report that the vaccine is well tolerated[206] with rare incidence of toxicity.[207] Minimal temporary side effects are primarily localized inflammation[208] or mild flu-like symptoms with fevers of up to 101°F (38°C).[209] The vaccine produces a positive immune response in 70 to 100 percent of patients tested.[210]

There are primarily two means by which viruses destroy their host cells: by inducing *lysis* as the cell wall of the tumor breaks down due to replication of the virus[211] and by programmed cell death *(apoptosis)*, in which cells are destroyed without toxicity to surrounding cells.[212] Activity observed by researchers included the following:

- T cells "loaded" with the NDV that targeted and destroyed tumor tissue[213]
- Increased activity by NK cells[214]
- Increased production of interferon in healthy cells, which protected them against the virus[215]

Stage II and III cancers. Equally impressive are the improved survival rates for patients treated with NDV for a range of cancers, particularly for patients treated in Stage II or III:

- *Melanoma, Stage II.* Ten years after treatment, over 60 percent of the eighty-three patients were alive and free of disease, compared with a typical survival rate of 33 percent.[216]
- *Melanoma, Stage III.* One study reported a survival time of five to seven years. Other research with a fifteen-year follow-up recorded a 55 percent survival rate with no adverse effects.[217]

Stage IV cancers. For patients with more advanced cancers, the vaccine still offers benefit:

- *Brain tumors.* Vaccine patients averaged a sixty-week survival, and without side effects.[218]
- *Renal cancer.* Disease-free survival of twenty-one or more months on average was reported in a study of 208 patients.[219]
- *Colon cancer.* Survival three times the norm was reported for colon cancer patients.[220]
- *Colorectal cancer with liver metastasis.* At eighteen months, approximately 40 percent of vaccinated patients had stabilized, compared with fewer than 15 percent of surgically treated patients.[221]
- *Advanced cancers.* Research on a range of advanced cancers showed that more than 50 percent of those receiving the vaccine stabilized or experienced tumor regression, compared with less than 10 percent of those in the control group.[222]

Support Your Own Health

One important question a patient needs to ask when exploring complementary cancer treatment options such as diet, botanicals, or vitamin infusions is, "Will this potentially support my immune system and health?"

In many cases conventional health professionals are hesitant to answer this question because they may be relatively unfamiliar with the technique. In numerous cases, although the research exists, there may be a limited number of double-blind, placebo-controlled clinical studies.

It is important to be a skeptical and wise consumer of all health care, whether mainstream or complementary, and to consider carefully all claims, including claims that the treatments are *not* efficacious. We encourage people everywhere to be active participants in their own healing process in collaboration with their physicians and health care providers.

Part III

SELF-CARE

●

Chapter 9

OPTIMIZING YOUR HEALTH

When I heard the diagnosis, my world crumbled. I felt myself spinning out of control. The cancer now ruled my life unto death, and there was nothing I could do about it. I felt overwhelmed by the loss of my health, which I had always assumed would just go on and on. It jarred my emotions. It overwhelmed my ability to make even the smallest decision.

PATIENT DIAGNOSED WITH COLON CANCER

When we hear the words, "You have cancer," thoughts of suffering, pain, and the possibility of death overwhelm us. We may find ourselves unable to respond or even to ask the most basic questions—we are at a complete loss of certainty and safety. All the trust we had in our own body and the expectation of a future seem lost.

A cancer diagnosis breaks the illusion that we are in control. In reality, none of us are in total control—the remarkable processes of birth, life, sickness, and death are beyond our control and ultimately beyond human comprehension.

The acceptance that we are not totally in control is part of the healing process. Despite the absence of certainty, we have choices—we can remain angry, overwhelmed, depressed, or hopeless—or we can take action to reduce our stress and support our own healing process. We can focus on the areas of our health that we *can* influence.

This chapter offers an overview of self-care strategies with an emphasis on the health-promoting actions you can take to support the self-healing potential of your body. The diagnosis is a time to initiate actions that will promote immune function and reduce cancer growth, while accepting that death is a possibility.

Holding these competing notions simultaneously (promoting healing while accepting the possibility of dying) seems counterintuitive. We want to avoid thoughts of death. How can we focus on living if we entertain the possibility of dying? Isn't that giving up? But from our own experience with cancer and our work with patients over decades, we know that the thoughts and fears of an uncertain future are part of the new reality of a cancer diagnosis. Spending our energy and worry focusing on what is beyond our control just isn't an efficient use of our efforts. Instead, we accept that death is a possibility and then focus on what is within our control. We make a conscious effort to quiet our anxiety so we have the ability to do what matters.

What we can do is to educate ourselves about aspects of lifestyle that support healing—good nutrition, gentle exercise, stress management, support from friends and family, choosing to do what you have always wished to do. The challenge is to increase our awareness, to accept the factors that are beyond our control, to focus on the areas where we do have control, and to act.

Dealing with the Diagnosis

If you or someone you love has recently received a cancer diagnosis, you'll probably find it useful to put the diagnosis in a broader perspective. The words, "You have cancer," are an immediate signal of *danger*. While we scramble to grasp the situation, our body mounts a stress response, which is either *flight/fight* or *freeze*. It is important to remember that these initial responses are normal. We need to give ourselves time to adjust to this new information and move out of the stress response.

The flight/fight response. This response prepares the body for immediate action. Stress hormones such as cortisol and norepinephrine flood our bloodstream. We may find ourselves sitting in the doctor's office, heart pounding, blood pressure up, and thoughts racing. At a time like this, most all of us regress to primitive survival patterns. Some "come out fighting" and lash out in anger. Others pull back and withdraw— or take off, get in the car, drive all night, and then return home to deal with the situation. During the immediacy of the stress response, we tend to react in a mode of pure survival—at that moment it is difficult to plan ahead and reflect.

The freeze response. A primal self-protective reaction is triggered when the word *cancer* translates in the brain as *life-threatening*. If this response is triggered, we freeze, begin shutting down, and do not act or move. This primitive survival response is triggered to avoid detection by our enemies and biologically to withdraw as if we are captured. Under this perceived threat of death, the body shifts to shutting down. This withdrawal numbs the body and evokes depression, which may account for the profound sense of detachment that is often experienced in trauma or tragedy. For the patient, this response can take the form of deep-seated fear, hopelessness, or resignation, and the inability to act. We may feel overwhelmed or blank out. At times we respond by curling up in bed for days, hiding until we can begin to mobilize our resources.

Difficulty with long-range planning. Both stress responses (fight/ flight and freeze) focus all our actions on immediate survival, and we respond out of pure instinct. From an evolutionary perspective, why regenerate or support self-healing when potentially you will become someone else's lunch (e.g., being eaten by a tiger)?[223] In the moment, it's almost impossible to do any thinking or planning, since rational thought occurs in the cerebral cortex, the area just behind the forehead. When our survival is threatened, we respond from deep within the "primitive brain." Given these typical reactions, you may want to temporarily defer major decisions and offer to get back to your physician when the overwhelming immediacy of the diagnosis has passed. Even a day or two will give you an opportunity to think more rationally.

Shifting Out of the Stress Response

When we shift into the stress response, our bodies have two choices: move into a combat mode or shut down. To be able to plan, you have to complete the stress response by being physically active. This allows the stress hormones that were released during the stress response to move through your system and for your system to re-balance. Once your body and brain get the message that the danger has passed, you can return to a place of safety and relax. At that point, the fight/flight or freeze cycle is completed, and regeneration and rational thinking can begin again. From an evolutionary perspective, this means having outrun, outfought, or successfully avoided a wild animal or an enemy. Once safe, you can access your rational mind (your cortex), so you can perform the sophisticated thinking and planning necessary to cope with a cancer diagnosis.

Shifting from stress to healing involves five components:

1. Being physically active and completing the stress response.
2. Making thoughtful decisions.
3. Tuning into your values.
4. Getting support.
5. Managing stress.

Being physically active. Do some form of physical activity, if possible, to complete the fight/flight response or move out of the freeze response. *Any* activity is better than *no* activity. Take a long walk—ideally in a natural setting, although even a city walk or a trip to the gym is better than sitting and worrying. Walk in a natural environment with someone with whom you feel "safe" and trust. Walk and talk, walk and talk, walk and talk. This movement completes the flight/fight/freeze response and dissipates the sense of helplessness that could sabotage your healing.

In between the thoughts of terror, fear of the known, and fear of the unknown, just keep walking. Focus on the natural beauty of your surroundings—trees and leaves, water, or the sky.

Making thoughtful decisions. Remember that the cancer probably has been present and growing for a number of years. This means that you usually have time to consider your present situation, reflect, and calmly choose what you want to do. Take your time to acknowledge your fears, your body's betrayal, the terrors, and the inability to know what to do. Focus your psychological energy on awareness, acceptance, and action.

Tuning into your own values. Find out what *you want to do* and not what your physician, family members, or friends tell you to do. Although you will want to know the opinions of your physician, your family, and your friends, it is your life—only you can live it, and only you will directly experience the consequences of the choices you make. So it is vital that you know what *you* want you to do. Not your doctor, not your family, not your friends. If you do not know what to do, use the diagnosis as the signal to begin this search and act on it.

Acknowledge that you feel unsafe. For almost all people, hearing the diagnosis scatters their sense of self, their trust in their body, and their personal sense of safety. Create within yourself and your community a feeling that you can be safe—safe to cry, safe to feel fear, safe not to know the answers, safe to just be, and safe to trust that you will make the right decisions.

Getting support.[224] Be with people and be part of, or create, a community upon whom you can lean in this time of need. If appropriate, let family, friends, and coworkers know that you have cancer and need support. Ask for specific kinds of support that you need, whether it means having meals cooked for you or your family, doing web searches for you, being your walking partner, or just sitting with you. This nurturing will encourage your sense of safety. Once you feel safer, your body is much more likely to shift out of the stress response into the relaxation/regeneration response. In this mode, the immune system will reengage, and the self-healing processes can be enhanced.

Managing stress. With the cancer diagnosis, realize that you have three primary goals: (1) to beat the disease, (2) to maximize your quality of life, and (3) to choose a path of development by building a meaningful life of wisdom, love, and faith. Within a matter of days, you're faced with a series of overwhelming decisions, large and small: Which treatment(s)? Surgery—and how extensive will it be? Chemotherapy? Radiation? Angiogenesis inhibitors (to slow growth of the cancer's blood supply)? Hormone blockers? Should I start conventional protocols, complementary and alternative treatments, or use the Gorter Model described in this book?

While making these seemingly overwhelming medical and life decisions, you also want to make lifestyle changes. Again, you're likely to find yourself overwhelmed. Should I exercise? How much? Should I change my diet—but what should I eat and what should I avoid? How much should I sleep? Can I stay out late? Can I have coffee? Is it OK to drink wine? We would like to offer some perspectives that will help you sort through the issues surrounding your cancer. You could call this an evolutionary perspective.

Taking the Long View: Getting Back in Sync

As humans, when we talk about "taking the long view," we may be thinking in terms of five or ten years. Biology is based on a much larger frame of reference. Evidence of the first humans dates to about 1.4 million years ago. We are genetically very similar to the hunters and gatherers who lived 40,000 years ago. Although our environment has changed, our genetics have changed very little, or not at all. Then, our

144

lifestyle included alternating between activity/movement and rest, and our diet consisted predominantly of fresh leaves, flowers and fruits, seeds, tubers, and a sprinkling of freshly killed meats or fish. For thousands of years, we probably ate an omnivore diet that we could digest easily. It is only in the last hundreds of years that we have radically changed our diets and activity patterns.

In terms of genetics, anything new to our bodies tends to be stressful. In defining "new," remember that new is measured over thousands of years. We are the result of evolutionary selection. Biological, psychological, and social traits that most enhanced survival and reproduction predominated through natural selection, and those traits that did not enhance or hindered reproduction were eliminated.

Yet, in the past 250 years since the advent of electricity, industrialization, and urban living, our entire lifestyle has changed radically. We live in cities of millions instead of smaller communities, exposed to thousands of novel chemicals, and thousands of microbes. Our food is made by machines—we eat processed foods and sugars. We experience long periods of inactivity on the job or at home. We're surrounded by electrical fields, we get jet lag and exposure to contagious illness from around the world brought by extensive travel, and much more.

It is challenging to think that 40,000 years ago a world existed where there were no electric lights, no TVs, no computers, no internet, no canned and packaged foods, no cars, bicycles, trains, or planes, no showers or flush toilets, no factories. . . .

The modern lifestyle has rapidly surpassed our genetics, and many of us pay the price. This most likely contributes to cancer, coronary conditions, stroke, diabetes, Alzheimer's and other diseases that are rare in traditional cultures. We are out of sync.

For a complex organism, adaptation to a new lifestyle usually engenders a biological cost.

Much of our food is manmade; most of us get very little exercise; we react constantly to noise and visual stimuli; and we are exposed to thousands of chemicals every year. Our technological progress, while beneficial in some ways, has had devastating health consequences for much of humanity.

The result is enormous stress on the body. This type of stress comes with a hidden cost that reduces the resources we have available for healing and has been directly linked to cancer. Take action now to reduce the stress on your system.

Taking Action

There are proactive steps you can take to reduce the biochemical and environmental stress—much of this self-care is relatively easy and can be done beginning *now*. You'll find that once you begin to take action, you feel less powerless—you shift into a sense of empowerment and hope. Research has shown that lifestyle changes contribute to cancer prevention, recovery, and the prevention of reoccurrences. But how can you know which changes will have the greatest benefit in your unique situation? Which changes are ideal for you?

The best approach is to simplify your lifestyle and reduce the factors that promote cancer.

These include reducing the toxins in the home, highly chemicalized personal care and beauty products, refined sugars in the diet, and heavy meat consumption. The next step is to begin reversing lifestyle patterns that are cancer promoting (smoking, high stress). This is also an opportunity to increase immune-enhancing lifestyle patterns (taking walks daily, sleeping at least seven to eight hours per night, eating more fresh fruits and vegetables, and getting sufficient vitamin D). Do anything that supports your immune system, brings you joy (whether it's sitting in the sun or watching a funny movie), and increases your energy level.

Start reducing anything that burdens or compromises your immune system and energy level (with the goal of eliminating as many toxins and as much stress as possible). Begin by nurturing your life with good, fresh nutrition, physical activity or exercise, and support from your social network and community. Use the diagnosis of cancer as an excuse or wake-up call to make necessary changes.

You can immediately begin rearranging you life so that it is more health promoting regardless what treatment options you will later choose; take your biography (and biology) into your own hands.

You may already be doing many of these health-promoting patterns—but it can be helpful to explore whether there is anything more you can do. Relatives, friends, health care providers, and your web searches will all suggest things to do, which will probably result in conflicting facts and opinions. The simplest approach is to implement a lifestyle in which cancer-initiating and -promoting factors are substantially reduced, and immune-enhancing lifestyle patterns are increased.

This does *not* mean that you caused your cancer or that others caused your cancer. Cancer is far too complex for a simple or single-cause explanation. Shift blaming into action. The purpose is to look at the present and future and encourage those actions that support your self-healing potentials. Also, resist a stoic or self-denial mentality. In other words, don't become so strict with your diet and exercise that you lose the flexibility to have joy and spontaneity in your life. Joy and balance are also immune enhancers.

As you begin your journey, remember that healing is not totally in our control; we can only contribute to the process, just as medical treatments can also contribute to healing. The question to focus on is not *Why do I have cancer?* but *What can I do to support my own self-healing process?* and *How can I live with my diagnosis?*

Make your choices among forms of treatment that are not harmful (there are very few scientific studies that have shown complementary and holistic techniques to be harmful and contraindicated). Open your boundaries and add to your healing and treatment strategies possibilities such as diet, massage, spiritual/energy healing, Chinese and anthroposophical medicine, imagery, love, and social support. These approaches are not intended as the sole approach to treatment, but we do know they support immune function and quality of life.[225]

Nutritional Support for Healing: Getting Our Nutrition in Sync

"We are what we eat." In the nineteenth century, many people shifted from eating predominantly brown rice to polished white rice and developed a vitamin B_1 deficiency disease called beriberi. This can result in difficulty walking, nerve damage, loss of muscle function, mental confusion, and eventually cardiac failure and even death. By removing the husks on the rice, which are rich in thiamine, people unknowingly created nutrient depletion and vulnerability to this disease. Had they simply continued eating brown rice, they would not have developed beriberi.

Similarly, sailors before the nineteenth century, who ate no fresh fruits or vegetables on their long voyages, often suffered from scurvy until it was recognized that fresh fruits, such as limes, would prevent the disease. British sailors became known as "limeys" because they ate limes to prevent scurvy.

The Western lifestyle and diet have been identified as contributors to the development of chronic and degenerative diseases such as cancer, cardiovascular disease, and arthritis. The most dramatic example today is the epidemic of type 2 diabetes due to excessive sugar intake from eating a diet of processed carbohydrates that are high in simple starches and sugars. Carbohydrates such as white flour, potatoes, and pasta test almost as high as white sugar on the glycemic index, an indicator of how rapidly they break down into glucose and raise blood sugar. These foods typically lack dietary fiber, antioxidants, vitamins, minerals, and other necessary micronutrients. Foods high in fiber, such as whole grains, are lower on the glycemic index, take longer for the body to digest, and thus raise blood sugar more slowly. In addition to problems like diabetes, a high-sugar diet triggers weight gain and chronic inflammation, both or which are associated with chronic diseases, including cancer.

The following tips will help you get your nutrition on track:

Eating more whole foods. Whenever you shop for food, buy foods that are real (rather than processed foods with labels of long, unpronounceable words or numbers). Include more fresh fruits and vegetables in your menus. The authors agree with Michael Pollan, the author of *In Defense of Food: An Eater's Manifesto,* that we should eat only the foods that our great-grandparents ate. So as a rule of thumb, eat only the foods that existed before the 1940s. Prepare your food fresh.[226]

Eating more fresh fruits and vegetables. Include generous servings of vegetables, fruits, nuts, and complex carbohydrates, both raw because they are rich in enzymes and cooked to obtain an array of nutrients. Antioxidants are the key ingredients in fresh fruits and vegetables, and they counter oxidative stress, which causes chronic inflammation and is cancer promoting. Oxidants are the products of stress in our body chemistry caused by everything from workplace chemicals and cigarette smoke to eating trans fats.

Cutting out free sugar. Are you tempted to boost your energy with coffee and sweets? Is your breakfast mainly sugary cereal out of a box? You'll find that you increase your energy and improve your health when you skip the sugar.

In the last fifty years we have shifted to foods and beverages containing exceptionally high amounts of sugar. Today in the United States, every man, woman, and child consumes on average 167 pounds of sugar a year. Sugar feeds cancer, so to optimize your health, you want a diet low in sweets and simple sugars. Emphasize foods that are absorbed into your blood stream more slowly, to keep your blood sugar stable. Reduce foods high in sugars, corn syrup, fructose, fruit juice concentrates, maltose, honey, maple syrup, and even agave (a natural sugar high in fructose, made from the agave cactus). That means cutting out sodas, juices, pastries, cakes, candy, sugary breakfast cereals, dried fruits, and other sources of sweets and increasing fresh fruits and vegetables that have a moderate rating on the glycemic index (see below).

Emphasizing whole grains. Reduce the white stuff. Eat foods made with whole grains instead of those made with white flour, white rice, potatoes, or corn. That means cutting way back on foods that are highly processed—those created in a factory and marketed in a box on the shelves of the grocery store.

Whole grains can be delicious—develop a taste for hearty breads, crackers, and whole-wheat products in place of foods made with white flour. Instead of white rice, learn how to prepare superb brown rice dishes (choosing between brown, basmati, long-grain, short-grain, wild rice, forbidden black rice, whole grain pilafs, or combinations such as rice and lentils). Replace genetically modified white potatoes with organic new potatoes, Peruvian potatoes, or Yukon gold.

Using the glycemic index.[227] Foods made with white flour or white sugar often cause a spike in your blood sugar. This is because simple carbohydrates break down quickly, flooding the bloodstream with glucose. Research has shown that a diet high in carbohydrates and simple sugars can cause obesity.

As a result, these foods are hidden causes of weight gain. This is especially true once we reach midlife, as lower hormone levels alter our metabolism. The chronic inflammation that results has been associated with diseases such as prostate and breast cancer. In addition, women with estrogen/progesterone positive breast cancer will want to focus on weight management since adipose tissue can be estrogen generating.

The glycemic index is a useful tool that indicates which foods raise blood sugar too high. This simple one-page table cuts through the confusion, making it clear which foods are likely to spike blood sugar and which ones won't. The international table of glycemic index and glycemic load values is available from numerous sources.[228]

Minimizing (or completely eliminating) meat. Reduce proteins derived from meat and increase proteins derived from plants. Large-population human studies have demonstrated a strong correlation between meat consumption and cancer.

An Italian study on meat and cancer correlation looked at data on ten thousand hospital patients and found a strong correlation between red meat and cancer. Although we strongly agree with the guideline to eat organic vegetarian nutrition, human beings are omnivores from a biological perspective. Thus, animal proteins were often part of the diet, although usually in a smaller percentage. We recommend eating organic and biodynamic food; and if animal proteins (fish and possibly organic poultry) are included, be sure they have been raised in the context of their evolutionary origins.

In addition, once cancer cells are present, the disease seems to progress more rapidly when the diet is derived from animal meat. This may be due in part to the fact that our foods are no longer raised naturally, but contain numerous chemicals, pesticides, hormones, preservatives, and other additives. A diet low in animal protein is associated with lower levels of cancer growth.[229]

Eating organic foods. Whenever possible, eat organic and biodynamic foods, and avoid those that contain pesticides or are genetically modified to be insect resistant. The additives in processed foods are another of the risks associated with cancer.

Products that have been sprayed, treated, or processed in some way all contain chemicals that need to be broken down and eliminated by our bodies. From an evolutionary perspective most of the pesticides used on food are unfamiliar to the human immune system, and we have not evolved to process them.

Even though the FDA and USDA report that nonorganic foods with the minute amounts of additives do not contain enough chemical residues to be harmful, most likely over a lifetime these chemical residues tend to build up in our bodies. This cumulative long-term exposure to chemicals may carry a cancer risk, since people who are exposed to pesticides frequently on their job show much higher rates of cancer. In addition, the very young, the very old, those with genetic vulnerabilities, and those with immune compromise appear to be more sensitive to the effects of additives.

Numerous lab studies have confirmed the development of cancer, birth defects, and eventually infertility in animals fed food additives. We can support our immune systems by reducing ongoing intake of these harmful substances. Consider that each time you eat or drink organic foods you are nurturing your body and supporting your body's self-healing processes.

Eating cancer-fighting vegetables and fruits. Extensive research has shown that people who eat antioxidant fruits and vegetables have at least a 50 percent lower risk of cancer. For men with early prostate cancer, a low-fat vegetarian diet has been shown to reduce PSA levels and stop the progression of cancer. This has been demonstrated in the research of Dr. Dean Ornish.[230]

Most cancer diets are predominantly vegetarian, in which most if not all of the proteins come from vegetables and fermented dairy products such as yogurt. Explore the following sources for diet recommendations:

Pollan, M. *In Defense of Food: An Eater's Manifesto.* New York: Penguin Press, 2008.
This book offers the basic rationale and general guidelines for what to eat.

Servan-Schreiber, D. *Anticancer: A New Way of life.* New York: Viking, 2009.

This provides a superb description of the anti-inflammatory diet and lifestyle based on solid scientific data from a renowned researcher who recovered from brain cancer.

Quillin, P. *Beating Cancer with Nutrition.* Carlsbad, CA: Nutrition Times Press, 2005.
This book gives detailed dietary recommendations on how to beat cancer through nutrition.

Beliveau, R., and D. Gingras. *Foods to Fight Cancer.* New York: DK Publishing, 2007.
This book gives some background and specific recommendations of foods to eat to fight cancer.

Individualizing Your Program

No one can totally predict the effect of specific lifestyle changes on an individual. Almost all research findings are based on group data and cannot predict how the finding will apply to a specific person. It can only predict that you belong to a risk group. This complicates decision making. No practitioner knows enough about the individual differences to be sure that the specific recommendations are 100 percent correct for every person. In nearly every study, there are some people for whom the guidelines are not effective or may even be harmful. Some people are lactose intolerant while others are not; some can eat massive amounts of simple sugars without developing type 2 diabetes; and some smoke every day and live to be a hundred years old. In most cases, the conclusions derived from research are that if you eat lots of processed foods or smoke, you become part of a higher risk group.

Notice what agrees with your body. If the suggested health-promoting actions or diet changes make you feel weaker or decrease your energy, *stop*. Do an experiment: eliminate the activity or food for a week and observe what happens. Then add the food or activity back into your routine, one step at the time, and observe its effect. Some people find it helpful to make just one major change a week, so they can invest their energy (and their money) in the efforts that prove to be the most beneficial.

Reducing Exposure to Toxins

The President's Cancer Panel was particularly concerned to find that the true burden of environmentally induced cancer has been grossly underestimated. With nearly 80,000 chemicals on the market in the United States, many of which are used by millions of Americans in their daily lives and are un- or understudied and largely unregulated, exposure to potential environmental carcinogens is widespread.

Environmental exposures that increase the national cancer burden do not represent a new front in the ongoing war on cancer. However, the grievous harm from this group of carcinogens has not been addressed adequately by the National Cancer Program. The American people— even before they are born—are bombarded continually with myriad combinations of these dangerous exposures. The Panel urges you [the president] most strongly to use the power of your office to remove the carcinogens and other toxins from our food, water, and air that need- lessly increase health care costs, cripple our Nation's productivity, and devastate American lives.

THE PRESIDENT'S CANCER PANEL[231]

Everywhere in our lives we are exposed to thousands of chemicals that did not exist even fifty years ago. Occupational cancer is now the num- ber one cause of worksite deaths worldwide, ahead of all other work- related diseases and accidents. The general consensus is that a majority of all cancers are either caused or promoted by environmental chemical factors; many of these are contained in food and the fluids we drink, the air we breathe, and the cosmetics we absorb in our skin.[232] These chemicals are distributed throughout the environment in our homes, gardens, workplaces, atmosphere, soil, lakes, rivers, and oceans.[233] Although you cannot control the toxins in the environment, you *can* reduce the toxins in your home. Go through all your closets and cabinets, reading labels and evaluating the products you use for their level of potential toxicity.

- Check your shampoos, conditioners, and makeup and discard those that contain parabens, bisphenol A (BPA), and other substances that act as hormone disregulators and contribute to cancer growth or interfere with healing.
- Cleaning products commonly used in the home are another source of toxins.
- Paints, paint thinner, chemical stripper, sealants, dyes, and products used in many hobbies are known to be carcinogenic.
- Mattresses, where we spend a significant amount of our time, are often made of substances such as foam rubber and other synthetic materials that contribute to exposure over time as the chemicals leach or outgas from the product.
- Use mainly organic substances with all natural ingredients whenever possible.
- Cigarette smoking triples or even quadruples the risk of many cancers.
- Formaldehyde, asbestos, and many other building materials are cancer causing, as is radon leakage, which can be identified through simple testing.

After clearing the toxins from your environment, explore the physical, social, emotional, and mental process that can enhance your immune functioning. In addition, explore the information on environmental exposures that increase our cancer risk. It is important to identify these exposures—particularly those that can be avoided or eliminated. Check the following resources:

National Cancer Institute (NCI) and the National Institute of Environmental Health Sciences (NIEHS). *Cancer and the Environment: What You Need to Know What You Can Do.* NIH Publication No. 03–2039, 2003. Available from www.niehs.nih.gov/health/docs/cancer-enviro.pdf

National Cancer Institute, National Institutes of Health, U.S. Department of Health and Human Services. *The President's Cancer Panel: Reducing Environmental Cancer Risk–What We Can Do,* available at http://deainfo.nci.nih.gov/advisory/pcp/pcp08-09rpt/PCP_Report_08-09_508.pdf

Schapiro, M. *Exposed: The Toxic Chemistry of Everyday Products and What's at Stake for American Power.* White River Junction, VT: Chelsea Green Publishing, 2009.

Steingraber, S. *Living Downstream: An Ecologist's Personal Investigation of Cancer and the Environment,* 2nd ed. New York: Da Capo, 2010.

Berthold-Bond, A. *Better Basics for the Home: Simple Solutions for Less Toxic Living.* New York: Three Rivers Press, 1999.

Greer, B. *Super Natural Home.* Emmaus, PA: Rodale Books, 2009.

Walking, Yoga, and Gentle Exercise

It can be helpful to think of exercise[234] as something that nourishes and restores you, rather than depletes you. Incorporate movement into your daily life. Find activities that leave you feeling relaxed and comfortable in your body, whether it's walking meditation or a brisk walk, Pilates, eurhythmy,[235] or qigong.

As hunters and gatherers, our ancestors were alternately physically active and then resting throughout the day. Only recently have we become stationary and immobilized all day, sitting in front of the computer or TV, or in a car. Immobility, except for regeneration during sleep or after activities, is deleterious. To facilitate venous blood and lymph return, we need to be physically active. Without the periodic muscle contractions of activity, the tissue stagnates, and venous blood and lymph fluids pool and circulate less. This may even result in some degree of edema. The harmful effect of inactivity is illustrated by the risk of edema and deep vein thrombosis (blood clots in the veins of the legs) experienced in long-distance air travel.

Research has shown the myriad benefits of movement and exercise for cancer patients, including immune system benefits, increased energy and better mood. Even when you feel tired and under the weather, getting out and moving around can be an excellent pick-me-up. The benefits are significant for survival, too. Doing moderate exercise for thirty minutes a day such as walking has been found to bolster the immune system significantly.[236] Women who exercise during chemotherapy have a lower risk of breast cancer recurrence.

When one becomes immobilized, energy drops and mood decreases. Respect your evolutionary origins and incorporate more physical activity during the day to regain energy. Many patients find it helpful to wear a pedometer (a step counter) to record how much movement they have achieved, which motivates them to stay active. Often if activities can be done with another person, one's mood increases significantly. You get the double benefit of social support and exercise.

For our bodies, immobility begets more immobility—think of it as *rest rust.* Consider the analogy of a stream of water. When water moves quickly, it is oxygenated, and often crystal clear—yet the moment the water stops flowing, the pool becomes stagnant. The health benefits of movement are well documented: longer lives, fewer degenerative illnesses, fewer heart attacks, fewer depressive episodes, and less cancer. Experience your change in energy when you do the following practice, "Pick the Flowers."

Pick the Flowers

Stand up and imagine that all around you are plants with flowers. Some are very high above your head, and others are far to the side. Now actually reach upward and then to the side or downward to pick these imaginary flowers to make a bouquet. As you reach out to pick the flower, reach way up, even stand on your toes, and as you reach, exhale, "Shhh . . ." Pick many flowers all around you, above you, to the side, and below you; rotate and pick the flowers behind you. Each time you pick the flower, put it with the others into the bouquet. Stop when you have collected a very large bouquet. Now imagine giving this to a friend you like.

After doing this practice, check how you feel. Almost everyone who does this practice reports an immediate increase in energy and positive mood. It works quicker than the caffeine fix of coffee.

To align your lifestyle with the patterns of our ancestors, if possible, incorporate twenty to thirty minutes of daily continuous movement such as walking, jogging, dancing, or therapeutic eurhythmy. People who walk or do aerobic exercise daily for about thirty minutes have significantly lower cancer rates than those who do not. They also have lower rates of heart disease, hypertension, and depression. Exercise is a much more successful long-term treatment for mild, moderate, and moderate/severe depression than is antidepressant medication, especially since the relapse rate for depression after a year was more than four times as high for the medication group as for the exercise group.[237] Staying active is one of the ways you can modulate the low mood and energy that tend to be so common from cancer and cancer treatment.

When doing movements, become aware of your own energy level. Listen to it without judgment and act upon it. When your energy level is low, be gentle, rest, and regenerate and then do some movement. Follow it up with some more movement and another pause to refresh and regenerate. Exercising does not necessarily mean going to the gym.

Do exercises that are fun. Go for walks in nature (alone or with a loved one); go dancing and be captured in the movement; join a class in yoga, tai chi, qigong, or therapeutic eurhythmy. Increasing movement can be as simple as leaving your car at home and using public transportation. Or it could mean parking your car a little bit further away from your destination and slowly walking the extra distance while looking up at the trees, clouds, and sky. If you have enough energy, walk up the stairs instead of taking the elevator or the escalator, or even walk up one flight and then take the escalator or elevator. Go outside and appreciate nature. Find a partner and learn a dance routine. If possible, work up to thirty minutes a day or more.

Always listen to yourself. Do not overexert. Allow plenty of time for regeneration. Give yourself permission to rest. Realize that the body does need time to regenerate after use. The research shows that cancer-related fatigue improves with exercise. This feels paradoxical to most patients. Thus gently push yourself despite the fatigue.

Cancer and Exercise

Patients often ask, "Is exercise safe for me? If so, what should I do? And will there be a real benefit—is it worth the effort?"

Researchers all over the world have tracked the effects of exercise on the well-being of cancer patients. To date, almost a hundred studies have evaluated the benefits of walking, and at least twelve studies have reported on yoga as a body-mind intervention. For the majority of patients, gentle exercise is a practical approach that is not harmful—the studies on yoga confirm improved quality of life and report major reductions in stress and fatigue.

Improved sleep. At least four studies have documented better-quality sleep and energy for cancer patients who do yoga.

- *Fewer sleep disturbances.* A study at the University of Texas on the progress of thirty-nine patients with lymphoma reported significant reductions in sleep disturbance.[238]
- *Significant improvement in fatigue.* At Wake Forest Medical School, researchers assessed the benefits of yoga for forty-four women with breast cancer, average age fifty-six years old. Some women participated in a ten-week yoga program while others were randomly placed on a waiting list. For those in the yoga program, the study reported "significant improvement in fatigue" and improved "mental health, depression, positive affect, and spirituality (peace/meaning)."[239]
- *Better quality of life.* From Albert Einstein College of Medicine, a study of 128 minority patients with breast cancer reported less fatigue and better social functioning following twelve weeks of yoga.[240]
- *Lower levels of pain.* Duke University research tracked the progress of thirteen women with metastatic breast cancer, which is usually fatal. The research reported significantly lower levels of pain and fatigue following an eight-week yoga class.[241]

Reduced stress. Yoga is well-recognized in the field of stress management, but these studies show that it also reduces stress for cancer patients. The research included lab tests for stress indicators such as cortisol.

- *Lower cortisol levels.* A study at the Tom Baker Cancer Center in Calgary evaluated cancer patients in programs for mind-body stress reduction. A study of fifty-nine breast cancer patients taking an eight-week class in mindfulness-based stress reduction found lower levels of cortisol.[242]
- *Lower levels of inflammation.* A second study at the Baker Cancer Center of 198 patients on this stress-reduction program found that patients had measurably lowered blood pressure, cortisol levels, and markers of inflammation. These patients continued to experience gains at the six-month and twelve-month follow-ups after a program of relaxation, meditation, gentle yoga, and daily home practice.[243]

- *Reduced nausea and vomiting.* A study at the Bangalore Institute of Oncology in India evaluated sixty-two early-stage breast cancer patients who were randomly assigned to yoga or supportive therapy. Following yoga, there was "a significant decrease in post-chemotherapy-induced nausea frequency and intensity... and anticipatory vomiting."[244]

- *Less mental disorganization.* Research at the University of Calgary evaluated the well-being of thirty-eight breast cancer survivors more than four years after their initial diagnosis. Improvements associated with yoga practice included lower cortisol levels in the afternoon with reduced digestive symptoms (diarrhea), and less mood disturbance, emotional irritability, and mental confusion.[245]

- *Lower levels of perceived stress.* A study at the National University of Singapore evaluated patients receiving radiation treatment. Researchers compared the benefits of a yoga intervention with the responses of a control group that had received treatment alone. Among the sixty-eight breast cancer patients who participated, those in the yoga group had a lower *Perceived Stress Scale,* whereas the control group did not show any change.[246]

- *Decreased anxiety.* Other studies at the Bangalore Institute evaluated approximately two hundred Stage II and III breast cancer outpatients who were randomly assigned to yoga or brief supportive therapy. The research evaluated morning levels of cortisol in saliva, which is a significant marker of anxiety and depression. Statistical analysis of morning cortisol levels showed an overall decrease in anxiety in the yoga participants compared with the patients in the control group.[247]

Researchers at the Baker Cancer Center report that mindfulness-based stress reduction enrollment "was associated with enhanced quality of life and decreased stress symptoms in breast and prostate cancer patients, and resulted in possibly beneficial changes in hypothalamic-pituitary-adrenal functioning." In the University of Calgary study, "initial findings suggest that yoga has significant potential and should be further explored as a beneficial physical activity option for cancer survivors."

Reducing Stress

Minimizing physical stress. To increase regeneration, reduce stress. Stress is a load on the body; and when cancer occurs, one's resources are limited and need to be available for mobilizing the immune system. Begin by identifying your negative stressors, and reduce and eliminate them if you can. Some stressors are not negative but come at a high cost to the body. For example, jet lag is highly detrimental as the body goes out of rhythm, and without those inherent rhythms, healing is reduced. Thus, respect the cost of jet lag. More importantly, regularize your rhythms of eating, sleeping, and physical activity. What is common among most people who live to a very healthy old age is that their lives have regularity—this does not mean boring lives. It does mean regularity with social support, such as eating breakfast at the same time with your partner—apparently it is irregularity that increases the stress. (See chapter 10 for resources on influencing your mood and energy through the mind-body connection.)

Managing emotional stress. Reduce and eliminate emotional and thought patterns that evoke a sense of powerlessness or depression, which can reduce immune functioning. Increase emotional and thinking patterns that are immune supportive and health promoting. The data suggest that a fighting spirit *(hope)*, optimism *(faith)*, and a supportive environment *(love)* increase survival while depression and helplessness decrease survival.[248] Begin assessing your energy drains and gains and then reduce the drains and increase the gains. This process takes a while to do; however, as you explore and act upon it, you are choosing to do more things that give you energy. (See chapters 10 through 13 for practical tools on managing stress.) The major theme is to develop a regenerative, health-promoting lifestyle (as illustrated in figure 9.1).

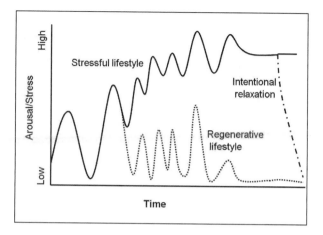

Figure 9.1. Comparison of a stressful, nonregenerative lifestyle. The stressful lifestyle can be interrupted through intentional relaxation and regeneration.

Learning stress management has a long-term effect on cancer recovery. For example, in an eleven-year follow-up study of 227 women with breast cancer, those who practiced stress management had a reduced risk of recurrence and premature death. The data show that the more patients practiced stress management, the better was their outcome.[249] The researchers also studied the biological stress responses and immune system responses of the women in the study and concluded that the beneficial effect of the stress management practice on the women's survival and lower risk of recurrence was likely achieved through a change in these mechanisms. (For more practices, see chapters 10 through 15.).

Reconnecting with Your *Self*

As you make your way through the shock of the diagnosis, the challenges of treatment, and the adjustment of life after treatment, ask yourself, "What is it that I really want to do?" And if you do not know what that is (many people don't, for most of their lives), start this exploration—it is an ideal time to live your dreams. Make time for regeneration and self-healing imagery, and use imagery to support the self-healing processes within you. Practice appreciation of the past, and gratitude for what's best in the present. In time it may even become possible to be grateful for how well your body has performed.

Most importantly, listen to yourself and take action. Some people—and this usually occurs much later—come to see the cancer as an opportunity, a second chance to engage in life, and to be who they really want to be. If possible, see the cancer as a wake-up call, and use the illness as an opportunity to make your own choices and live a life that is meaningful to your own values.

Notice what agrees with your body. If the suggested health-promoting actions or diet changes make you feel weaker or decrease your energy, *stop*. Do an experiment, and eliminate the activity or food for a week and notice what happens. Then add the foods or activities back one at the time and observe its effect. Remember, life is very complex, and often the effect occurs only through multiple interactions.

Be critical but remain open-minded. Take a skeptical attitude toward the guidelines and recommendations of the FDA and USDA, as most of their administrators have held or will hold positions in the future in either international food, agribusiness, or pharmaceutical companies.

Consider a healthy skepticism if a food, drug, or chemical has not coexisted with us for thousands of years and contributed to our evolutionary selection. If it is a new product or is used in a totally new way, then there may be a chance that your body will experience it as metabolic stress. Consider these examples:

- Mad cow disease was spread by feeding cows (which are plant eaters) ground-up meat and fish-waste products (which happened to contain contaminated nerve tissue with prions). The disease was stopped when a ban was instituted on feeding meat products to cows.
- Clothing and furniture containing fire retardants substances (per-fluorooctanoic acid [PFOA] and perfluorooctane sulfonate [PFOS])

reduces fertility in woman by more than 30 percent. New state laws now outlaw the use of these specific substances in clothing.

- Hydrogenated fats (trans fats) have been standard fare in fast food, despite the fact that they raise the risk of heart disease and decrease healthy cholesterol (HDL) levels. Many states now prohibit the use of trans fats in foods.

- Cigarette smoking was once considered healthy, and for many years physicians were primary spokesmen for the tobacco companies.

Each of these were approved and lauded by the official U.S. government agencies such as the FDA and USDA and for years were advertised as being healthy— despite the fact that they were beyond the evolutionary experience of the animal or human. Cows never ate meat; PFOA and PFOS have never existed in the environment; trans fats are rare in nature; cigarettes and the chemicals they contain bathe the lungs in carcinogens with every use. The list goes on and on.

Genetically modified corn is a case in point. In terms of foods, consider genetically modified corn, which was genetically engineered to contain novel insecticide (two different Bt toxins used as insecticides) so that pests would not harm the corn. These genetically produced substances are now produced by the corn plant and are present in the corn you eat. Monsanto received USDA approval that it was safe as a food and could be planted by farmers. Monsanto has the patent for this plant; the company financially prospers by selling this seed to farmers. However, their data were based on measuring potential harmful effects for a very short-term study, and short-term studies usually do not show long-term effects. Just as smoking a few cigarettes usually causes no harm, smoking them for years can be distinctly harmful. Similarly, when researchers fed rats this genetically modified corn for ninety days as part of the rat's diet, there were negative effects to the liver and kidneys and damage to the heart, adrenal glands, and spleens of the animals.[250]

From an evolutionary perspective, because these are chemicals foreign to our bodies, the detoxifying pathways of the body are challenged as they cope with these novel substances—a process that may create biological stress.

When cancer is present, your body is under stress. Instead of increasing the stress, help your body heal by simplifying what you eat and eliminating toxins in your environment to match your biological heritage.

Chapter 10

GETTING YOUR LIFESTYLE IN SYNC

For cancer patients, even before they get diagnosed, many aspects of their day-to-day lifestyle are out of balance, and the rhythms of the body (especially sleep) are frequently disturbed. Since cancer affects at least one in three people, this may be an indication that contemporary lifestyle is at odds with our biology. One of the things that can come with a cancer diagnosis is a reminder to bring our lifestyle in harmony with our genetics.

How We Got Out of Sync

Taking another look at our genetics, the fact human genes haven't changed in the past 40,000 years means we're encoded to live a simpler life. Consider a basic aspect of lifestyle such as sleep, seen from the perspective of a hunter-gatherer:

The hunter-gatherer's mind-set. It's twilight, the time when predators roam, so I need to be in a place that's safe and secure. A cave offers this protection. With the small entrance, there's only one area in my living space where I am vulnerable, where I must be vigilant. Our small clan curls together for warmth and sleep. As the sun sets, it becomes totally dark inside, and even the light from the moon and stars does not illuminate the back of the cave. The only sounds are the rustling and breathing of my family. Our leader is sleeping near the entrance on guard, ready to awaken and respond to any sound or change in light. The rest of the family sleeps secure, with no light or noises to disturb us. Only the bright sunlight reflecting off the walls of the cave in the morning awakens us.

Compare this with a typical night in almost any bedroom in any modern city:

Contemporary lifestyle. *I start to drift into sleep, but the screeching of brakes pulls me back to startled awareness. What was that? I wonder. Not hearing anything else, the speed of my jumbled thoughts slows down, and once again I begin drifting downward into sleep. Sometime later I'm awake, without knowing why. It's still night. A translucent glow radiates through the curtain, and the street lamp illuminates a ribbon of light at the bottom edge of the window. On the dresser, the light from my alarm clock pierces the night. Even in this relative darkness, I can see all the objects in the room. Once again, I close my eyes and allow myself to fall into the emptiness of sleep. Just as everything begins to fade, bright lights move across the wall, and I'm aware of a truck going down the street. . . . When the alarm clock goes off, I am jolted out of bed. As I stumble into the day, I find myself wondering, Why can't I seem to get a good night's sleep?*

The modern bedroom experience is far removed from the hunter-gatherers' environment. In our nighttime world, there are many sources of light glowing or flashing—the alarm clock or the phone next to you on the night stand, the light on a power strip, on the TV or a computer, the flashing lights on a modem, or the glow of a night-light.

Every light source triggers a tiny cascade of brain activity that can interfere with the depth of our sleep. Our skin, which responds to light during the day, also reacts to lower levels of light at night, affecting our *pineal gland*. The pineal regulates rhythms of sleep and waking through the production of *melatonin,* which controls our circadian rhythms. Light and noise tend to be underappreciated factors in disrupted sleep and disturbed biological rhythm. No wonder forty-three million prescriptions for sleeping pills are written every year in the United States.

The more we move away from our biological hardwiring and assume an artificial lifestyle, the more our bodies must compensate. In the case of sleep, we're built to sleep in total darkness, after sunset. Think of how much light exposure we typically experience in the evening.[251]

Loss of sleep tends to drain our energy and also reduce the amount of energy we have for healing. Interrupted sleep is just one common example of how we live out of synchrony with our genetics and our evolutionary roots. When we can become attuned to our natural patterns and fit them to our lives, most people experience a boost in energy and noticeable improvements in their health. By improving sleep, there is generally an increase in immune function and mental focus, as well as a reduction in pain and fatigue.

Life Rhythms and Cancer

There is a link between disturbed rhythm and cancer, and higher cancer rates have been documented in occupations that involve disrupted sleep. Shift workers, such as nurses or factory workers, and people who experience frequent jet lag or irregular sleeping habits, tend to have higher cancer rates. For example, female airline attendants have double the incidence of breast cancer compared to the rest of the population. (Their risk factors include varied patterns of sleeping and eating, frequent jet lag, and exposure to cosmic radiation in flight.)

Our bodies have a number of rhythms and cycles that are multiyear, annual, seasonal, monthly, daily, and hourly, as well as shorter repeated cycles, like heart rate. Circadian rhythm is the twenty-four-hour cycle of all living beings, which is affected by light.[252] These rhythms are encoded within almost all life-forms.[253] When these rhythms are disturbed, illness may occur.

Cancer tissues have disrupted biological patterns. As the number of cancer cells increases, normal twenty-four-hour circadian patterns throughout the body go out of synchrony, as has been demonstrated in disrupted temperature rhythms. Biological rhythms that are affected include

- Sleep patterns
- The rise and fall of body temperature
- Heart rate and heart rate variability and its interconnection with the breathing patterns
- Patterns of cell and tissue growth

Sleep patterns. Insomnia is well documented in cancer patients. Research has confirmed poor sleep quality in cancer, not just due to the stress of illness, but also due to disturbed circadian rhythm.[254] The body's output of melatonin (the hormone that controls our circadian rhythms) can also be lower or even absent in cancer patients. In addition, some treatments for cancer, such as steroids and endocrine therapies, can contribute to disrupted sleep.

Body temperature. Cancer patients have a lower core body temperature, and often the absence of temperature rhythm. In healthy adults, circadian rhythm rises from a low at about 6 AM in the morning to a high at about 5 PM in the evening.[255] The range of temperature variation is about 1°F (0.5°C). However, most cancer patients do not experience this daily gradual rise and fall in temperature—their bodies remain at the low end of the temperature range. In practically all cancer patients, core temperature is 97.5°F (36.4°C), which is nearly 1.0°F (0.5°C) lower than that of healthy normal patients. The disruption of the temperature rhythm is an indicator of a decrease in health and immune function and seems to precede the manifestation of cancer. Most cancer patients report that for several years before their diagnosis, they often felt chilly and suffered from cold hands and feet.

Heart rate and heart rate variability. Rhythms embedded within the heart beat are described as heart rate variability. These patterns reflect the balance between the systems that are associated with the stress response (sympathetic mode) and the relaxation response (parasympathetic mode). When the balance between these systems is lost, it becomes more difficult for the body to regenerate and repair. Reduction in heart rate variability has been identified as a risk factor for cancer and as a predictor for cardiac disorders.[256]

Abnormal cell development. Cancer cells initially divide slowly, as long as their metabolism is limited, and they are not connected to a blood supply. However, if angiogenetic factors are secreted, the cancer forces the body to develop new blood vessels. These factors promote increased blood flow to the tumor and allow it to grow more rapidly in a disorganized, chaotic pattern. This tissue no longer follows the patterns of normal tissue development. An expanded network of blood vessels develops, which supports the growth of the cancerous tissue at a dangerous rate (as far as we know, none of the normal mechanisms of the body that regulate growth are present to limit the growth of these kinds of tissue).

What You Can Do

Rhythm brings balance as the body alternates between activity and restoration (breaking down, or *catabolism,* and building up, or *anabolism*). Whenever the body's rhythms are disturbed and the rhythms no longer provide this balance, it sets the stage for illness. It is not the momentary disturbances that are harmful—it is the chronic ongoing disturbance that sets the stage for disease.

In order to counter this effect, pace yourself. Look for the harmonious patterns that bring simplicity and richness to your life—long, deep sleep, refreshing exercise, and profound regeneration. What you want is that sweet spot where everything feels right (despite your illness).

Sleep and Cancer

From the moment we wake up in the morning, we begin using our body's resources, and causing a certain degree of wear and tear on our bodies. (This is true even if we're simply sitting with a book at the rim of a swimming pool all day.) This process of breaking down, or catabolism, can be defined as a form of stress. After a day of consciousness and alertness, we crave sleep to restore the resources that have been used up or worn down during the day. We need to rebuild, to restore our body and mind through relaxation and deep sleep in a process of anabolism. Deep sleep is essential for repair, healing, and good health. Health and the process of healing are a balanced, rhythmic alternation between being fully awake and productive and experiencing deep, rejuvenating sleep.

In most cancer patients, the patterns that underlie sleep are out of sync. When we are healthy, the body produces melatonin, which promotes natural sleep. In some cancer patients, the body's output of melatonin is significantly lower, whereas others produce no melatonin at all. In breast cancer patients, melatonin release is not synchronized with the body's inner twenty-four-hour clock. This can be a key factor in both insomnia and poor-quality sleep. Restorative sleep is a key to our capacity to heal. Our quality of life is also profoundly affected by the depth of our sleep and therefore the quality of our conscious awareness when we are awake.

The effects of chronic exhaustion. Often cancer patients report that long before they received a cancer diagnosis, they suffered from insomnia in one form or another, with constant fatigue and sometimes feelings of depression or loss of control. We need to honor the rhythms of the body. Constant activity is exhausting, making us vulnerable to infection, burnout, or injury (this is a well-know phenomenon observed in elite athletes and even students who become ill after their exams). Sleep deprivation and insomnia are well-recognized symptoms that precede physical and psychological dysfunction. The goal is to explore the causes of dysfunctional sleep in order to restore our natural rhythms.

What about sleeping pills? Essentially all synthetic sleeping medications put a person in a less-conscious state (surrogate sleep). As a result, the medications do not provide deep and regenerating sleep. Sleep medications tend to disturb the body's ability to repair and rebuild. The consensus of sleep researchers is that sleeping medications are not helpful and are probably harmful if used on an ongoing basis. Patients who habitually use sleeping medication have a 25- to 36-percent increased death rate, while those who take them occasionally have at least a 15-percent increased mortality.[257] They are acceptable as a crisis treatment for a few days, but not for extended use, as they can be harmful.

What You Can Do

Resetting your internal clock. Reset your circadian rhythm by reducing the exposure to light at bedtime. These rhythms are set by the exposure of full sunlight during the day and then total darkness at night, which provides the basis for the twenty-four-hour (diurnal) rhythms of our bodies.

The production of melatonin, triggered when it gets dark, can be disrupted by light exposure. To avoid this, limit exposure to light after bedtime. This means turning off and unplugging night-lights, TVs, and computers to limit light exposure. If you want to "reset your inner clock," you'll also want to limit computer work and TV after a certain nightly hour.

Given modern lighting, even in a seemingly darkened room, there may still be enough light to interrupt one's biological rhythms. Although we can cover our eyes with a sleeping mask, our skin may also be a potent light receptor, and it sends sensory and hormonal signals when exposed to even the smallest amount of light. Wearing a sleep mask helps, but it is usually not enough to enter a deep and relaxed sleep.

Sleeping in a state of total darkness duplicates the lifestyle of our ancestors, when night was often experienced without any source of light and was also cooler than the day. You can explore for yourself the difference in your sleep quality from sleeping in a cooler room, totally darkened, without the stimulation of light photons on your retina or your skin. Sleeping in absolute darkness, many people find that their sleep becomes deeper and less interrupted.

To fully darken your bedroom, consider window shades that block all the light in the room. To control the light from electrical appliances, it can be helpful to plug all appliances into a power strip and simply turn off this power strip at bedtime (or unplug them). This has triple benefits: it darkens the room completely; it lowers the subtle electromagnetic energy given off, and it reduces the residual power drawn by devices that are plugged in but not operating.

Balancing your body chemistry. Cancer and cancer medications can interfere with the metabolism of essential nutrients. In other cases, difficulty sleeping may simply reflect a higher requirement for a particular nutrient. For example, some people need a light protein snack in the evening to sleep through the night. Others find a calcium supplement helpful. These needs are specific to your metabolism and may be identified by a physician who practices integrative or nutritional medicine.

Cultivating peace of mind. In many cases, insomnia is triggered by fear and worry. It is understandable that you worry—if you have cancer, by definition you have just cause for worry. However, worry is counterproductive and could interfere with your progress. We encourage you to tap resources such as cognitive restructuring or mindfulness practice.[258]

In other cases, the mind is overstimulated at bedtime. Watching daily news just before going to bed often induces insomnia. Use the bedroom for sleeping and not for watching TV, reading a gripping thriller, or arguing with your partner. Choreograph the time before going to sleep with peaceful music, videos, or uplifting reading. Allow an hour to relax. Even laughter, as Norman Cousins[259] reported years ago, reduces pain and discomfort. Explore the following practices to develop self-awareness and mental and emotional balance.

Practice 1: Reviewing the Day

A powerful meditation from the tradition of anthroposophy is *retrospection*. At the end of each day, sit or lie down, relax, and remember your day as vividly as possible in visual images, but go *backward* in time! Thus, starting from the present moment, you stop to review your day until the moment you woke up. This meditation should not take you more than ten to fifteen minutes in total.

Benefits. Many people report that when they do this daily practice for several weeks, they feel more at peace, become more self-aware, and tend to be less judgmental and less reactive to stressors. It is as if you have seen your own reactions before and can develop a compassionate acceptance of your own pattern. Thus change is more possible.

Practice 2: Making Your Mind Stop

Worrying at night, going back over the what-ifs and if-onlys, and then the lonely terrors at two in the morning.... I am waiting for the dawn to come to drive the fears away.

Try the following practices to help you relax at night. Begin your bedtime ritual by enjoying inspirational reading or listening to soothing music. Since your goal is to calm your mind, it's probably a good idea not to watch the ten o'clock news. So the first step is to reduce the stimulation. Once you get in bed, take a moment to acknowledge that despite the fears, the unknowns, and the pain, you can choose when you want to worry. Before you lie down, put an audio recorder or a notepad and a pen next to the bed, and schedule a specific thirty-minute period the next day when you will sit quietly and focus on the concerns that you had recorded or written down as you were going to sleep.

Once you've scheduled time for worrying, bedtime becomes your time to relax. Lie down, begin relaxing, and focus on your breathing. Each time you exhale, whisper the sound "Haaaaa," very softly. Let the air flow slower and slower as you exhale. Imagine the air flowing outward like a wave on the ocean. As you exhale, imagine healing energy going through your body and out your arms and legs. Each time you exhale, feel the air flowing outward.

Initially, you may want to pair this imagery with touch. In that case, sit up in bed in a relaxed position. To sense the air flowing through and out of your body, take a breath; and then as you exhale, stroke your arm from the shoulder to the hands. As you exhale the next breath, stroke one of your legs from your hip to your foot.[260] Keep focusing on the flow of energy through your arms and legs, drawn by your breath.

If you start worrying, shift your focus of attention back to your breathing. If the worry persists, and takes more and more of your attention, you can record your concerns or write them down on the notepad and say to yourself, "I will definitely sit down tomorrow—just as I promised—and go over these issues." Now lie down again and go back to breathing. Again imagine the air flowing down and out your arms and legs. When another worry surfaces, bring your focus back to your breathing. Again if it stays, record it or write it down and tell yourself that you will give this your undivided attention tomorrow at a certain time, but right now, this is your time to relax. Be gentle but firm with yourself, recording any worries that arise, and then quietly insisting that this is your time to relax.

The next day, at the time agreed on, sit quietly and reflect on the concerns you recorded or wrote down last night. For thirty minutes give these issues serious attention, and reflect only upon those items. While you are problem solving, you may be tempted to daydream, but keep gently bringing your focus back to the issues on your list. You can also use one of the imagery techniques in chapter 14 to encourage solutions. After thirty minutes, get up and do something physically active—take a walk, do some yoga, or just shake the stress off (see Practice 2 in chapter 13).

Benefits. Many people report that when they do this exercise and keep their promise to review their concerns the next day, their worries decrease, and sleep comes easier. Even if sleep does not occur, the breathing practice encourages regeneration. Interestingly, often when the people look at their list of nighttime worries the next day, they are surprised to find that the concerns are not as important as they had thought. They may be tempted to consider it a time waster to reflect on the issues that caused them to lose sleep the night before. However, it is important to follow through with the reflection exercise and spend the concentrated effort during the thirty minutes to think about your concerns. If you skip the reflection time the next day, you are telling your subconscious mind, *Don't trust what I tell you; I don't keep my promise,* which sets the stage for more worry the next night. Sometimes we learn that thoughts that seem so important during the night turn out to be *not worth thinking about* in the light of day. This helps us put things in perspective when we're tempted to start worrying at night and allows us to more easily refocus on our breath.

Waking Up in the Middle of the Night. Some people wake up in the middle of the night due to low blood sugar. One solution is to have a protein snack at bedtime to sustain your blood sugar level throughout the night.[261] Another is to have a protein snack when you wake up. Other people find that taking calcium supplement helps them sleep better. What is important to remember is that each of us has a unique metabolism—be open to explore to find out what works for you. You may want to try the following practice.

Practice 3: Prayer and Meditation

When you're wide awake at 4 AM, don't worry about being unable to sleep. Instead, capitalize on this opportunity and use the time to quiet your mind, since a quiet and peaceful mind regenerates the body.

As you lie in bed, begin to meditate or say a prayer. For meditation, you could repeat a word or phrase such as *love* or *I am at peace,* say a peaceful prayer, or recite an inspirational poem. Keep repeating the phrase, prayer, or poem. Softy say it out loud or to yourself (so as not to disturb your sleeping partner). Keep bringing your attention to the meaning of the phrase, prayer, or poem. When other thoughts arise, let them drift away, and refocus your attention on what you are saying. Continue this for thirty minutes.

Benefits. Many people report that doing this practice allows them to stay restfully in bed, and sometimes sleep returns. Ultimately, prayer and meditation are the essence of any practice: *faith,* the belief that there is meaning to everything; *hope,* the sense that ultimately, I will be OK no matter what; and *love,* the knowledge that I will continue to care for myself and others. These are themes we'll explore in greater depth in chapters 11 through 15.

Explore a wealth of scientific articles on the subject,[262] or consider the following resources on getting your body in sync:

Ancoli-Israel, S. *All I Want Is a Good Night's Sleep.* New York: C.V. Mosby, 1996.
This classic book offers very pragmatic and helpful strategies to improve sleep.

Jacobs, D. *Say Good Night to Insomnia.* New York: Holt, 2009.
This book outlines useful self-management approaches for overcoming insomnia and is based on university and clinical research protocols.

Smolensky, M., and L. Lamberg. *The Body Clock Guide to Better Health: How to Use Your Body's Natural Clock to Fight Illness and Achieve Maximum Health.* New York: Holt, 2001.
This very useful book helps readers understand the biological rhythms that control and underlie our physiology.

Chapter 11

THE ROLE OF THE MIND IN HEALING

In the mirror, a raised scab, just below my hairline. Did I hit something? I don't remember. It's getting worse, an angry-looking red scab. Has my melanoma returned? My stomach tightens. I can't seem to let go of the fear. Although I can see that it looks different from my first melanoma, the doubt nags at me. I Google melanoma—the pictures look just like the scab on my forehead. Panicked, I call my doctor for an appointment. "I would like an appointment," I say calmly. But my brain is yelling, "I want it NOW!!" "Sorry, the appointment calendar is filled; the next open appointment will be Thursday at 2:40 PM." Two days from now. "Yes, I'll take it." For two days, the angry welt seems to grow as fast as my fear.

Inhale, exhale, and keep breathing. I imagine my body filled with healing light. I try to practice all the techniques I teach my students. Yet I continue to feel unsettled. I can't seem to return to inner peace. Finally it's Thursday, and I'm sitting in the waiting room. I force myself to read the paper. I keep reading the same story over and over. The doctor comes in, and I begin talking in a calm voice that masks my anxiety, "I have this scab that doesn't seem to heal. I'm worried that it could be melanoma." A quick look; "It is most likely shingles," he says. To be sure, he gives me a referral to the dermatologist. A massive weight falls from my shoulders for the first time since I noticed the scab. I feel unburdened, safe, quiet, hopeful.... The anxiety is gone. By evening, I am totally exhausted. I go to bed early, and for the first time in four nights sleep without interruption.

179

Cancer—or any other life-threatening diagnosis—challenges our sense of safety on the most basic level. To my surprise, the experience of having cancer deeply affected my trust in my own body. Once I recovered, I panicked at the sight of any changes in my skin. Every change seemed to automatically trigger a deep sense of insecurity. An itch was no longer just an itch, but possible melanoma.

ERIK PEPER

Will the Worry Ever Go Away?

A major challenge facing almost every patient who has cancer is that the basic trust that we once had in our bodies has been lost. This sensitization has certain benefits—it encourages us to visit our doctor for an earlier diagnosis (and therefore possibly more successful treatment). There is also a down side—it may trigger fear and even avoidance of seeing the doctor. If the fear and worry win out, they also activate the stress response and can suppress the immune system.

The challenge is not to be caught up in these feelings, in the inevitable doubts and fears that accompany any serious illness. How to let go of these reactions? How can I learn acceptance that somehow whatever happens, things will work out OK? Even if the final prognosis is death, there is still a sense of acceptance—an acceptance of hope and a sense of the rightness that occurs when we are actual participants in our own lives.[263]

The purpose of this chapter is to illustrate how thoughts can affect our body and health and offer some exercises on how to use our thoughts to enhance immunity and support our health—or if health is not possible, to experience wholeness. Healing from cancer usually includes at least two basic approaches: medical procedures that treat the cancer and self-care to mobilize the immune system. This chapter takes a closer look at the mind-body connection, illustrates how thoughts affect the body, and offers practices that can be implemented. From our perspective the common factors of empowerment include

- Finding meaning
- Experiencing greater love of life
- Embracing illness as an opportunity to grow and change[264]
- Being proactive
- Taking control

The Mind-Body Connection: A Holistic View

A holistic perspective assumes that mind, body, emotions, and consciousness (spirit) are all part of the whole and affect and are affected by each other and by the external environment. Similarly, our immune system is affected by and affects every part of us. The process of mind and body linkage was originally labeled "the psychophysiological principle" by two well-known biofeedback pioneers, Elmer and Alice Green.[265] They stated,

Every change in the physiological state is accompanied by an appropriate change in the mental emotional state, conscious or unconscious and conversely, every change in the mental emotional state, conscious or unconscious, is accompanied by an appropriate change in the physiological state.

As long as we are alive, every part affects every other part, and the whole is more than the sum of its parts. A cadaver is essentially a piece of meat; whereas a live human being is something more. We embody consciousness. As living human beings we can act—we have the option to think, to feel, to make choices, and to take action through will.

When we are *struck down* by cancer or have a heart attack, the language implies that it is an event totally beyond our control that induced the illness. Yet, does our heart *attack* us; does cancer *strike* us? It appears as if we had nothing to do with the illness.

The present 24/7 world so captures our attention that we tend to become disconnected from ourselves. We may be unaware of how our bodies, minds, and emotions are interlinked. Instead of being guided by our physical and emotional experiences, we only take action when we hurt or stop functioning. The first step is to increase our awareness, then to explore options and new solutions, and finally to implement those solutions.

The Power of Positive Emotions

Our thoughts and emotions significantly affect our bodies.[266] Positive emotions actually activate and mobilize the immune system. These qualities include hope, love, purpose, and passion, as well as belief in a positive outcome for one's self and the world.

Holding empowering thoughts and acting on health-promoting beliefs are associated with remission of cancer. Healing is promoted by active involvement in life and by doing things that offer a sense of efficacy and control, and give purpose. (See table 11.1.)

How Thoughts and Images Affect Us

We tend to be unaware of how thoughts and images affect our health. In a world flooded with visual images from TVs, cell phones, and computer games, what we think and what we imagine becomes the template of our lives. Thoughts we have held in the past shape our present, and those we hold today contribute to create our future. We develop a desire, a thought, an image, and then, whether it's positive or negative, we tend to move toward actualizing that image and thought.

We think of mind and body as separate—in medicine the body is treated by physicians, and the mind is treated by psychologists and psychiatrists. Study of the interaction between the mind, the nervous system, and the immune system has shown that they are actually intrinsically

Belief in a positive outcome	75%
Having a fighting spirit	71%
Seeing the disease as a challenge, yet accepting it	71%
Taking responsibility for the disease and its outcome	68%
Positive emotions, renewed desire and will to live	64%
Faith in a higher healing power and renewed sense of purpose	61%
Changing unhealthy habits and behaviors	61%
Making lifestyle changes and having a sense of control	59%
Self-nurturing	57%
Good social support	50%

Table 11.1. The most important psychospiritual factors associated with remission of cancer. Adapted from R. Daniel, *The Cancer Directory* (London: Harper-Collins, 2005); C. Hirschberg and M. Barasch, *Remarkable Recovery: What Extraordinary Healings Tell Us about Getting Well and Staying Well* (Darby, PA: Diane Publishing Company, 1999).[267]

interconnected (this field of study is called psychoneuroimmunology, also known as PNI). There is no separation between body, mind, and emotions. Every thought or feeling is reflected in some aspect of the body— in brain and brain chemistry, inflammation, muscle tension, and circulation—as well as in life choices. Every physical event is linked to some change, however subtle, in thought, feelings, and awareness. These responses are different for every person. Although stress is a significant risk factor for everyone, we each interpret and experience the stressors and the physical reactions differently. Our responses are the interplay of genetics, temperament, family upbringing, cultural beliefs, and the environment. Nevertheless, people with high workloads, excessive stress, and lack of control over their own lives experience up to three times as much illness as do those with less stress and a sense of control.

Mind-set also plays a role. A tendency to chronic frustration or perfectionism can have a detrimental influence on our bodies. For example, when we're anxious, angry, or frustrated, most of us tighten the muscles at the back of the neck. This may produce tense shoulders or a stiff neck—"raising the hackles on the back of our neck." We may also have this experience when we feel insecure or afraid or when we feel that our future is threatened. When threatened and under stress it is normal to anticipate potential problems. Although this is a normal pattern of thinking, anticipating the worst can make us depressed, which tends to make us a little more vulnerable to illness.

The first exercise will give you a sense of the direct effect of your thoughts or mental images on your body. This practice demonstrates the immediate effect of our thoughts and imagination on our physical responses. You can read this image to yourself or have someone read it to you, and it just takes a few minutes.

Practice 1: Slicing a Lemon

Gently close your eyes and imagine a lemon. Notice the deep yellow color, and the two stubby ends. Imagine placing the lemon on a cutting board and cutting it in half with your favorite kitchen knife. Notice the pressure of the knife in your hand as you cut the lemon. Feel the drop of lemon juice against your skin. After cutting the lemon in half, put the knife down and pick up one half of the lemon. As you look at it, notice the drops of juice glistening in the light, the half-cut seeds, the outer yellow rind, and the pale inner rind. Now get a glass and squeeze this half of lemon so the juice goes into the glass. As you squeeze, notice the pressure in your fingers and forearm. Feel droplets of lemon juice squirting against your skin. Smell the pungent, sharp fragrance. Now take the other half of lemon and squeeze the juice into the glass. Now take the glass in your hand. Feel the coolness of the glass and bring it to your lips. Feel the juice against your lips, and then sip the lemon juice. Taste the tart juice and swallow the lemon juice. Observe the pulp and seeds as you swallow.

What did you notice? As you imagined this, did you notice that you experienced an increase in salivation, or that your mouth puckered? Almost everyone who does this exercise experiences some of these physical changes. The increase in salivation demonstrates that these thoughts and images have a direct effect on our bodies. Similarly, when we have thoughts of anger, resentment, frustration, or anxiety, they similarly affect our bodies. Unknowingly we may tighten our shoulders or our abdomen. We may unconsciously hold our breath or breathe shallowly. This response interferes with our ability to relax and heal. If this kind of tension is a constant habit, it reduces the body's ability to regenerate.

Although we may dismiss our experience when we did the imagery exercise with an imaginary lemon—it was only an imaginary lemon, after all—it is fundamentally important. Every minute, every hour, every day, our bodies are subtly affected by thoughts, emotions, and images. Just as the image of the lemon caused us to salivate, our thoughts and emotions also cause physiological change.

These imperceptible changes can be compared to water rushing down a riverbed. At any given moment, there is almost no perceptible effect. However, as the stream grows, it becomes wider and deeper. As the water flows, year in, year out, it will scour the ground and carve a deeper and deeper riverbed. Eventually, the river changes the landscape.

In a similar way, over time, our patterns of thinking influence every aspect of our lives, both our internal health and also the types of experiences that we focus on. This includes the friends we make, the career opportunities that come to us, and the lifestyle that we live. So, just as drops of water over the years can create a streambed where there was none, so your thoughts ultimately shape your life. If you get cancer, the way you think will influence your quality of life from that point on, and may influence your potential for healing.

Practice 2: How Our Thoughts Affect Our Strength

In the following exercise, notice how changing your thoughts from negative to positive (or the reverse) can affect your physical strength.

This exercise needs to be done with a partner or a friend. Take turns, but begin by identifying who is the subject and who is the tester.

- Begin by standing facing each other. First test the strength of the subject's arms (see figures 11.1a and 11.1b).
- The subject extends his left arm straight out to the side and holds it in a horizontal position so his arms are in the same position as the cross on the letter T. The tester places his right hand on top of the subject's left wrist and gently applies downward pressure while the subject resists. The tester slowly increases the pressure until he senses when the subject can no longer hold the arm in a horizontal position.
- Relax, and repeat the test with the subject's right arm.
- Identify which arm appears stronger and more able to resist the downward pressure.
- Now let the subject relax. Then have the subject mentally evoke a past memory or experience in which he felt either (1) hopeless, helpless, and powerless or (2) empowered, positive, and successful.
- The subject should not reveal to the tester which memory is chosen.
- Encourage the subject to think about the memory and make it as real as possible—feel it, hear it, and so forth. The goal is to experience that memory as vividly as if it were happening in the present moment.
- At that point the subject extends their stronger arm straight out to the side. The tester once again tests the strength of the arm by pressing downward on the wrist.
- Now relax and have the subject focus on the opposite memory, again making it as real as possible. Once the subject feels the experience, he should raise the same arm again, and the tester will test the strength of the arm by pressing down on the wrist.

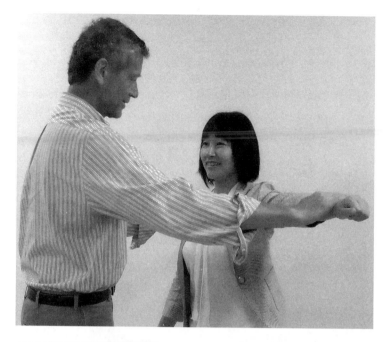

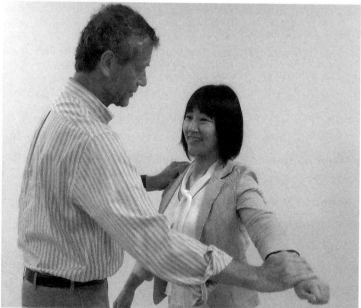

Figure 11.1a and 11.1b. Testing how a subject can hold his arm up and can resist the downward pressure

- Reverse roles. The tester becomes the subject and repeats the same exercise.
- Now share and compare your experiences.

What did you notice? In almost all cases, when people think of hopeless, helpless, or powerless memories, they have significantly less strength than when they think of empowering, positive, and successful memories.

With hopeless, helpless, and powerless memories, it's much easier to press down the subject's arm. The subject experiences a lack of energy and feels unable to resist the pressure, as if the energy has just drained from their body.

In about two percent of people who do this exercise, the arm feels stronger. In most of those cases, the person was actually evoking a memory that included anger and resentment instead of hopelessness and powerlessness.

When the person thinks about the empowering, positive, and successful memory, the tester typically needs to apply more pressure to the subject's arm to lower it. The person experiences a sense of increased energy and greater ability to resist the pressure.

This subjective experience of the change in strength and resistance is the metaphor for how positive/empowering or helpless/powerless memories affect the immune system. When feeling empowered and hopeful, our immune system is more competent, and our body can cope better with challenges.[268] Even seeing inspirational movies, such as a documentary about Mother Teresa, will increase immune competence.[269]

Without conscious awareness, our thoughts and images form the template of our future. Many of these thoughts and images are derived from the covert hypnotic suggestions given by our family, friends, and culture—suggestions that can limit our potential unless we make an effort to think otherwise.

If we become aware of, accept, and change habitual thought processes that act as hypnotic suggestions, we may be able to expand our health and potential. It is truly amazing to witness the tenacity of a thought pattern. Deepak Chopra, a well-known Ayurvedic physician, states in his book *Quantum Healing* that our mental patterns are largely responsible for creating our bodies: "Memory must be more permanent than matter. What is a cell, then? It is a memory that has built some matter around itself, forming a specific pattern. Your body is just the place your memory calls home."

Practice 3: How Our Posture Affects Our Mood

When we feel happy, we sparkle and walk erect with a bounce to our step. When depressed, we tend to slouch and "feel down," and sometimes our vision appears to have less color and is flatter. Emotions and thoughts affect our posture and energy. Conversely, posture and energy affect our emotions and thoughts.

In the following practice, explore how posture affects recall of memories.[270] Not only do thoughts and emotions affect the body, but the body equally affects thoughts and memory.

- Sit comfortably at the edge of a chair and then collapse downward so that your back is rounded like the letter C. Let your head tilt forward and look at the floor between your thighs as shown in figure 11.2.

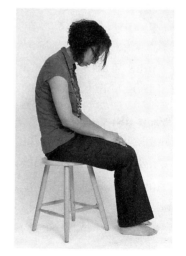

Figure 11.2. Sitting in a collapsed position (photo by Jana Asenbrennerova)

- While in this position, bring to mind many hopeless, helpless, powerless, and depressive memories one after the other for thirty seconds.
- Then, let go of those thoughts and images and, without changing your position and still looking downward, recall empowering, positive, and happy memories one after the other for thirty seconds.
- Shift position and sit up erect, with your back almost slightly arched and your head held tall while looking slightly upward as shown in figure 11.3.
- While is this position, bring to mind many hopeless, helpless, powerless, or depressive memories one after the other for thirty seconds.

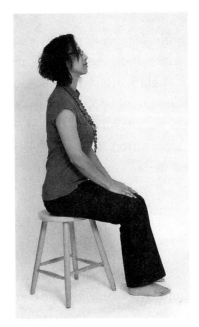

Figure 11.3. Sitting in an upright position (photo by Jana Asenbrennerova)

- Then, let go of those thoughts and images and, without changing position and while still looking upward, recall as many empowering, positive, and happy memories one after the other for thirty seconds
- Ask yourself: In which position was it easier to evoke negative memories? In which position was it easier to evoke empowering, positive, and happy memories?

What did you notice? Most people report that the collapsed position looking downward facilitates recall of negative memories, while the upright position and looking up encourage recall of positive and empowering memories. In many cases, when people looked down, they could not evoke *any* positive and empowering memories at all. Similarly, for most it was impossible to recall negative, hopeless, helpless, or powerless memories while looking up. It is no surprise that when people feel optimistic about the future, they say, "Things are *looking up.*"

Lightening your mood. When feeling down, acknowledge the feeling and say, "At this moment, I feel overwhelmed, and I'm not sure what to do" or whatever phrase fits the felt emotions.

When your energy is low, again acknowledge this to yourself: "At this moment I feel exhausted," or "At this moment, I feel tired," or whatever phrase fits the feeling. Acknowledge the feeling as it is at that moment. As you acknowledge it, be sure to state "at this moment." The phrase "at this moment" is correct and accurate. It implies *what is* occurring without a self-suggestion that the feeling will continue, which helps to avoid the idea that *this was, is, and will always be.* The reality is that whatever we are experiencing is always limited to this moment, as no one knows what will occur in the future. This leaves the future open to improvement.

Remind yourself that you can begin to shift your emotions by changing your posture. When you're outside, focus on the clouds moving across the sky, the flight of birds, or leaves on the trees. In your home, you can focus on inspiring art on the wall or photos of family members you love and who love you. When you hang pictures, hang them higher than you normally would so that you must look up. You can also put pictures above your desk to remind yourself to look up and to evoke positive memories.

After acknowledging the feeling, do not keep looking down and ruminating, worrying about what will happen—especially over things you cannot control. Do not "veg out" in front of the TV. In most cases when you sit for prolonged periods in front of TV, your body collapses as you sit on the couch or recliner. The longer you collapse and watch, the more your energy is drained, and the more you feel exhausted. Also, do not reach for a soda, coffee, or that sugary snack; instead, go for a short walk and look upward at the scenery. (In controlled research studies, Robert Thayer has shown that after short exercise, your sub-jective energy is higher.[271])

How our bodies affect our moods. When we're exhausted, depressive thoughts become more prevalent. When we're hungry, we tend to be more irritable, since low blood sugar increases irritability and may allow more negative and impulsive thoughts. In many cases, cancer makes us more vulnerable to fatigue, so knowing this can help us take better care of ourselves.

Practice 4: Tuning In to Your Inner Dialogue

Our internal world involves how we think and how we process information. Our thoughts or cognitions can be compared to a set of eye-glasses. They are the lenses through which we perceive reality. Do we see the world through rose-colored glasses or through dark lenses that cast a shadow on everything? (In fact, our thoughts and cognitions are actually more like contact lenses than they are like glasses, because we are usually unaware of possible distortions.)

Language shapes and structures our perception of reality. How we experience reality is determined in large part by how we talk and describe reality to ourselves, consciously and unconsciously. The first step in becoming attuned to your self-talk is to begin listening to your automatic inner language. The more clearly you can hear the dialogue, the easier it is to identify distortions and shift them.

Know that you can train yourself to shift from negative self-talk to positive reinforcement and stream-of-consciousness. Frequently, we respond unknowingly and automatically to situations. Most of us are completely unaware of how conditioned we are in our responses and reactions. When people say that something *pushes our buttons,* it means that we are reacting negatively, without thinking. Instead, we can take control by noticing—and shifting—our inner dialogue to a more positive train of thought.

Some of our self-talk echoes messages from our family, especially those from our childhood. Often these messages are embedded deep within our psyche and seem to hold us with hypnotic power. As an adult, how often have we said, "I sound just like my mother" or "I sound like my dad, and I promised myself I would never do that." The inner voices also include messages from our culture. Once conveyed mainly by priests, doctors, and teachers, today the media is a powerful source of the messages we internalize.

The inner dialogue and cancer. With a cancer diagnosis, our thoughts and emotions can run rampant. How we speak to ourselves, how we describe our condition, can have an effect on our ability to cope and to heal. The internal dialogue can empower or undermine us. Do we describe our condition with a glimmer of hope, take a fatalistic stance, or toss our diagnosis off with dark humor? This can backfire because it may create negative and helpless thoughts that do not support optimal immune function.

Experience it. Observing and changing your thoughts is a good place to start, because this is an area of your life that you can use to influence your health and well-being—and it is something you can begin working on right now.

To a surprising degree, coping is a reflection of how we describe our experiences in our own internal dialogue rather than the actual experiences themselves. Our perspective also influences how we interact with the world.

Many people have a habit of focusing on negative experiences and disregarding positive ones. This kind of thinking can result in generalizations like "The world is a dangerous place," "Men are no good," or "I have an 80 percent chance of dying from cancer." In some situations, our emotional distress is colored by our interpretation of the situation.

Although your thought process seems beyond your conscious control, know that it is a dynamic that you can shift. This is a learnable skill.

Over time, you can gently train yourself to focus on what is working, on the positive. Remember Philippians 4:8:

Whatever is true, whatever is noble, whatever is just, whatever is pure, whatever is lovely, whatever is admirable ... think on these things.

The first step is to acknowledge your fears and then focus on what you want. Knowing what you want, you will become more attuned to self-talk that does not serve you, and listen in on the inner dialogue. That will enable you to reframe your experience, to help you focus on what you want. As you begin to rewrite the internal script of your self-talk, you may find that you also rebuild your self-esteem.[272]

Practice 5: Reframing an Experience

Reframing, a term used in neurolinguistic programming (NLP), is the process of shifting our perception from negative images and self-talk to a more positive perspective.

If our thoughts are a series of *can't do* and *no way,* we are likely to perceive ourselves as helpless victims. When our internal language is a barrage of *should* and *must,* we are likely to feel boxed in by a set of obligations, medical appointments, tests, and procedures. Approaching cancer from a negative perspective also calls up worst-case scenarios—with images of suffering and death, making us forget that in every case of cancer, there is always hope and the potential for some quality of life.

I took a different attitude toward my illness. I refused to say things to myself such as, "I am never going to get better." Once I began doing that, I felt better. I feel that this was due in part to controlling the panic I usually feel whenever I get sick.

PATIENT DIAGNOSED WITH CANCER

Experience it. Every time we say, "I should," or "I can't," that disconnects us from our energy, we can practice reframing the situations to reconnect with our own personal power.

194

Step 1. Feeling the impact of negative self-talk. Explore the following practice and notice how changing your inner dialogue also changes your mood and energy.

- Sit comfortably and gently close your eyes.
- Now think of a task or a skill you want to learn that seems a bit challenging. Choose an activity that would automatically trigger self-doubt, whether it's learning Japanese, cooking, web design, or martial arts.
- Choose a real-life situation and just keep repeating a "can't do" phrase for about one minute—"I can't learn ... I can't learn Japanese. I couldn't even learn Spanish," or, "I can't cook," or, "I'll never be able to do martial arts. I'm so uncoordinated." You can substitute any other negative phrase here.
- Repeat the same phrase over and over for a full minute. Now stop and observe how you feel.

Step 2. Problem solving. The statement "I can't" often has multiple interpretations. It can be useful to have a rational conversation with yourself, to track down some of these misconceptions. When you said, "I can't," did you mean one of the following?

- *It is impossible to do.* If that's the case, you might just accept the situation and focus on things that you *can* do.
- *I have not taken the time to learn how.* What about finding a tutor or taking a class?
- *I do not really want to do it.* This is an opportunity to acknowledge that you do not want to do the task. You could problem solve and find a workaround—or simply say *no.* If it is an essential task, it may be possible (and surprisingly easy) for others to do it.

Whatever you intended, rewrite your phrase positively, such as, "I want to learn Japanese. I'll find a tutor on Craigslist and set the time aside on my calendar," or "I haven't taken the time to learn Japanese," or "I choose not to learn Japanese, and if I ever need it, I will hire a translator," or "I will attend films and events at the Japanese Cultural Center, or go to the Zen Center for morning meditation."

Step 3. Feeling the impact of positive/revised self-talk. Choose one of the revised phrases and repeat it over and over for a minute.

- Stop and notice how you feel. Now compare the feelings evoked by the negative and positive perspectives.

What did you notice? When people reframe the task from hopeless, powerless, and helpless to possible, they often feel lighter, as if a weight has been lifted from their shoulders. They feel more optimistic and have a greater sense of possibility.

Reframing in real life. In a familiar example, suppose everyone around you seems to be coming down with the flu. If you find yourself worrying, your self-talk might sound something like, "I always catch everything that's going around," or "Just my luck—I'll probably be next." However, reframing this situation so you take action might involve thought patterns such as, "Everybody's coming down with the flu. I'd better get some extra sleep tonight," or "Afternoon break—time for some water and vitamin C."

This philosophy can also be applied in more sobering circumstances. Even when facing death, the focus can be on how to live in the time you have left, how to focus on meaningful activities, and how to say goodbye or thank the people in your life who have done things that have improved your life.

Reframing practices increase our choices. We can continue to react and think in the same old ways, or we can choose to do something differently and think in new ways. Life is change. Thoughts, even though they may seem permanent, can change as we grow. Making changes in habitual thought patterns requires patience with oneself, flexibility, openness, and, above all, a sense of humor. By changing our internal language we can create a shift in our reality. As the Buddha Gautama said,

We are formed and molded by our thoughts. Those whose minds are shaped by selfless thoughts give joy when they speak or act. Joy follows them like a shadow that never leaves them.

Practice 6: Decreasing Energy Drains and Increasing Energy Gains

Begin by observing your subjective energy level. Do you still have the same vitality as when you were a child or when you were in love? Curiosity, excitement, and expectation are part of the child's experience—described in Zen as *beginner's mind*. Remember the excitement of going fishing or skiing for the first time, or starting on your first cross-country road trip? Remember waking up at five in the morning, filled with anticipation?

The goal of this exercise is to free up your energy by releasing some of the situations that drain you and increase those that enhance your energy. Energy is the sense of feeling alive and vibrant. An energy gain is an activity, task, or thought that makes you feel better and more alive—things you *want to do* or *choose to do*. Health is created by filling your life with activities that contribute to your energy and minimizing those that drain you.

An energy drain is the opposite—it makes you feel depressed or less alive. Drains may also be things you *have to* or *must do* that you do not really want to do. An energy drain can be an energy gain for someone else and vice versa.

An example of an energy drain might be doing the dishes and feeling resentful that your partner or children are not doing them. To reduce this drain you could trade tasks with others in your household.

Drains may also involve people who seem to suck your energy—you feel a loss of energy after spending time with them. You may want to limit your time with these people but increase time spent with people who add to your energy. Other examples of energy gains can be going for a walk in the woods, or finishing an important project.

- *Gains:* Although I only talk to Sharon once in a while, every time I do, I feel as if a twenty-five-pound weight is lifted. Now we talk nearly every day, and the deepening connection means a great deal to me.
- *Drains:* I just hated doing the weekly data entry, but when I talked to one of my coworkers, I found out that he actually doesn't mind doing it. We've traded tasks—he does the data entry, and I do the filing—and it's working out just fine.

Energy drains and gains are always unique to the individual. The challenge is to identify your energy drains and gains and then explore strategies to decrease the drains and increase the gains. Begin the practice by first observing, identifying, and recording your specific energy drains and gains at home using table 11.2. Then repeat the process for other environments where you spend a lot of time. At that point you're ready to develop a program that optimizes your energy.

At this point, take another look at your entries. Identify one energy gain from all the entries that you would like to increase. Be very concrete and specific. It is not an abstract concept such as "I want more energy." It is specific, such as "When I talk to Dr. Z., I feel hopeful" (an energy gain) or "When I listen to Mozart, I feel at peace and quiet with more energy." Then identify one energy drain from all the entries, such as "When I see Dr. Y., I leave depressed" or "When I clean the bathroom, I am exhausted."

Now develop a strategy to reduce the energy drains. Be very concrete and develop a realistic scenario by which the energy drain is reduced. For example,

I talked to my husband about how exhausted I felt after cleaning the bathroom. We explored options and finally decided that he would do

Tracking what builds your energy and what drains it at home:

Energy Gains (Sources)	Energy Drains

Tracking what builds your energy and what drains it at work:

Energy Gains (Sources)	Energy Drains

Tracking energy gains and drains associated with cancer:

Energy Gains (Sources)	Energy Drains

Table 11.2. Data sheet to record energy gains and energy drains

it for the next month. And that would give us time to find the right cleaning person, someone who would come in every two weeks.

If you feel stuck and cannot develop a new strategy, take a look at the problem-solving strategies in Appendix A.

When you explore how to reduce the drain, be sure to indicate exactly how you will do it—when, where, how often, and with whom. For example if talking to Dr. Y. drains you, do not run away from it. Develop options such as bringing a friend with you as a medical advocate, sharing your concerns with the doctor, or requesting a change of health providers. There are many options. However, you may decide that you do not want to change, and in that case, another option is to develop acceptance. You may also decide to do something that increases your energy immediately before or after a visit with the doctor.

Similarly, in planning to increase an energy gain, be very specific. Plan it, and incorporate it into your life and schedule it on your calendar. If talking to Michelle increases your energy, call her more often. If taking a short walk or looking at plants and flowers increases your energy, plan to go for a short walk with friends or ride through the park if you are too tired to walk.

After having created a detailed plan of how you will decrease the drains on your energy and increase the gains, mentally review the factors that could interfere with these plans. Consider how you would overcome the obstacles. Then begin to implement the plan through action. Keep a log and periodically monitor your drains and gains since they will change over time.

What did you notice? When people practice this, they usually experience a noticeable increase in subjective energy. Many report that it made them realize how much of the time they were doing things they really did not want to do. Knowing this encourages them to explore what increased their energy and sense of purpose in life.

Practice 7: Developing Acceptance and Appreciation

Being grateful is an opportunity to shift the focus from feelings of hopelessness to feelings of appreciation. This can be challenging with cancer since so often it is difficult to find hope: "I feel that my body has betrayed me. The treatment was even worse than the cancer, and I am just a shadow of my former self. I have no energy to even be angry."

Gratitude to your body. Find ways to be grateful to your body for the good service it has given you without complaint in the past despite the many abuses that you unintentionally inflicted (working at the computer for hours without taking a break, falling off your bicycle and then getting up and continuing to ride, going on a walking tour of New York in spike heels, eating out at all-you-can-eat restaurants, etc.). When you think of your body, appreciate what it has done for you over so many years (allowing you to run on the beach, give a massage to your partner, drive your car without thinking, etc.). Remember how it felt to learn to ride a bike, to dance, or to throw a football and how much pleasure your body gave you without ever asking for reward. Whenever you are tempted to judge yourself, thank and appreciate your body for having done all it did for you. If these thoughts bring thoughts of grief for having lost so much or regrets over not making other choices in the past, redirect thoughts to focus on gratitude for what you had and still have.

Releasing blame. It's a temptation to continue searching for the causes of the cancer. Self-blame and self-inflicted pressure are not helpful. Remember, the cause of the cancer and the outcome were not, are not, and will not be completely in your hands. There are many factors that contribute to the development of cancer and to its progression or remission. Clearly it does no good to blame yourself for either not anticipating the future—none of us are omnipresent and God—or for doing the wrong things. The important concept to remember is that thoughts and emotions are reflected through the body. Thinking hopeless thoughts shifts the body into a more immune-compromised state.

Freeing yourself. Instead of honest emotional sharing, we give the superficial answer, "I am OK" to the question, "How are you?" This superficial response for the sake of *harmony* and *not making waves* also separates one from others and from oneself. The internal isolation masked by being helpful and continually trying to be in charge can be exhausting. The struggle of putting on a happy face in which the deep emotional feelings and wariness are not shared distances us from close friends and family. It makes us feel as if we are living in a glass bell jar, emotionally separated from others and from our own unmet dreams. This disconnect often leads to exhaustion.

True acceptance. To promote healing, an attitude of acceptance without resignation will support your sense of security. A sense of safety always mobilizes the immune system. The challenge is to accept, and remind ourselves that our destiny is not in our hands. We can only work on that over which we have control.

Practice 8: Projecting Goodwill[273]

Just thinking of Mark, my ex-husband, the anger wells up. How could he have treated me like that? Why did I let him? We were so in love once—what happened? And how could he have turned out to be such a jerk?

For the events and stresses over which we have no control, you may find the following exercise helpful. During the day, use anger, resentment, or frustration as the cue to project goodwill.

Experience it. Thoughts, events, and people over which we have no control automatically can trigger feelings of frustration, powerlessness, irritation, anger, resignation, depression, or other negative sensations, which get expressed physically as tension. At times, we may even think that our family members and medical staff are selfish, don't care, or don't want to help. These negative thoughts are normal, especially when we are exhausted and at our wit's end; however, they increase tension and decrease our energy.

There are times when forgiveness is called for, as much for your well-being as for that of the other person. It is absolutely true that people make mistakes, act incompetently, and let us down. You will probably find that this exercise is quite useful. It is especially beneficial for situations in which you have no control over the event or the person who caused grief. You don't have to like or condone what they have done in order for you to be able to forgive them. Obviously, if there are things that can be done to resolve the conflict, do those first. So often, we have no control over others or situations, but we can have control over how we respond in our bodies and minds. In the following practice, every time the thought or memory surfaces, use that as a cue, a reminder to send goodwill.

- Sit quietly and for a moment focus on deep, relaxed breathing. Let your exhalation grow slower and slower.
- As you breathe slowly, think of a past memory where you felt loved and safe. Continue breathing slowly and put your hands on your heart.
- Then as you exhale, imagine that as you blow your breath out, your breath carries the feeling and intent of goodwill to a person or an event that triggers negative feelings.
- You can also use this process to project goodwill toward a future event, such as a procedure that you may be dreading. As you exhale, open your arms outward and send goodwill like a wave on the ocean. (See figures 11.4a, 11.4b, and 11.4c.)
- Every time when you think of someone with whom you are having difficulty, or a challenging event, send the person goodwill as you exhale.

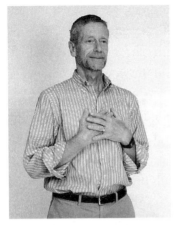 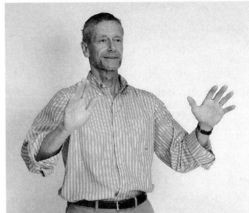

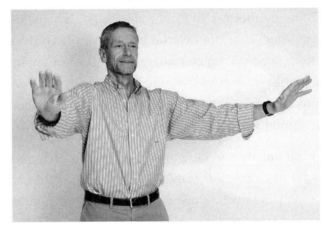

Figures 11.4a, 11.4b, and 11.4c. Illustration of hand movements while sending goodwill (photos by Jana Asenbrennerova)

- Practice it every time you are reminded of that person or the event and when you anticipate or think of any situation that produces conflict.

What did you notice? When practicing this for a few weeks, most participants are surprised by how much they have changed and also how the person with whom they had the conflict has changed. They realized that the very act of choosing to focus their attention on sending goodwill seems to change the energy and the negative situation.

Practice 9: Gratitude Visit[274]

Tears came to my eyes. I felt totally touched when Margaret shared how helpful it had been that I brought over a pot of soup and a salad when her husband passed away. I had totally forgotten that I had done this. She confided that it had helped her not feel so alone, and it gave her the courage to go on. Her thoughtful comments rekindled a much deeper friendship between us. For days, I felt more human, more caring, and much more connected to Margaret.

When we're thankful, every day can bring unexpected joy. Yet when one gets a diagnosis, it's difficult to feel positive. This is a time to remember that we can only work on that over which we have control. One of the gifts we still have, as long as we can speak, write, or sign, is to share our appreciation with others of what they have done for us. None of us knows how much time we have, whether you have cancer or not. Use the time you have to share your gratitude with others for what they have contributed to your life.

Experience it. The focus of this practice is to remember people who did something important for you that changed your life in a positive direction, who you have never had a chance to thank. Take the time to thank them for contributing to your life. Reflecting on people who did something positive for us tends to make us feel better. And, when we thank them, it gives them a good feeling, and we feel better as well.

Adapt the exercise depending upon your situation. If you have time, energy, and resources, visit them in person. If that is not possible, call them by phone or write them a personal note. It is the positive intention and the effort of focusing outward, and sending love, that allows our energy to expand and regenerate.

- Make a list of all those people who have done something for you and whom you have never had the opportunity to thank. They could be family members, ex-partners, neighbors, coworkers, childhood friends, teachers, or even strangers.

- Choose one of them and write a 300-word testimonial—a brief thank-you note—in which you share how their specific actions positively affected your life. Describe what the person did for you. Describe how it changed your life in a positive direction. In the testimonial, detail the impact of their act of kindness and how it has improved your life and convey that you want to thank them for it.
- Call them on the phone and ask them that you would like to visit them without really explaining why you want to see them.
- Visit them and then as you meet them, read them your testimonial aloud.

What did you notice? Almost everyone reports that the person to whom they read the testimonial was deeply touched and grateful. It created a genuine, deep emotional bond of friendship and love. In many cases, the tears flowed—tears of love and joy. In the process of giving gratitude to others, we ourselves feel more peaceful and whole.

In some cases, this practice is impossible to do because the person is far away or cannot be visited. If possible, do the exercise using Skype or some similar technology. The mutual connection tends to deepen the feeling. If a video connection is not possible, then use the phone. Generally, do not use email or regular post (snail mail), because the immediacy of a real-time connection deepens the experience, and our voice can express a range of emotional nuances.

If the person has already died, create a ritual. Write the testimonial, then go to a peaceful place, read it out loud, and then burn the letter, or tear it into little pieces and cast it on the water or into the wind. Imagine that the message will be carried by the air or the water to the spirit of the departed person.

By sharing our appreciation of others and how they have contributed to our own development and growth, we nurture the human spirit.

These positive feelings are contagious, affecting and nurturing both the giver and the receiver. They ripple outward like waves from a pebble touching the water. The same positive wave of appreciation spreads outward, evoking immune-enhancing effects.[275]

Healing Includes Many Aspects of Your Life

The essence of self-care has been summed up by Steven James in this tongue-in-check little guide, originally written to encourage preventive self-care for patients with AIDS.[276] We have adapted his guidelines for patients with cancer. James used humor to point out (1) how to get sick—the factors that tend to hinder the immune system and thus may initiate illness, (2) how to get sicker if you are already sick, and (3) how to stay well or get better, if you're not so well to begin with. Beneath the dark humor, there is a great deal of wisdom about health.

Steven James's Totally Subjective, Nonscientific Guide to Illness and Health: Ten-Step Programs

How to Get Sick

- Don't pay attention to your body. Eat plenty of junk food, drink too much, take drugs, have lots of unsafe sex with lots of different partners—and, above all, feel guilty about it. If you are overstressed and tired, ignore it and keep pushing yourself.
- Cultivate the experience of your life as meaningless and of little value.
- Do the things you don't like, and avoid doing what you really want. Follow everyone else's opinions and advice, while seeing yourself as miserable and "stuck."
- Be resentful and hypercritical, especially toward yourself.
- Fill your mind with dreadful pictures, and then obsess over them. Worry most, if not all, of the time.
- Avoid deep, lasting, intimate relationships.

- Blame other people for all your problems.
- Do not express your feelings and views openly and honestly. Other people wouldn't appreciate it. If at all possible, do not even know what your feelings are.
- Shun anything that resembles a sense of humor. Life is no laughing matter!
- Avoid making any changes that would bring you greater satisfaction and joy.

How to Get Sicker (If You're Already Sick)

- Think about all the awful things that could happen to you. Dwell upon negative, fearful images.
- Be depressed, self-pitying, envious, and angry. Blame everyone and everything for your illness.
- Read articles, books, and newspapers, watch TV programs, surf the net, and listen to people who reinforce the viewpoint that there is NO HOPE. You are powerless to influence your fate.
- Cut yourself off from other people. Regard yourself as a pariah. Lock yourself up in your room and contemplate death.
- Hate yourself for having destroyed your life. Blame yourself mercilessly and incessantly.
- Go to see lots of different doctors. Run from one to another, spend half your time in waiting rooms, get lots of conflicting opinions and lots of experimental drugs, starting one program after another without sticking to any.
- Quit your job, stop work on any projects, give up all activities that bring you a sense of purpose and fun. See your life as essentially pointless, and at an end.
- Complain about your symptoms, and if you associate with anyone, do so exclusively with other people who are unhappy and embittered. Reinforce each other's feelings of hopelessness.

- Don't take care of yourself. What's the use? Try to get other people to do it for you, and then resent them for not doing a good job.
- Think how awful life is, and how you might as well be dead. But make sure you are absolutely terrified of death, just to increase the pain.

How to Stay Well (Or Get Better, If You're Not So Well to Begin With)

- Do things that bring you a sense of fulfillment, joy, and purpose, that validate your worth. See your life as your own creation and strive to make it a positive one.
- Pay close and loving attention to yourself, tuning in to your needs on all levels. Take care of yourself, nourishing, supporting, and encouraging yourself.
- Release all negative emotions—resentment, envy, fear, sadness, anger. Express your feelings appropriately; don't hold onto them. Forgive yourself.
- Hold positive images and goals in your mind, pictures of what you truly want in your life. When fearful images arise, refocus on images that evoke feelings of peace and joy.
- Love yourself, and love everyone else. Make loving the purpose and primary expression of your life.
- Create fun, loving, honest relationships, allowing for the expression and fulfillment of needs for intimacy and security. Try to heal any wounds in past relationships, as with old lovers, and with your mother and father.
- Make a positive contribution to your community, through some form of work or service that you value and enjoy.
- Make a commitment to health and well-being, and develop a belief in the possibility of wholeness. Develop your own healing program, drawing on the support and advice of experts without becoming enslaved to them.
- Accept yourself and everything in your life as an opportunity for

growth and learning. Be grateful. When you screw up, forgive your-self, learn what you can from the experience, and then move on.

• Keep a sense of humor.

Consider the following resources on mind-body health:

LeShan, L. *Cancer as a Turning Point.* New York: Plume, 1999.
This book was written by a master clinician using case studies to show how listening to yourself and doing what you truly want improves your quality of life and may sometimes lead to cancer remission. This book provides numerous useful practices.

Kabat-Zinn, J. *Full Catastrophe Living.* New York: Delacorte Press, 1990.
This very helpful manual describes the basis of mindfulness mediation that is used with many patients and offers background information and practical exercises.

Luskin, F. *Forgive for Love: The Missing Ingredient for a Healthy and Lasting Relationship.* New York: HarperOne, 2009.
This book offers a very useful approach to develop and maintain loving and nurturing relationships as demonstrated by the numerous case studies.

Peper, E., K. H. Gibney, and C. Holt. *Make Health Happen: Training Yourself to Create Wellness.* Dubuque, IA: Kendall-Hunt, 2002.
This book presents a sixteen-week, structured stress-management and healing approach with detailed guided instructions that help us live with our bodies—a path that offers emotional, physical, and spiritual strength through changing our internal language, images, and somatic responses

Seligman, M. *Learned Optimism: How to Change Your Mind and Your Life.* New York: Free Press, 1998.
This superb pragmatic text details how to observe, assess, and change your internal language.

Chapter 12

BREATHING FOR HEALING

I was afraid to move—I couldn't seem to find a position that felt comfortable. With every breath, I could feel the skin being pulled apart on my chest where my breast had been removed. The skin felt tight and clammy. Trying to turn onto my side, I anticipated the pain and held my breath. The waves of pain were excruciating. With every movement, it felt like sharp hooks were pulling on the incision. Each new sensation triggered a deep sense of fear—did they really get all the cancer?

To calm myself, I shifted my thoughts back to the coaching I'd gotten on managing the pain. I relaxed and began breathing deeper. Before I moved again, I inhaled into my stomach, and then as I softly blew out the air, I rolled onto my side. It still hurt, but it was tolerable. I realized that I had an effective defense against the pain—and with that realization, I felt something deep inside me relax.

A PATIENT AFTER CANCER SURGERY

Cancer and cancer treatment almost always involve a certain amount of pain. If we're in pain, it's instinctive to hold our breath and tense our muscles. Unfortunately, that usually makes the pain worse. Over time, shallow breathing and tension can continue to aggravate our aches and pains. If we're afraid that the slightest movement will increase pain, that triggers the freeze response—a primal survival reflex.

When your goal is to reduce pain, there are a number of effective body-mind techniques that you can use. These techniques will not *cure* cancer, but they can be a helpful complement to treatment. You'll probably find that these approaches also quiet your mind and emotions. As

211

that occurs, you'll find that your body shifts out of the stress response into a more healing mode—the regeneration response.

Minimizing pain. Once we tense up, the freeze response takes over, and we become hypervigilant—and hypersensitive. Even minor sensations are amplified. Instead of holding our breath and tightening our shoulders, we can learn to use our breathing to minimize pain. The trick is to exhale whenever you feel or anticipate pain—for example, when you need to change position or have blood drawn. Most people are amazed at the degree to which the pain is reduced.

Distracting yourself from pain. You can also learn to use breathing exercises to shift your focus away from pain. Remind yourself that your brain cannot focus on two things at once. The human mind processes one thing at a time, which is why multitasking has been shown to be so counterproductive. We process information in a sequence, not in multiples or in parallel patterns.

So if you're thinking about your breath, you can't worry about the cancer. If you focus on the rhythm of your breathing, you're not focused on the pain. We can use this fact to distract ourselves from worry using breath work or physical activity. This chapter includes several breathing techniques that may help you cope with pain and discomfort.

Breathing for Life

Breathing is essential to our survival. We can live more than fifty days without food and about seven days without water. But without oxygen we cannot survive more than about five minutes. In many cultures, breath *(qi, chi, prana)* is considered the vital link to energy, awareness, composure, and ultimately to transcendence.

Your breathing is a bridge between body, mind, and mood. Changes in our breathing patterns occur unconsciously all the time and reflect our emotional, mental, and physical states. Breathing is under both conscious and unconscious control—it occurs automatically, yet we can also voluntarily change it. Examples of this control include holding your breath, slowing your breathing or breathing faster, and changing the pattern of your breath when you are speaking or singing.

The exercises provided here will help you deepen your control over your breathing and your ability to use breath to support relaxation and healing. This is not a form of treatment, but rather good self-care.

Your ability to influence your breathing provides a leverage point for influencing automatic functions such as heart rate and blood pressure. You can affect aspects of the involuntary nervous system by managing your breathing and bring greater balance to these involuntary systems. By changing your breathing pattern, the nervous system and immune function move out of a state of stress into the relaxation response. Benefits of regenerative breathing include the following:

- *Breathing more comfortably.* These brief practices offer insight into what it feels like when your breathing is harmonious and effective.
- *Turning on the relaxation response.* The focus here is on using your breath to switch into a state of relaxation, which may activate a suppressed immune system and quiet an overreactive system. As you become skilled at effortless breathing, you will be better able to reduce discomfort when you're having a procedure done.
- *Quieting your emotions.* This chapter will look at several ways in which breathing affects moods and emotions. Quieting your breathing will soothe your emotions and thought patterns, and also calm your body. You'll be able to learn breathing techniques that will help you manage stressful situations and soften the effects of unavoidable stress on your body.
- *Improving your frame of mind.* It's generally easier to influence your mind through your body than it is to create a mental shift by changing your thinking. A body-mind approach provides you with a leverage point when you're under stress, a way of intervening when you feel

yourself slipping out of balance. The quickest way to stop the stress response is not meditation, because that takes at least twenty minutes, even for an accomplished meditator. However, brisk walking will reduce stress within a matter of minutes. This is why mental and emotional conditions such as depression can often be effectively treated with exercise.

We encourage you to explore the practices in this chapter with an open, playful mind-set. Most are very short and can be done anywhere, anytime. A few take about fifteen or twenty minutes and involve the use of a guided script. Practice each one and then integrate the concepts and practices into your lifestyle to create your own unique practice. The purpose of the longer practices is to encourage the immune response through the use of breathing and relaxation.

Breathing for Health

What happens when we don't breathe deeply enough? Or when we hold our breath without realizing it? These are two common dysfunctional breathing patterns—incomplete exhalation and breath holding. You can safely experience these patterns in the first two practices.

Practice 1: Why Breathing Matters

Purpose and benefits. When you don't fully exhale, that may cause brain fog or nervousness, and even exaggerate aches and pains. By noticing these patterns, you can change them whenever you find yourself breathing too shallowly. Often, breathing more deeply will help you clear your thinking and reduce fear or panic. In terms of cancer treatment, some patients find that breathing exercises also reduce the experience of "chemobrain," which reportedly can cause some patients to feel spacey, unfocused, disoriented, or forgetful.

Experience it. This practice will give you the immediate experience of how your breathing affects your sense of well-being.

- Sit comfortably and breathe normally.
- Now inhale normally, but exhale only 70 percent of the air you just inhaled.
- Inhale again, and again only exhale 70 percent of the previously inhaled volume of air. If you need to sigh, just do it, and then return to this breathing pattern again by exhaling only 70 percent of the inhaled volume of air.
- Continue to breathe in this pattern of 70 percent exhalation for about forty-five seconds, each time exhaling only 70 percent of the air you breathe in. Then stop, and observe what happened.

What did you notice? Within thirty seconds, more than 98 percent of people report uncomfortable symptoms. For most, the sensations include lightheadedness, dizziness, anxiety or panic, tension in their neck, back, shoulders, or face, nervousness, an increased heart rate or palpitations, agitation or jitteriness, feeling flushed, tingling, breathlessness, chest pressure, gasping for air, or even a sensation of starving for air. This exercise can also aggravate symptoms that already exist, such as headaches, joint pain, or pain from an injury.[277] If you're feeling exhausted or stressed, the effects seem even worse.

How to change the pattern. It's easy to shift into a rapid, shallow breathing pattern when you're under stress—for example, during a visit to the doctor or if you're worried about an impending treatment. The goal is to become aware of this shallow, incomplete breathing. Whenever you experience dizziness, or any of the other symptoms you may have experienced in this exercise, remind yourself that these symptoms could be triggered by the way you are breathing. An easy solution is to shift into deep, effortless breathing and more complete exhalation, to regain your mental focus and reduce stress. We'll explore two simple breathing patterns you can use to combat stress in Practices 3 and 4.

Practice 2: Eye Snap

Purpose and benefits. This practice amplifies the breathing patterns that often occur when we feel fearful. Breath holding often occurs beneath our level of awareness when we're under stress. For example, the moment we anticipate pain, most of us tend to stop breathing and hold our breath. Once we become aware of how easily we are triggered to hold our breath, we can take steps to change the pattern. The goal of this exercise is to help you anticipate situations in which this is likely to occur—and then notice when you are actually holding your breath. With this awareness, you will be better able to change the pattern. You can use that awareness as a cue to exhale. Exhaling initiates the relaxation response associated with healing.

Experience it. To do this exercise, sit comfortably.

- Cover both ears with cupped hands. Now move both your hands away from your head, about one foot to the left and to the right, over your shoulders.
- Create a snapping sound by alternately snapping your thumb and index finger with one hand and then the other hand.
- With each snap, dart your eyes rapidly in the direction of the sound—without moving your head.
- As soon as you look in one direction, snap your fingers on the other side of your head and rapidly dart your eyes in that direction.
- Perform this exercise in a state of hypervigilance as if you were startled or searching for a source of danger. Repeat the process as quickly as possible back and forth, snapping the fingers of your right and left hand alternatively for about five to ten seconds.

What did you notice? Almost everyone holds their breath, stops blinking, and tenses their body when their eyes dart rapidly to the extreme right and left. Often we tend to hold our breath, without realizing it, when we are reacting to sounds, visual changes, or emotional triggers.

Once you become attuned to this, you'll notice that you hold your breath in many situations—hearing your cell phone ring, getting up from a chair, changing the channel on the TV set, or even stopping to think.

In sports, we usually hold our breath when we hear the instructions "On your mark. Get set. Go!" Breath holding tends to amplify negative emotional experiences or pain sensations. When we hold our breath, we get captured by the event, and it holds our attention. Breath holding activates the fight/flight/freeze response, reduces healing and regeneration, and tends to increase the sensation of pain, stiffness, anxiety, or fear.

What you can do. To reduce the stress response and evoke a regenerative mode, try to become more aware of when you hold your breath. As soon as you realize you've stopped breathing, exhale slowly to shift back into effortless breathing. Many patients report that learning to exhale and to breathe more naturally becomes a technique they use consciously whenever they feel nervous or afraid. Over time, most learn to shift into the relaxation response in a matter of minutes.

Practice 3: Using Breathing to Reduce Pain

This practice is useful whenever you anticipate pain—for example, when getting an IV inserted or having blood drawn. You can also use this technique if you've had recent surgery, for example to reduce discomfort whenever you roll over in bed or get out of a chair. If you want to use this breathing technique during a medical procedure, first practice it at home so it will be easier to do when you need it, as shown in figure 12.1.

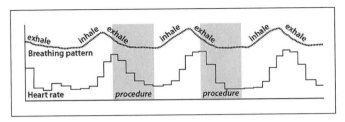

Figure 12.1. Graphic representation of the relationship between beginning exhaling and the beginning of a potentially painful procedure or movement

Experience it: Reducing the pain during a procedure. Note: It is easier to do this breathing pattern if you coordinate with the health professional doing the procedure. Have them coach you, by coordinating their breathing with yours and guiding you verbally. Since exhaling relaxes us and reduces pain, ask your provider to inhale and exhale with you while they are doing the procedure. Ask if they will make a sound as they exhale to guide you.

It is the process of exhaling that reduces the sensation of pain and relaxes you. Consider a simple blood draw:

- Coordinate with the health professional providing the procedure.
- Relax. Then inhale just before the procedure begins.
- Right after you both begin to exhale, the practitioner initiates the procedure.
- As you exhale, relax your shoulders.
- If the procedure is brief, such as an injection or an IV insertion, one breath may be sufficient. But if it is longer than a minute, ask the provider to pause the procedure briefly while you inhale a second time, and then continue just after you start to exhale again.

Experience it: Minimizing the discomfort of movement. If physical movement causes you pain, you can use this same process with your breathing to minimize the pain when you are rolling over or moving, such as following surgery.

- In preparation, first exhale. Then allow the air to come in, exhale again, and relax your shoulders.
- Now allow the air to flow in, in an effortless inhalation.
- Once you start the next exhalation, move while you exhale.
- If the movement takes more than one breath, pause while you inhale again. Then as you exhale, resume the movement. Let your exhalation flow out softly and slowly.
- If you practice this breathing pattern, you'll probably find that once you repeat it several times, it will become easier and more automatic.

Let's apply this breathing technique to the example of getting up from a chair (for example, when one is postsurgery or has back pain). This technique often reduces the sensation of pain.

- Exhale and then allow the inhalation to flow in easily. As you as exhale the second time, move from a relaxed position to sitting erect in the chair.
- Stop moving and allow the inhalation to occur—if possible, always stop the movement while you inhale and continue the movement while you exhale.
- During the next exhalation, slide your body forward on the chair until you're sitting on the edge. Stop the movement and allow yourself to inhale. (Now you're in a position that makes it easier to go from sitting to standing.)
- Begin exhaling and then stand up.

Whenever you anticipate pain during movement, do the movement as you exhale. Keep exhaling as you move. When you need to inhale, if possible stop the movement and resume the movement once you start to exhale again.

How we know it works: Exhaling fear and pain. When we experience a sharp pain, our natural instinct is to gasp and hold our breath. However, holding our breath triggers the stress response—which amplifies pain sensations. The stress response can also impede healing. Research has shown that in patients who are stressed, skin lesions heal at least 24 percent more slowly.[278]

This self-healing is graphically illustrated by our work with Mr. Kawakami, a Japanese yogi, who uses breathing and mental patterns to reduce pain sensations (as shown in figure 12.2).

He pushed the skewers through the skin of his body only during the exhalation phase of breathing.[279] He reported no pain when he exhaled while self-skewering. When he pulled the skewers out, again during the exhalation phase of breathing, there was no bleeding, and the wounds healed very rapidly and were not visible the next day. During these demonstrations, we carefully monitored his heart rate, skin perspiration, and brain wave activity—and found no changes. In other words, his body showed no sign of pain or distress.

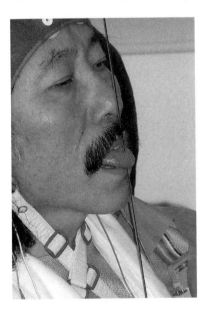

Figure 12.2. Photo of Mr. Kawakami, a yogi who inserted an unsterilized skewer through his tongue without experiencing pain, bleeding, or infection. He inserted the skewers during the exhalation phase of breathing (used with permission from Peper et al., 2006).

Effortless Breathing

Babies and young children tend to breathe effortlessly in an instinctive natural mode of diaphragmatic breathing. Most of the movement associated with their breathing occurs primarily in the abdominal area, which expands and decreases in diameter without effort, and is rhythmically pumped by the diaphragm. Similarly, when dogs and cats rest on their side, they breathe diaphragmatically—their stomach and lower abdomen rise and fall while the chest shows limited movement. When they inhale, the stomach expands; and when they exhale, the stomach drops.

The diaphragm is the primary muscle involved in breathing. This dome-shaped layer of muscle is located just below the lungs and above the abdomen. It separates the chest cavity from the abdominal cavity, creating a horizontal "floor" just below the lungs, like the skin across the bottom of a drum. However, we are totally unaware of its movement, as it tightens and relaxes, except by noticing its effect on the body in the abdomen.

Although your lungs are located in your chest, relaxed breathing occurs as if there were a balloon in the abdomen that expands when we inhale and contracts when we exhale. The diaphragm has an action comparable to a piston inside an engine. When we inhale, the piston goes down, passively increasing the space for the lungs so air flows into the lungs—and the abdomen is pushed outward. When we exhale, the abdomen contracts, pushing the organs and liquid content of the abdomen upward, pushing the diaphragm upward like a piston. The air is pushed out of the lungs, and we exhale as shown in figure 12.3.

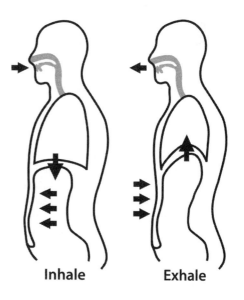

Figure 12.3. In effortless diaphragmatic breathing, the abdomen widens and expands during inhalation, and the abdominal wall tightens and pulls inward during exhalation.

Inhale   **Exhale**

Experience it. With ideal breathing, the amount of effort involved is imperceptible. To improve your breathing, keep your focus on your abdomen, since you want less movement in the chest than in the abdomen.

How it works. Why do so few of us breathe effortlessly? As children, we all used diaphragmatic breathing, but by the time we are adults, most of us no longer breathe in this healthy, regenerative pattern. Many people breathe high in their chest—and either slouch or hold their abdomen rigid ("stand up straight and suck in your stomach!"). That means that when they breathe, they use excessive effort to lift their chest as they inhale and tend to breathe rapidly and shallowly.

Practice 4: Designer Jeans Syndrome

Why it happens. For many people it is challenging to breathe diaphragmatically, and it may feel totally unnatural and awkward. Some common reasons for this include the following:

- *Restricting our breathing with tight clothing.* We wear restrictive clothing such as skinny jeans, panty hose, girdles, belts, or tight pants, inducing "designer jeans syndrome." In the nineteenth century, upperclass women were known for their fragility and fainting spells, probably caused by the tight corsets that compromised their breathing (shown in figure 12.4).

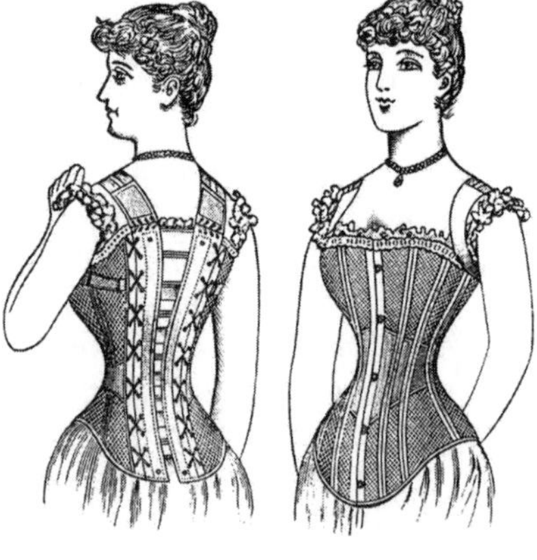

Figure 12.4. Example of a properly corseted lady during Victorian times. Women often fainted after mild physical exertion due to thoracic breathing (hyperventilation). We can surmise that the fallacious belief that women fainted under stress was, in fact, due to the Victorian version of the designer clothes (corset) syndrome.

- *Tightening the abdomen to project an image of beauty.* We may develop the habit of pulling in our "abs" (simulating "six-pack abs"), since a flat stomach is considered highly desirable.
- *Tensing the abdomen unconsciously when we're under stress.* This is a natural reflex in response to both physical and emotional stress.
- *Avoiding abdominal pain.* We may minimize movement in an effort to reduce pain due to a surgical incision, ulcers, chronic infection, severe menstrual cramps, or sexual insult. The abdomen is tensed to avoid any activity that would increase the pain. This protective response, which works well in the immediate moment, often becomes habitual. Chronic tension also tends to inhibit natural movement. As a result, tension can maintain an illness because it impairs normal circulation and adequate lymph flow.

Experience it. Try the following:

- Pull your stomach way in, and if you're wearing a belt, pull the belt as tight as possible (women, imagine that you are wearing a laced corset).
- Now stand and move around, continuing to hold your stomach in tightly, while trying to breathe normally.
- Do this for about one minute, and be sure to stop if you become too uncomfortable.
- Now release your abdomen fully, loosen your belt completely, and allow your breathing to occur in your abdomen again.

What did you notice? When we hold our stomach in, most people find that it takes more effort to breathe, although for some it feels almost normal, because they habitually have almost no abdominal movement as they breathe. Most feel a sense of pressure in their head or light-headedness. Some experience abdominal discomfort, and others develop a sense of anxiety, panic, or nervousness.

Notice how quickly the effect occurred. Yet many people unknowingly live with this type of restricted breathing all day long. This can contribute to chronic discomfort and interfere with healing.

After you've loosened your belt and let your abdomen relax completely and begun breathing normally, the symptoms fade. You'll probably find your breathing easier than before, and you'll probably find yourself much more relaxed.

When we restrict our abdominal movement, our breathing pattern shifts from regenerative diaphragmatic breathing to rapid, shallow breathing in the upper chest that can induce subtle hyperventilation. This is referred to as "subclinical" hyperventilation because it occurs below the level of conscious awareness. This shifts us into a low-level chronic stress response. Hyperventilation occurs when the dissolved carbon dioxide (CO_2) in the blood is reduced, which increases the risk of muscle twitchiness, light-headedness, sensations of panic, fear, or cold hands and feet.

How effortless breathing supports healing. Relaxed breathing is also a tool you can use to reduce panic or nervousness. During regenerative breathing, the breath slows down to a rate of six to seven breaths per minute, and exhalation is about twice as long as inhalation, with most of the movement of breathing occurring in the abdomen rather than in the chest.

When people can breathe around six breaths per minute, the rhythm of the heart rate tends to parallel the breathing—it increases with inhalation and decreases with exhalation. Slow, relaxed breathing promotes a balance between two primary aspects of the nervous system—the sympathetic nervous system (which controls the stress response) and the parasympathetic nervous system (which controls the relaxation response).

Practice 5: Regenerative Breathing

Getting started. You can practice regenerative breathing in any position—lying, sitting, or standing. Begin by practicing diaphragmatic breathing while you're lying down once or twice a day for fifteen to twenty minutes (see figure 12.5). Lie flat on the bed or the floor with pillows under your knees, back, and head. If you're wearing clothing that is tight around your waist, loosen it. Close your eyes if that feels comfortable.

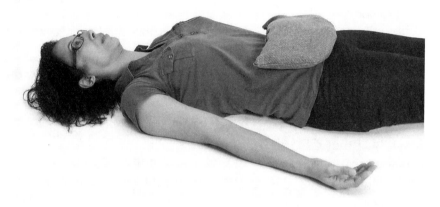

Figure 12.5. Lying comfortably with a weight on the abdomen (photo by Jana Asenbrennerova)

- First, place a two- to five-pound bag of rice or beans on your abdomen.
- Relax and then become aware of your breathing. Each time you inhale, push the weight on your abdomen upward and away from you.
- As you exhale, allow the weight to gently press on your abdomen, so the weight controls the exhalation. Let the air flow very softly out of your mouth while whispering "Haaaaa." Allow the breath to flow out very slowly. Do not force the inhalation or exhalation.
- At the end of the exhalation, just wait until you feel the urge to inhale.
- Again inhale so that you are pushing the weight up and away from

you. Do it without effort. Be gentle. Then let the pressure of the weight guide your exhalation.

As you inhale, imagine a white light coming in through your head, and feel your stomach rising. As you exhale, imagine the air going down your arms and out your hands and fingers. On the next exhalation imagine the air flowing through your hips, thighs, lower legs, ankles, and out through your feet. Continue to breathe in this pattern. Feel the breathing occur through the expansion and passive contraction of your abdomen. Imagine that the light brings healing energy throughout the body.

If your attention wanders, bring it back to your breathing each time. During inhalation, be aware of the weight on your abdomen moving upward and away from you. During exhalation, focus on the air flowing down and out your arms and feet as healing light.

Continue for about fifteen to twenty minutes. Allow the rate of your breathing to slow. Let each exhalation become slower so that in time you are breathing six or seven breaths a minute without any effort. Then allow yourself to go to sleep or take a deep breath, open your eyes, wiggle, stretch, roll to your side, and gently get up.

Optionally, there are many ways to use imagery and to focus your attention as you're breathing. For some people the image of light makes sense—others experience energy flow. Some find it helpful to imagine that they are breathing from their feet upward, pulling air (or energy or light) in through the soles of their feet to their abdomen as they inhale and then, as they exhale, experiencing the flow downward, from their abdomen to their toes and beyond.

What did you notice? Most people report feeling refreshed and peaceful. You may even fall asleep during the exercise. Often, the world looks sharper and brighter. Initially, it can be challenging to keep your focus on the flowing sensations going down your arms and legs. Many people report that their hands and feet have warmed. The weight on the abdomen usually feels comfortable and secure, and the weight also helps to keep the attention on the abdominal area without effort. Practice makes perfect, and over time it will become easier and easier.

Common challenges. Below are some of the challenges you may face in this practice.

- *Wandering thoughts.* Most people find that their attention wanders. Just keep gently bringing your attention back to your abdomen during inhalation. You may want to do this exercise with a partner and have him or her guide your breathing through touch. This can be an effective focusing technique and a distraction from pain.
- *Mild hyperventilation.* Some people do these exercises with too much effort and unintentionally hyperventilate. A few people experience light-headedness or find that their hands become a little clammy and cold. To avoid this, breathe with less effort, and as you exhale, simply allow the air to flow out more slowly. Then pause until you need to inhale, and at that point let your abdomen push the weigh upward with minimal effort. In short, inhale less air, exhale more slowly, and breathe with less effort.
- *Negative associations.* Occasionally a patient reports that the flowing imagery reminds them of the sensation of chemotherapy and the neurological symptoms induced by chemo. In that case, it is helpful to bring attention back to the abdomen and then, as one exhales, to imagine the air soothing and healing the tissues.
- *Not feeling any awareness or sensation in the arms and legs.* If possible, have a partner stroke your arms and legs in rhythm with your exhalation. You can also perform this practice yourself. (These two practices are described below.)

Experience it: Doing the exercise with a partner. In many cases, this practice is easier to do with a partner. The sensation of touch tends to hold your attention without effort.

- As you exhale, have your partner stroke your arms in rhythm with your exhalation so that as you exhale, your arms are being stroked from the shoulder to the fingertips and beyond (as shown in figures 12.6a, 12.6b, and 12.6c).

- Inhale, and then during the next exhalation, have your partner stroke the sides of your legs from your waist and hips down the sides of your thighs, your calves, your feet, and your toes. Be sure your partner applies a steady pressure so that you feel the sensation (see figures 12.7a, 12.7b, and 12.7c).

- Have the person who is stroking you exhale audibly in unison with you, whispering "Sheeee." Repeat the stroking six to ten times, each time in unison with your exhalations. Ask your partner to stroke you gently and slowly as if his or her hands are moving through molasses. Usually, one downward stroke takes about one exhalation if you are breathing at a rate of about six or seven breaths per minute.

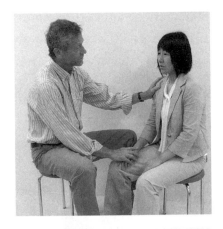

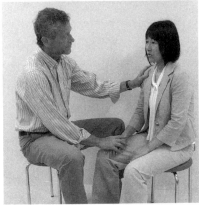

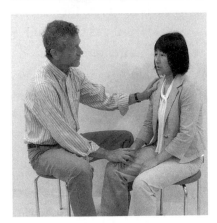

Figures 12.6a, 12.6b, and 12.6c.
Stroking down the arms

228

- If you are breathing rapidly, then have your partner do one downward stroke for every two breaths (have your partner begin the downward stroke, gently stop when you inhale, and then continue again when you exhale).

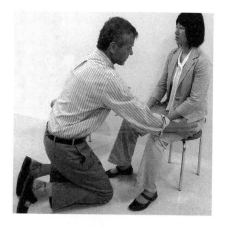

What did you notice? Most people report that it is much easier to feel the sensations in their arms and legs as they exhale. They also report that being touched helps focus their attention. After the practice, you may find that your hands and feet have become pleasantly warm. Usually pain is significantly reduced.

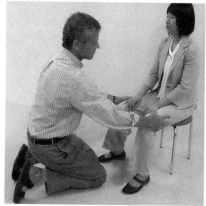

Doing the practice on your own. If a partner is not available, stroke your own body as you exhale. To do this exercise, you'll want to be either sitting or lying down with your knees bent. Place your right hand on your left shoulder, and then as you exhale, stroke down your left arm past your hands and fingers. Usually, it is helpful to use gentle but firm pressure or squeeze slightly as you

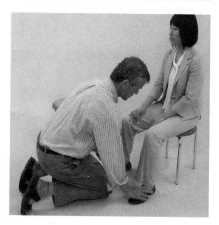

Figures 12.7a, 12.7b, and 12.7c.
Stroking down the legs

stroke down so you can consciously feel the sensation. Repeat stroking your left shoulder and arm with your right hand. Then shift your attention to your legs. Place your right hand on your right hip and your left hand on your left hip and as you exhale, stroke down your right leg and left leg past your feet. Again apply firm pressure. (Note that occasionally when we practice breathing, old emotions or memories surface. Although this may be momentarily uncomfortable, it is a wholesome form of clearing. Simply let the emotions go. Do not focus on them or amplify them. Just acknowledge them as you would a thought or an emotion in a mindfulness practice, and then return your focus to your breathing.)

Keep Breathing

Breathing is an unappreciated process that contributes significantly to health and healing. It is the boundary between the conscious and unconscious that reflects all our body's physical and emotional patterns. Breathing is also a leverage point for influencing our physical, emotional, and mental being.

The most important part to remember is that healthy breathing is the ability to respond to the body's needs. Sometimes you need to be able to breathe rapidly to escape danger. At other times, you want to be able to breathe slowly to relax and regenerate. This chapter has offered a few exercises to help you become attuned to patterns that interfere with healing and others that support your natural healing process.

Consider the following resources on breathing:

Farhi, D. *The Breathing Book: Good Health and Vitality through Essential Breath Work.* New York: Henry Holt, 1996.
This book describes in detail a series of thoughtful breathing and movement practices derived from a yogic perspective.

Peper, E. *Breathing for Health*. Montreal: Thought Technology Ltd., 2008. Available from www.mindgrowth.com/.

This CD set has been designed to explain the importance of breathing and teach effortless diaphragmatic breathing. The CDs include instructions on how to recognize and transform unhealthy breathing patterns. The guided exercises will enable you to become quiet and relaxed, control stress, enhance wellness, and optimize performance.

Chapter 13

PHYSICAL RELAXATION

I lay there trying not to move. All I could hear was the loud clicking sound of the MRI. My heart was in my throat. My hands and feet were cold, and the even the air in the room felt cool and clammy. I could hardly breathe—I kept wondering what they would see on the MRI. Has the tumor grown? Has it shrunk?

It only took about twenty minutes, but it seemed like hours before they rolled me out of the MRI chamber. I felt exhausted and stiff. Although the procedure was over, I still couldn't relax, and my mind kept racing, obsessed with the question, "What did they find?"

A PATIENT DIAGNOSED WITH CANCER

Cancer and cancer treatment almost always involve a certain amount of discomfort, both physical and emotional. To reduce pain, calm the mind, and encourage healing, there are several body-mind techniques that can be quite useful. These techniques will not *cure* cancer, but they can be an effective complement to treatment. You'll probably find that these approaches quiet your thoughts and emotions and shift you out of the stress response into a more healing mode, the regeneration response. This occurs when your body is relaxed and your mind and emotions are at peace—once you have reestablished a sense of safety and are able to shift your focus away from pain or discomfort.

To let go of thoughts, quiet the emotions, and move the body to the regeneration response, shift the focus of your attention into the present moment. Focus on the sensations and feelings that occur while doing the practice. These types of exercises are referred to as somatic practices because they combine training to master relaxation with new skills to change breathing patterns. The goal is to evoke regeneration and inhibit pain by practicing a process of focus and awareness. This will help you develop mindfulness and promote self-healing.

Regeneration includes relaxation and regeneration of the physical, mental, emotional, social, and spiritual aspects of your life. It includes establishing a sense of safety, allowing relaxation, and quieting your mind. This chapter focuses on integrated body-based approaches to reduce pain and promote the regeneration response.

Tools for Coping

Dealing with cancer brings many challenges into our lives. One of those challenges is how to access our own healing abilities—not just to fight the cancer, but also to deal with the pain and exhaustion caused by the testing and treatment.

Cancer diagnosis and treatment often involve physical and mental tension. Many procedures, such as MRIs and CT scans, require us to remain in the same position without moving for extended periods of time. Being confined in a restricted space to think with time on our hands can be a double whammy, increasing exhaustion and pain. When we're immobilized, and have no way to work off the stress, it's a temptation to just keep worrying. It can be difficult to relax and stop one's mind from working overtime, unless we train ourselves through a relaxation practice.

Recovery from surgery often requires even longer periods of inactivity. After surgery, we attempt to protect the incision. We quickly learn not to move and usually keep the injured area of the body immobile. We are sore and tired, and our primary goal is to guard against pain. This avoidance is an automatic reflex—comparable to how we learn not to touch a hot stove as a child.

As a result, we may find ourselves substituting awkward patterns of movement for our usual balance and poise. However, these new patterns of movement can soon become habitual. Our muscles react to the stress as we distort our movements to compensate for the injury.

We may also unknowingly tighten muscles we're not using—for example, hunching our shoulders or holding our breath. This misdirected effort is usually unconscious, and unfortunately, it can lead to fatigue, soreness, and a buildup of additional muscle tension.

This chapter offers brief, simple practices to avoid and reverse dysfunctional patterns of bracing and tension and reduce discomfort. Practicing healthy patterns of movement can reestablish normal tone and reduce tension and pain. The relaxation practice at the end can be useful in mastering deep relaxation to promote regeneration and support better sleep.

Breaking the Cycle of Muscle Tension

To reduce discomfort and encourage healing, there are several relaxation and stretching techniques that you can use.

- *Regaining your poise.* These techniques can help you regain your composure following treatment.
- *Quieting your emotions.* You'll also probably find that these practices quiet your thoughts and emotions.
- *Shifting out of the stress response.* These exercises will provide you with additional tools for shifting into a more healing mode.
- *Relaxing.* A shift into the relaxation response occurs when your body is relaxed and your mind and emotions are at peace—once you have reestablished a sense of safety.
- *Distracting yourself from pain.* You can use these practices to refocus away from pain or discomfort.
- *Regaining flexibility.* You'll probably be surprised at the degree to which the practices increase your flexibility and help you relax.

- *Becoming attuned to your patterns of movement.* These brief practices will also help you recognize adaptive patterns of bracing or tension.
- *Reestablishing normal patterns of movement.* As your awareness increases, awkward patterns of movement are reduced by restoring balanced ways of moving.
- *Promoting deep release.* Relaxation exercises can support an ongoing practice of deep release, so you can cope with the tension and worry and heal more quickly.
- *Improving sleep.* You can also use these practices to help you sleep better.
- *Coping with the tension that builds up during inactivity or confinement.* Being confined during treatment or convalescence can cause cumulative tension, unless we learn to consciously relax. Normally we would work off the tension by walking, working out, taking a shower, or getting a massage. Exercises to reduce muscle tension give you another option for coping.
- *Breaking the domino effect of tension.* Chronic muscle tension may result in other aches and pains. In our efforts to compensate, we can become even more knotted up. The goal of these practices is to increase your awareness of tension and how reduce it.

The practices show that brief exercises, performed without effort or exertion, can relax you and release the tension that tends to build up in the neck, shoulders, or back. They are tools for interrupting the pain-tension-pain cycle, and to quiet the voices of worry in your head. During and after cancer treatment you can use these targeted, gentle exercises as effective tools that help you face the ongoing challenges.

To make these practices easier and more playful, you can download an audio file from www.medical-center-cologne.com or www.biofeed-backhealth.org that will guide you though each brief exercise step-by-step.

Practice 1: How Tension Interferes with Simple Tasks

Goals and benefits. Muscle tension can be a major contributor to fatigue. Most of us are unaware of how much tension we actually carry. The following short exercise is designed to show how tension interferes with your ability to move comfortably. Chronic, low-level muscle tension tends to impede circulation and also restricts the flow of lymph, which carries the immune factors essential for healing.

- Sitting comfortably, place your hands on your lap.
- Now raise and tighten your shoulders.
- Keeping your hands on your lap with your shoulders tensed, now tighten your arms.
- Holding your shoulders and arms tight, move your fingers as if you were typing rapidly on an imaginary keyboard in your lap. Then stop the typing motion and relax your shoulders and arms.
- Now lift your arms about a foot above your lap and then let them drop loosely in your lap like a rag doll. Feel the pull of gravity and totally relax your arms and hands.
- With your shoulders and arms relaxed, again type on the imaginary keyboard in your lap, moving your fingers rapidly as if you are typing. Now relax.

What did you notice? Most people report that when their shoulders and arms are tight, their fingers move much more stiffly and slowly. In addition, some even notice the beginning of achiness in their neck, shoulders, and arms. You can use this increased awareness of tension as a reminder to consciously relax.

If we're under stress, we commonly tighten many muscles not necessary to perform the task—for example, clenching the jaw or neck or raising our shoulders and frowning. In terms of physiology, these are unnecessary efforts (termed *dysponesis*) that often initiate pain. The tension can contribute to exhaustion and can cause headaches or pain in the neck, shoulders, back, hips, arms, joints, or legs. Often we are totally unaware of the tension that is building up until we experience the sensations as pain.

Yet if we can become aware of the tension and relax the muscles not needed for the task at hand, we won't get tired as quickly, and we'll have more flexibility.

Practice 2: Playful Relaxation—Wiggle

Goals and benefits. It's human nature to brace against pain. When we reduce bracing and relax tense muscles, our flexibility is enhanced, and we experience less discomfort. This practice demonstrates the benefits of relaxing.

- Try this in a spirit of playfulness. This light relaxation exercise can be done lying down, seated with headphones, or standing. Try it with music on your iPod, the radio, or a CD.
- Listen to some of your favorite dance music (especially music you enjoyed when you were in your teens or early twenties). Begin to wiggle and shake every part of your body in rhythm with the music. Do whatever feels right and is fun. You might even wiggle your hips and do a lying-down hula.
- The movements can be very small—for example, if you're resting in bed, you might just move your hands and feet or your fingers and toes. You can even move just your head, your tongue, or your eyes. You'll probably find that "wiggling" lifts your spirits in a matter of seconds.[280]

Practice 3: Relaxing before a Procedure

Goals and benefits. While sitting in the waiting room before a medical procedure, you can practice "invisible exercises" to reduce the tension by simply tightening and relaxing your muscles.

- For example, tighten and relax your glutes (your buttock). Hold for about five seconds, and then relax.
- Now tighten and lift the balls of your feet about an inch off the floor and curl your toes toward your knees. Hold for five seconds. Relax, and then relax even more.
- You can continue doing this type of exercise with other muscles using the same approach.

When getting an MRI or CT scan, since you will need to lie totally still, use mental visualization practices to relax. Several options for visualization are described at the end of this chapter and in chapter 14.

Practice 4: Taking a Minute to Get Centered

Goals and benefits. If you find yourself tensing up or starting to worry, it's helpful to relax. Focus your attention on the feeling of releasing the tension systematically in various sets of muscles. You can do these anywhere—in the car, at the doctor's office, or at work. Remember that you usually have the option of slipping off to the bathroom to take a minute to get centered. The easiest way to tighten a muscle is to move one of your joints:

- *Shoulders.* To relax your shoulders, raise them, roll them back, and then drop them.
- *Hips.* Raise one hip and then lower it. Use the same motion on the opposite side of your body.
- *Feet.* Lift your heels a few inches off the floor and then drop them.
- *Hands.* While you're sitting, lift your hands a few inches above your lap and drop them.

Each time you relax an area of your body such as your hands or feet, let it be so completely relaxed that when it drops, it seems to bounce. One way to relax any group of muscles is by tightening them and then releasing them. Another approach is to practice opposing movements, and this works especially well with the muscles of your neck and trunk.

Practice 5: One-Minute Stretch

Goals and benefits. This is a great tension reducer once you return home after an appointment or a long drive:

- Lying down, take just a minute to stretch. Inhale, and then as you begin to exhale, flex your feet so your toes are pointing toward your knees. Tilt your head forward and look toward your feet. When you begin to inhale, point your toes away and tilt your head backward, looking as far up and back as possible. Repeat this sequence five times.

Practice 6: Regaining Your Natural Coordination

This exercise involves several steps—you can listen to this script on the web or download it to your computer or an iPod.

Goals and benefits. Diagonal movements underlie all human coordination. If you're right-handed or left-handed, that tells your nervous system how to respond quickly, whether you're pulling a hot pan off the stove or catching a baseball. When you walk, if you are right-handed, and right-side dominant, when your right foot goes forward, then your left arm swings forward.

If your coordination is in sync, this will happen as a reflex without thought. There are many examples of these basic reflexes, all based on diagonal coordination. To restore this coordination, we use exercises that emphasize diagonal movements.

This will help you reverse unnecessary tension and use your body more efficiently (reducing "sensory motor amnesia"). Remember to do the practices without straining, with a sense of freedom, while you continue relaxed breathing. If you feel pain, you have gone too far, and you'll want to ease up a bit. The following exercises can be done while you're sitting or lying down.

Preparation. This is a light series of movements that involve tapping your feet and turning your head. You'll be able to do the entire exercise in less than twenty seconds.

- Sit erect at the edge of the chair with your hands on your lap and your feet shoulders' width apart, with your heels beneath your knees.
- First, notice your flexibility by gently rotating your head to the right as far as you can. Now look at a spot on the wall as a measure of how far you can comfortably turn your head and remember that spot. Then rotate back to the center.
- To become familiar with the movement, lift the balls of your feet so your feet are resting on your heels. Lightly pivot the balls of your feet to the right, tap the floor, and then stop and relax your feet for just a second. Now lift the balls of your feet, pivot your feet to the left, tap, relax, and pivot back to the right.
- Just let your knees follow the movement naturally. This is a series of ten light, quick, relaxed pivoting movements—each pivot and tap takes only about one or two seconds.

Doing the brief sequence. At this point, add head movement. Turn your head in the opposite direction of your feet. This series of movements provides effortless stretches that you can do in less than half a minute as shown in figures 13.1a and 13.1b.

- When you're facing right, move your feet to the left and lightly tap.
- Then face left and move your feet to the right and tap.
- Continue the tapping movement, but each time pivot your head in the opposite direction. Don't try to stretch or force the movement.
- Do this sequence ten times. Now stop, face straight head, relax your legs, and just keep breathing.

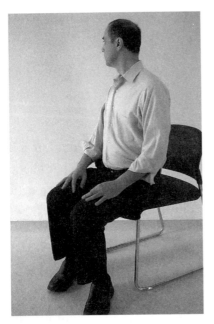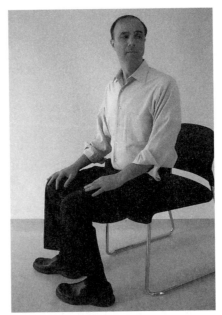

Figures 13.1a and 13.1b. Rotating the feet and head
in opposite directions (photos by Gary Palmer)

- Rotate your head to the right as far as you can see and look at a spot
  on the wall. Notice how much more flexibility/rotation you have
  achieved.

What did you experience? Almost everyone reports being able to
rotate significantly farther after the exercise than before. They also
report that they have less stiffness in their neck and shoulders. This
type of exercise can be done anywhere. Now that you have the concept,
you can also create brief exercises to use while lying down to counter
stiffness and relax you.

Practice 7: Mini-exercises

Goals and benefits. Here are a number of short practices that will
help you loosen up your muscles, reduce tension, and encourage a
sense of restfulness.

Head and feet diagonals. Lie on your back with your arms along your sides and your feet shoulders' width apart. Simultaneously roll your head to the right and your feet to the left; then roll your head to the left and your feet to the right. Remember to exhale at the beginning of the rotation.

Arm and leg diagonals. Lie on your back with your arms along your sides and your feet shoulders' width apart.

- Simultaneously lift your right arm and left leg about six inches and then let them drop and relax, and then relax even more for about ten seconds. As you relax, notice how the tension in your muscles is fading out.
- Then lift your left arm and right leg up and let them drop, relax, and again relax even more for ten seconds. Repeat five times, alternating by lifting the opposite arm and leg and then dropping and relaxing them.

Head, arm, and leg diagonals. Lie on your back with your arms along your sides and your feet shoulders' width apart.

- Inhale, and then while exhaling, bring your right arm over your abdomen and reach toward your left knee.
- Rotate your head to the left while rotating your feet to the right.
- While inhaling, return to a relaxed position on your back, with your right arm along the side of your body.
- Now repeat the rotation with your left arm. While exhaling, bring your left arm across your abdomen and reach downward toward your right knee. At the same time, rotate your feet to the left. While inhaling, rotate back so that your left arm is along the side of the body. Repeat five times.

What did you experience? Many people report that performing these small movements reduces stiffness and increases their sense of energy and aliveness. They can also be used to shift attention back to the present moment.

Practice 8: Increasing Flexibility

It's human nature to brace against pain. When we reduce bracing and relax the muscles that we're holding tense, our flexibility is enhanced, and we often experience less discomfort. This practice demonstrates the benefits of relaxing your muscles.

Goals and benefits. You can increase your energy level and flexibility without effort when you practice a range of different movements. These movements involve tensing and relaxing the muscles of your neck and shoulders. This can significantly decrease neck and shoulder tightness and increase your range of motion and often interrupts or reverses the cycle of pain-tension-pain. When doing simple tasks, learn to relax the muscles that you don't need for the task.

Do this exercise in a standing position. Give yourself enough space, so that when you lift your arms to shoulder level and rotate, you don't touch anything. Continue to stand in the same spot during the exercise as shown in figures 13.2a and 13.2b.[281]

- Lift your arms and hold them out, so that they are at shoulder level, positioned like airplane wings.
- Gently rotate your arms to the left as far as you can without discomfort. Look along your left arm to your fingertips and beyond to a spot on the wall and remember that spot.
- Rotate back to center and drop your arms to your sides and relax.
- Again, lift your arms to the side so that they are like airplane wings pointing to the left and right. Gently rotate your trunk, keeping your arms fixed at a right angle to your body. Rotate your arms to the right and turn your head to the left. Then reverse the direction and rotate your arms in a fixed position to the left and turn your head to the right. Do not try to stretch or push yourself. Repeat the

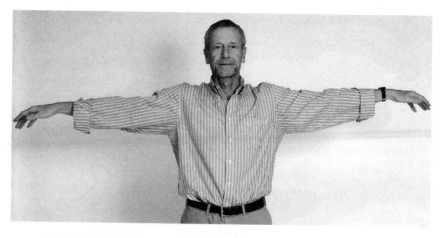

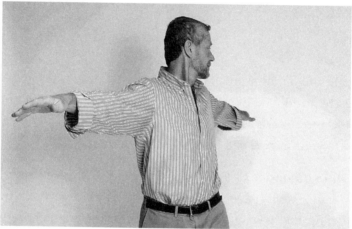

Figures 13.2a and 13.2b. Rotating the arms as far as is comfortable (photos by Jana Asenbrennerova)

sequence three times in each direction and then drop your arms to your sides and relax.

- With your arms at your sides, lift your shoulders toward your ears while you keep your neck relaxed. Feel the tension in your shoulders, and hold your shoulder up for five seconds. Let your shoulders drop and relax. Then relax even more. Stay relaxed for ten seconds.
- Repeat this sequence, lifting, dropping, and relaxing your shoulders

two more times. Remember to keep breathing; and each time you drop your shoulders, relax even more after they have dropped.

- Repeat the same sequence, but this time, very slowly lift your shoulders so that it takes five seconds to raise them to your ears while you continue to breathe. Keep relaxing your neck and feel the tension just in your shoulders. Then hold the tension for a count of three. Now relax your shoulders very slowly so that it takes five seconds to lower them. Once they are lowered, relax them even more and stay relaxed for five seconds. Repeat this sequence two more times.

- Now raise your shoulders quickly toward your ears, feel the tension in your upper shoulders, and hold it for the count of five. Let the tension go and relax. Just let your shoulders drop. Relax, and then relax even more.

- Finally lift your arms up to the side so that they are at shoulder level and are positioned like airplane wings. Gently rotate without discomfort to the left as far as you can while you look along your left arm to your fingers and beyond to a spot on the wall.

What did you notice? Almost everyone reports that when they rotate the last time, they rotated significantly further than the first time. The increased flexibility is the result of loosening your shoulder muscles.

Regenerative Relaxation[282]

Learning relaxation means quieting your body so you can become aware of the automatic reactions that are occurring within your mind and body. When your body is relaxed, by definition your mind will also be relaxed. As both body and mind relax, regeneration can occur. Many people find it helpful to do these practices for twenty minutes at least once a day or more. Although there are many strategies for learning to relax, you may want to adapt these exercises to your own personal needs so they work best for you. We have seen that people who personalize the exercises report even more benefit.

Listen and practice the relaxation script. It is much easier to either listen to an audio of the script or to have a family member or friend read it to you and guide you through it. This specific script can be downloaded as an audio file from www.medical-center-cologne.com or www.biofeedbackhealth.org. You may want to use earphones if the room is noisy.

Setting the Stage

Adapting the script. If you're going to have the script read to you, you want to first read it over and edit it to make it fit for you. Once you've tried it, you can vary the script if you'd like, inserting a detailed description of your favorite personal memory or peaceful imagery. In the script, an ellipsis (...) means a pause. Wait about ten seconds or so before continuing. Give yourself time. Do not hurry—remind yourself that you are worth it.

Create a healing environment. Begin by creating a supportive environment where you will not be interrupted. Make yourself comfortable while sitting in a recliner or lying down. If possible, lower any bright lights or wear a sleep mask, reduce the sounds you can control or else use headphones, take off your shoes, and loosen clothing such as a tie or bra and waistband so that nothing constricts your body.

Steps in the relaxation practice. This process integrates three key components:

- Using a ritual to begin the relaxation
- Practicing tightening and relaxing muscles while breathing effortlessly
- Recalling a personal memory from a time when you felt happy, healthy, and whole

Developing a ritual. Always begin your practice with the same ritual. The ritual will become a cue to which you become conditioned. Each time you use the ritual, it will evoke and deepen your relaxation and feeling of safety.

The ritual can be any sequence of practices that you repeat each time, such as thoughtfully loosening your clothing, using a refreshing taste such as a peppermint, or using a fragrance such as lemon, incense, or a scented candle. Taste and aroma are powerful conditioning cues. Other rituals could involve music, which could range from soft classical music to Buddhist chanting or nature sounds, such as a recording of waves on the beach. Still others could include snuggling up with a teddy bear as shown in Figure 13.3.

It is helpful to develop a ritual that you can use anywhere, so if you want to use music or sound, you may want to load it on an iPod or a cell phone. Each time you begin your practice, begin with the same ritual. After you've gone through the sequence many times, the ritual will automatically initiate conditioned relaxation. As you become more practiced, this can enable you to evoke the relaxation when you are waiting for a medical appointment or having a procedure done.

Using your ritual to evoke the relaxation response. Whenever you need to relax, we encourage you to use the ritual to evoke a state

Figure 13.3. Patient holding a toy dog as a mascot to evoke the feeling of safety and hope (photo by Jana Asenbrennerova)

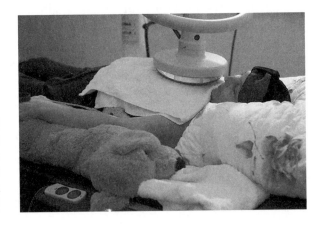

of deeper relaxation. You can adapt parts of the relaxation practice to the specific situation. For example, while sitting in the waiting room before a medical procedure, you can begin with the ritual and then practice invisible exercises (discussed earlier) to reduce the tension. When having an MRI or CT scan done, you can use your initial ritual followed by images of a peaceful memory. For these tests, you'll want to omit the muscle relaxation, since the scans require that you lie absolutely still.

Tuning in to your body. This is an opportunity to become aware of the automatic reactions, sensations, thoughts, and feelings that are occurring within your body. Also notice your reactions to all the external stimuli in your environment that you are seeing and hearing (e.g., bright lights, the ringing of a cell phone, a beeping IV pole, the sound of a TV, or the voices of other people in the room or nearby).

The practice of muscle relaxation. To begin the relaxation, sit in a relaxed position or lie down. The script will guide you to systematically tighten and relax different muscles. While tightening a specific muscle, feel the sensations of that muscle. At the same time, keep all your other muscles as relaxed as possible. Hold the specific muscle contraction for about ten seconds and then relax and let go for about ten to twenty seconds while passively noticing the sensations of relaxation in the muscle as the tension fades. If your attention wanders to your mental list of things you have to do, to physical sensations, noise, or other distractions, gently bring your focus back to the specific muscle you are tightening or letting go. When you relax the muscle, just let it go. Always listen to your inner guidance. Do not force either tightening or letting go. If the tension causes discomfort, skip those muscles and tighten and relax others. Be gentle with yourself and continue to breathe.

Recalling a personal memory. In the guided script, there is a time when you will be asked to recall a positive, joyful memory. You want a memory that is about a time or an experience when you felt happy, healthy, or whole—or when you felt safe, joyful, peaceful, or loved. The more you practice recalling that memory, the more real it will become. The process of remembering activates the same biological processes of wholeness or health that you felt during that actual experience. The process is similar to the practice of imagining a slice of lemon that was presented in chapter 11. Just as the imagery of the slice of lemon made your mouth water, your personal memory of wholeness will activate biochemistry in your body. In this case, the chemistry is intended to support the healing processes.

When you recall a personal memory, picture it in your mind's eye and fill in all the details of your original experience. See the colors, the shapes, and the textures that you delight in—feel the texture of the ground under your feet and the temperature of the air on your skin. Make the experience vivid—so vivid that you can hear the sounds of the place or feel the stillness. Are there any flavors or fragrances that you associate with this memory? Can you smell and taste them? Experience the imagery playfully without forcing it, and without effort.

If possible, bring a little reminder of your healing memory—an object or a photo, or something that you associate with the memory. You want to pair the cue with the experience of relaxation—and the memory with the experience of health and well-being. Think of tangible objects, such as an old teddy bear, a shell from the beach, a favorite song, or a certain perfume—as mentioned, taste, touch, and smells can be especially powerful cues. Be creative in finding items that will help you to remember that time. This process can be compared to the cues that children unconsciously use to put them in the right frame of mind to go to sleep, such as a teddy bear or a special blanket.

Overcoming challenges to relaxation. When evoking your personal memory, there two common challenges often occur: (1) the memory may be bittersweet, and (2) one may feel unable to recall a joyous childhood memory. A bittersweet memory evokes both positive feelings and also a sense of loss because the joyous time has disappeared or the loving person may no longer be in our lives. In this case, be appreciative that you have had this positive experience, gently release the feeling of loss, and use a different memory.

It is very common not to be able to recall a personal memory when one is ill because of the stress and discomfort. If it is difficult to evoke an actual memory, create your own imaginary positive memory, use the structured image included in the script below, or ask someone you feel close to if they would describe a positive memory that you could use—for example, making sand castles on a warm beach while hearing the sounds of the surf.

Before you begin, go over this checklist:

Checklist for Relaxation Practice

_____ Phone and cell phone unplugged or turned off (if possible)

_____ Pet(s) out of the room

_____ "Do Not Disturb" sign on the door or family informed

_____ Lighting turned low/drapes pulled

_____ Temperature adjusted for comfort

_____ Sweater or blanket available if the room is cool

_____ Pillows for your knees and head

_____ Object associated with your personal memory

_____ MP3 or CD player

_____ Remember to use the bathroom

_____ Remove your shoes

_____ Loosen your clothing (especially at the neck and waist)

_____ Take off your glasses or contact lenses

Relaxation Script

Set aside about twenty minutes for this practice. As you are guided through the script, remember to bring your attention back to your body whenever it drifts. Listen to the relaxation practice on audio or have someone read the script to you.

Begin by performing your personal ritual ...

Sit comfortably in a chair or lie on a sofa or bed. (If you're lying down, you may want to put a pillow beneath your knees and under your head). Wiggle around and make yourself comfortable ... Loosen any constricting clothing, loosen your collar, take off your glasses, take off your watch, remove your wallet and keys from your pocket. If you wear hard contacts, you might want to take them out because it's difficult to relax your eyes completely while wearing them. Be sure to loosen your belt and the buttons and zipper on your pants.

Gently close your eyes and begin relaxing your muscles ... First, raise both arms about a foot above your body. Tighten your fists and tense your arms while continuing to breathe ... Study the tension ... Let the rest of your body stay relaxed ... Now relax and let your arms drop like those on a rag doll ... Let go and relax ... Just become aware of any sensations in your arms and hands ...

Now hunch up your shoulders toward your ears and tighten your neck, while keeping your legs, glutes, abdomen, and jaw loose ... Continue to breathe easily ... Let go and relax. Allow your shoulders to drop down ... Feel the relaxation flowing from your shoulders, down your arms into your hands and out your fingers ... Allow your breath to flow down your arms ...

Squeeze your eyes shut tight, press your lips and teeth together, and wrinkle up your nose ... Feel the tightness in your whole face while keeping your neck and shoulders relaxed ... Notice any tension that may creep back into your upper body and let go of that tension ... Let it go and relax ... Allow your face to soften, feel the sensations of your eyes sinking in their sockets, your cheeks relaxing ... Allow your breath to flow in and out effortlessly ...

Press your shoulders back and tighten your chest and stomach. At the same time, keep your jaw and thighs as relaxed as possible ... Let go and relax ... Allow your body to sink comfortably into the surface on which you are resting ... Feel yourself being pulled down by gravity ... Allow the breath to flow through your arms and out your hands and fingers ...

Tighten your bottom, and your thighs, calves, and feet by pressing your heels into the bed or the floor while curling your toes and squeezing your knees together ... Feel the tension as you continue to breathe while keeping your face, shoulders, and arms relaxed ... Let go and relax ... Allow relaxation to flow through your legs ... Imagine inhaling the air up through your legs and then exhale the air down your legs and out your feet ... Feel the sensations of letting go ...

Feel the deepening relaxation, the calmness and the serenity ... Observe the ease with which your breath is flowing ... Let the feelings of relaxation and heaviness deepen as you relax even more ... Notice the developing sense of inner peace ... a calm indifference to external events ...

Let your entire body become more and more relaxed. Let the feeling of relaxation, calmness, and serenity deepen for a few minutes while continuing to breathe slowly. At this point, imagine that each exhalation is flowing out your arms and legs ...

Pause and continue breathing slowly, deeply. Now recall a personal memory when you felt happy, healthy, or whole ... Imagine being there and experiencing joy, peace, or love ... Take a few minutes to be fully in that memory ...

If you do not want to explore a personal memory at this moment, the script will guide you through a series of peaceful natural images.

Imagine that you are walking in a mountain meadow after having emerged from a nearby forest. Here and there, the green grass is dotted with brightly colored wildflowers in hues of pink, yellow, red, and purple. Touch the delicate petals of a flower and inhale its fresh, sweet fragrance. Remove your shoes and socks and let your feet feel the moist softness of the thick grass. Feel the sun overhead warming your shoulders and arms. A gentle breeze tousles your hair and soothes your forehead. In the distance you can hear the occasional clear note of birdsong breaking the silence. A butterfly lazily dips and floats among the flowers and grasses. Smell the grass and a faint scent of pine needles.

As you walk along, enjoy the feel of the grass under foot, become aware of the sound of a brook, which grows a little louder as you approach. For a while, watch the flow of the water over the shining stones. The sun glistens brightly on the moving water. Leaning over, let your fingers dangle for a moment in the clear, cool stream. Now relax and settle back comfortably for as long as you would like . . .

Gently let go of the images or memories and know that you can return to this peaceful place any time you choose to do so . . .

When you are ready, take a deep breath, gently stretch your body, open your eyes, move, and wiggle.

What did you experience? Many people report that they feel much more relaxed and at peace following the relaxation and the imagery. For some, tension headaches or aches and pains decrease. Others fall asleep, and when they open their eyes, the world looks brighter. Many report that the more they practice, the more intense the personal memory becomes, and that additional positive memories come forth. Many use it to quiet their ongoing internal dialogue. It takes a great deal of practice to take charge of the "monkey mind," which floods the brain with thoughts and images. Evoking a peaceful memory often decreases mental intrusions. With each intrusion of thoughts or sensations, return your attention back to the process of relaxation, the flow of your breath, or the memory or imagery.

Sustaining Your Practice

Learning relaxation skills takes time and practice. Remind yourself that when you first learned to drive a car, it seemed almost impossible, yet after a few weeks of practice, you could drive almost anywhere. You'll find that this process of learning is true of relaxation as well. Give yourself at least two weeks of daily practice to experience the benefits of your practice.

Practice the relaxation many times so that it is overlearned and becomes automatic. At that point, it will available to you when you are awaiting a medical procedure or experiencing pain or stress. Through daily practice, you will be able to condition your mind and body to relax at your suggestion.

This practice can be helpful when it is difficult to go to sleep or when you wake up at three in the morning. Bring your focus on the specific muscles, feeling the breath flowing down your arms and legs. Use the practice as an opportunity to channel your attention—it is a mindfulness meditative practice that uses the body and memory as a reference. As your body becomes quiet and relaxed, regeneration is supported.

At times you may find that the level of stress is so great that even this practice is beyond what you can handle. If that occurs, you may also use a prayer or meditation that has given you solace and comfort at other times in your life—for example, the Lord's Prayer, the Rosary, St. Francis's Prayer, mantras associated with yoga and meditation, Buddhist chants, Native American prayers, or passages from the Old or New Testament, the Koran, the Tao, or the Upanishads. Poetry and inspirational quotes can be helpful. As an alternative, you may want to look at a picture of a loved one or of a spiritual image that has great personal meaning to you to sustain you.

Consider the following resources on physical relaxation:

Hanna, T. *Somatics*. Reading, MA: Addison-Wesley, 1988.
This classic describes how dysfunction can be the result of the triggering of the alarm reaction and contains outstanding simple practices to improve mobility, flexibility, and health.

Schneider, M. *Movement for Self-Healing: An Essential Resource for Anyone Seeking Wellness*. Novato, CA: New World Library, 2004.
This outstanding resource book provides many movement practices and concepts to reduce pain, increase flexibility, and return to health.

Chapter 14

HEALING VISUALIZATION

I woke up in a panic. I have chemo again today. Waves of anxiety and nausea washed over me when I thought of driving to the hospital. My thoughts kept running. Is this worth it? I've already lost my hair; I have diarrhea almost every day; and I'm exhausted all the time.... I could feel myself getting more and more upset, so I focused my thoughts on my relaxation practice. I looked out the window and made it a point to appreciate the crocus pushing up through the snow. I did my relaxation practice and decided to relive some childhood memories this morning—building a sandcastle with my grandfather on the warm sand at the beach, while my grandmother brought me a cookie.

Later that day, sitting for the chemo drip, I did another practice, relaxing my whole body and focusing on my breathing. With every breath I imagined cleansing and healing liquid washing through my body, down my arms and legs, and out my hands and feet. I imagined the air was coating every healthy cell while the cancer cells were killed by the chemo.

A PATIENT DIAGNOSED WITH CANCER

After a cancer diagnosis, our emotions tend to be triggered by any new symptom. Even the simplest medical procedure can remind us of what we've been through and trigger our fears anew. For some patients, almost any sensation associated with the cancer or treatment tends to evoke worry and fear.[283] The purpose of the exercises in this chapter is to give you tools you can use to interrupt the cycle of stress associated with cancer and support healing. Whenever you are tempted to start

257

worrying, you can use imagery to interrupt negative thinking and shift into a more positive frame of mind.

What Is Healing Visualization?

Visualization was initially developed as a psychological strategy to support healing. It has been successful utilized as an adjunct of treatment with thousands cancer patients over the past thirty years.[284] The term *visualization* is often interpreted as a visual experience; however, it may be applied more broadly. For many people this approach is experienced as sensations of sound, taste, touch, or movement, rather than vision. For example, one could imagine and even feel blue water flowing through the area of the tumor and washing all the tumor cells away. You can even apply the principle of visualization by acting out the image. In this example, you actually gently brush your hands across your body, imitating the flow of water and imagining the water washing the cancer cells out and away from the body.

The components of effective imagery include the following:

- Relaxing
- Exploring the problem, illness, or area of discomfort
- Accessing images of wholeness and health
- Engaging in a self-healing process that transforms the area of discomfort into health or wholeness
- Integrating visualization into your life
- Imagining yourself as whole and healthy

After doing the visualization, it is helpful to draw or paint the imagery that came to mind. These drawings can be done after each practice, and you will probably notice the content change over time. They provide an external expression of your visualization practice.

Relaxing. The practice begins with guided relaxation derived from the regenerative relaxation practice (see chapter 13). The purpose is to relax deeply, so that the critical mind becomes less active, allowing a more dreamlike consciousness to emerge. The relaxation opens the nonverbal communication channels between the unconscious and the autonomic nervous system.

Exploring the problem. Without preconceptions, mentally examine your health concerns with an attitude of openness, as if this were the first time you've ever explored them. Imagine what the issue (cancer) looks like *at this moment in time*, not how you remember it from the MRI image, from your doctor's description, or from the illustration seen on a web page. Imagine how it is right now. Some patients imagine their tumors as a raw piece of hamburger, others as dark red cells expanding like yeast rising, still others as animals getting bigger.

When you inspect the area of concern, be open to any image that may emerge, however bizarre. Sometimes a very clear image occurs, and in other cases, especially when you're forcing yourself to imagine something, nothing occurs. If nothing emerges spontaneously in your thoughts, just make up something that could represent the disease process. At times, the image may relate to emotional or psychological experiences rather than to the disease itself. Simply accept whatever emerges, regardless of whether your thoughts focus on the experience or on the disease itself.

Accessing images of wholeness or health. Imagine how the area might look when it becomes whole or healthy, without preconceptions. Again, allow spontaneous images to simply occur, and if none occur, make something up that could represent the area being whole and healthy. Images commonly used to indicate healthy tissue include normal cells, or even images from nature, such as clear flowing water or sunlight. If no self-healing images occur, you can simply make up something, or ask a friend to suggest images that represent the healing process. We'll offer suggestions for encouraging a flow of positive images later on in the chapter.

Engaging in a self-healing process. Develop a dynamic image that transforms the area of concern into one of wholeness or health. Create or imagine a process in which what you saw when you initially viewed the problem is transformed into your image of wholeness and health. Always be open to unexpected associations, images, or feelings that may arise. An active healing process allows images of disease to be transformed and eliminated.

One patient imagined his cancer as dark red cells being washed away with a strong flow of bright, white, healing light. Another young patient imagined his brain tumor as "dumb hamburger." During the healing process, he saw his white blood cells as Pac-Men, like the video game, eating up the cancer cells, until there was no cancer left. Research has shown that when patients use visualizations of their cancer that intuitively portray the cancer as weak or powerless—or see their healing process as much more powerful than the cancer—their clinical outcome is significantly better.

Integrating visualization into your life. Run the self-healing imagery continually in the background, in the back of your mind, as much as possible. Imagine that this healing process will continue even when you are not actively focused on it. If you realize that you are worrying, use that as a cue to shift your attention back to the imagery.

Imagining yourself as whole and healthy. Imagine yourself as whole. Imagine your illness as resolving, and your body healing. Acknowledge that you are supporting your own healing process and be open to any images that may occur.

Challenges in Performing Visualization

A number of challenges can occur during a visualization practice. These challenges can usually be overcome by your own creativity or by a few suggested techniques. In other cases you may want to ask for support from friends, family, a health provider, or other patients with cancer. You can also use the problem-solving process that's described in Appendix A. Some of the common challenges that occur are highlighted below.

Lack of time. Making personal time is challenging, especially when so much of the diagnosis and treatment depends on others. However, most patients find they are able to set aside twenty minutes a day to do this type of practice. If you find it difficult to set aside time for yourself, the issue to address here is, "Am I worth it?—or is my worth defined only by responding to the needs of others?"

Negative images from the past. The imagery always reflects the present moment. Each time you do your practice, inspect the area of concern or illness as if you have never seen it before. If a frightening image occurs, acknowledge it and let your thoughts move on. If the image is a memory of an MRI or a CT scan, acknowledge it and say that's just how you were when you took those tests. If it's a doctor's comment that comes to mind, just remind yourself that that was in the past, that's what he said then, and make it clear that you are here now, updating those images.

No images. At first, many people report that it is difficult to visualize anything. If no image or association emerges, you have the option of viewing the cancer as a dark red blob. Ask yourself if that's the right image. If you answer yes, then you have the right image. If you answer no, see if another image emerges. If you respond with the sense that you have no idea what one means by an image, then imagery may not be the right process for you.

In our experience, everyone is able to create some form of image.

For some, the image is very biological, very specific—for example, draw-ings of cancer cells. For others the cancer is represented by animal shapes or by colors. There are many ways to access the images as you explore your condition and the healing process and imagine your body becoming healthier and your spirit returning to wholeness.

Not being able to see yourself as healthy or whole. Accept that at this moment you may not know how to imagine yourself as healthy. This is normal—the shock of the diagnosis and treatment can make it difficult to see ourselves being healthy or whole again. In some cases, health may not be possible, and you may sense that you are dying. One healing strategy is to work on acceptance, however challenging. Imagine what it will be like when you are whole and at peace. In addition, ask yourself: What do I still want to do in the time I have left? What can I do to support my quality of life and make the eventual transition to death as peaceful and nurturing as possible?

The Visualization Process

Practicing self-healing imagery means that you are playing an active role in your own healing. It means influencing your unconscious mind to optimize your health. The themes that underlie this process include the following:

Using imagery as a tool for healing. This can be an opportunity to take control and shift from hopelessness, powerlessness, and helplessness to proactive involvement in your own healing.

Keeping an open mind. Be open to the occurrence of any unexpected image, feeling, association, or memory that may be related to the disease or the healing process. Whatever image comes up is the image you want to work with at that moment in time, as long as it feels safe. Be open to the image, no matter how bizarre, illogical, or biologically inaccurate, in a literal sense. The thoughts that emerge in imagery can bear a certain resemblance to the quality of images in our dreams, and that is because our subconscious often accesses important information for us through mental and emotional images. Although these images may not make sense immediately, they may be metaphors for some aspect of our condition. For example, they may relate to past events in our lives. Trust and explore these images as long as that feels safe. It is possible that these images are messages from your unconscious. You will probably find that some images are universal or essentially archetypes, while others may have very personal individual meaning.

Developing "beginner's mind." Each day, see your life beginning anew. The goal is to explore and experience the healing process in that moment, with as few preconceptions as possible. Obviously, if no new images emerge, you can use a previous image. It can be challenging to let go of a negative image especially when there are intense emotional experiences connected with the image or the symptoms. There's a tendency to either hold onto the image or to reject it aggressively. Ideally, you want to encourage an attitude of passive attention toward the image as you would in mindfulness practice. You can take the attitude: I notice this image, I acknowledge it, and I am not invested in it or attached to it. Surprisingly, this attitude of passive acceptance and open exploration may allow the image to shift and change.

Creating positive imagery to guide your thoughts. You can support your well-being by holding an image of the healing process as a constant background in your thoughts. Like humming a favorite song, keep the healing imagery in the back of your consciousness at all times. It will take some time to integrate this habit into your thinking and to gain a clearer sense of how the healing imagery actually works. The ultimate goal is to imagine the healing taking place and then feel the healing occurring. Throughout the day place your awareness and love on your body and especially on the injured area.

Selecting healing images that make sense. The healing is not magic. There is a logical transition from the problem as it is at this moment to the transformation through healing. The transition does not need to be realistic or literally possible, but it needs to make sense to you. Allow the healing process to be stronger than the disease process.

Examples of powerful images. For example, if a person imagines the cancer as spreading sticky cells, having a magical wand that makes them disappear may be stronger and more magical than the power of the cancer itself. An even more powerful image might be sunlight that dries up the sticky mess, which can then be simply swept away with a broom or even eaten by Pac-Man cells. One young boy with leukemia kept the cancer at bay with thoughts of gorillas that clubbed the unwanted cells, creating an image that prevents against future illness. One patient imagined a healing light filling her immune cells, making them bigger and stronger. Then she imagined them actively searching for the cancer cells and killing them. Another patient combined imagery with her chemo treatment. She imagined all her healthy cells closing up like hatches on a ship, leaving all the cancer cells with open hatches so that they received the chemo and were destroyed.

Making the image real. A common way to make the image concrete is to draw or paint each of the steps involved in your healing journey. If you are doing drawings, you might portray (1) what you see at this moment, (2) the healing process that you have developed in your mind's eye, and (3) yourself as healthy and whole. If drawing or painting feels difficult, try a collage of images selected from magazines. It can be helpful to do the visual representation before writing or talking about the image. Otherwise, the images may stay on the intellectual level as if they are simply thought forms. Additional options can include the following:

- Describe the images verbally to others.

- Use a dream board to convey a series of images in a form similar to a collage.
- Take digital pictures of objects or clipart or landscapes that represent the problem, the healing process, and a return to health and wholeness. Put these positive visual images on your computer desktop or cell phone screen.
- Sculpt images in clay that represent the problem, the healing process, and health and wholeness.
- Talk to a family member or friend and ask them to join with you in creating images to represent each of these phases.
- Record music that reminds you of the healing process.
- Create spontaneous sounds or select three musical compositions that represent healing images. For example, one woman described her melanoma as a steak sizzling on a grill. A man with prostate cancer selected three music themes and kept humming the theme that reminded him of healing throughout the day.
- Act out the images physically involving others if you would like. For example, one or two people could represent the area of illness or injury, and others could play the part of the healing process. You become the director in the play. This is especially appropriate for a support group.
- Take photos that represent the images you saw in your exploration of the healing process. This technique is especially useful for people who find it difficult to find their own images internally, or to express them.
- Take a walk in a natural setting, focusing on natural objects such as flowers, rocks, or clouds that symbolize the images in your healing process.

There is no right way to experience an image. Respect whatever images occur in whatever form they take. Often the images that you resonate with will provide you with valuable information. Be willing to allow new images to replace those that are not working for you. Use the imagery process with an attitude of openness toward any intuitive associations that may relate to your healing.

Imagery Script for Relaxation

Listen and practice the relaxation script. It is much easier if you do not read the script yourself (how can you really relax if you have to continuously focus your attention on the page?). Instead, you can make an audio file of the script to which you can listen, or have a family member or friend read it and guide you through it. Or you can simply download the audio file from www.medical-center-cologne.com or www.biofeedbackhealth.org so that you can just listen to the instructions. You may want to use earphones if the room is noisy.

Before you begin, you may find it helpful to go through the relaxation script in the previous chapter. There you'll also find a checklist of suggestions on preparing for relaxation.

Sit comfortably in a chair or lie comfortably on a sofa or a bed (when lying down, make sure you have a pillow beneath your knees and under your head). Loosen any constricting clothing; loosen your collar, take off your glasses, take off your watch, remove your wallet and keys from your pocket (if you wear hard contacts, you might want to take them out as it is difficult to relax your eyes while wearing them). Be sure that your pants are not confining you— loosen your belt, the buttons, and zipper. Wiggle around and make yourself comfortable ...

Gently close your eyes ... Now, tense both arms by making fists, and extend them straight ahead, while continuing to breathe ... Study the tension in your arms, but let the rest of your body remain relaxed ... Now relax and let your arms flop down like a rag doll ... Let go of the tension and relax ... Just become aware of any sensations in your arms and hands ...

Raise your shoulders toward your ears and tighten your neck, while keeping your legs, buttocks, abdomen, and jaw loose ... Continue to breathe easily ... Let go and relax. Allow your shoulders to drop down ... Feel the relaxation flowing from your shoulders, down your arms into your hands, and out your fingers ... Allow your breath to flow through your arms and out your fingertips as well ...

Squeeze your eyes shut ... Press your lips and teeth together, and wrinkle up your nose ... Feel the tightness in your whole face while keeping your neck and shoulders relaxed ... Notice any tension that may creep back into your upper body and let go of that tension ... Let it go completely and relax ... Allow your face to soften, feel the sensations of your eyes relaxing, and allow the muscles around your mouth and in your cheeks to relax, and then relax again ... Allow your breath to flow effortlessly in and out ...

Now press your shoulders backward, and tighten up your chest and stomach at the same time ... Let your jaw and thighs be relaxed ... Let go and relax ... Allow your body to sink comfortably into the surface on which you are resting ... Feel yourself being pulled down by gravity ... Allow your breath to flow down and through your arms and out your hands and fingers ...

Tighten your buttocks, thighs, calves, and feet by pressing your heels down into the bed or the floor while curling your toes and squeezing your knees together ... Feel the tension as you continue to breathe while keeping your face, neck, shoulders, arms, and hands relaxed ... Let go and relax ... Allow relaxation to flow through your legs ... Imagine exhaling the air through your legs and out your feet ... Be aware of the sensation of letting go ...

Feel the deepening relaxation, the calmness, and peace ... Observe the ease with which your breath is flowing ... Imagine each exhalation; feel it flowing down and through your arms and legs ... Let the sense of relaxation and heaviness deepen as you relax more ...

Let your entire body become more and more relaxed. Let the feeling of relaxation, calmness, and serenity deepen for a few minutes while you continue breathing slowly, and feel the exhalation flowing through your arms and legs and out your fingertips and toes ...

... As you exhale, imagine the warmth flowing down your body ... Let each breath be slower and longer ... Let your breath slow down ... If your attention wanders, let the distraction be a reminder to breathe slowly and regularly while feeling the air going down your arms and legs ... Become aware of the throbbing of the pulse in your fingers ... Feel your hands warming as your breath moves down and through your arms ... Continue breathing easily for the next few minutes.

Now recall your personal memory when you felt happy, healthy, and whole ... Just imagine again being there and experiencing the joy, the peace, and love ... Take a few minutes to be in that memory ...

... Let go of your memory and attend to your breathing ... Let your breathing slow down and deepen. For the next few minutes allow your attention to go to your area of concern ... As your breath slows down, know that you are mobilizing your health.

Begin to inspect your area of concern as if you have never looked at it before ... Just look and feel inside to see what this area looks like at this moment in time ... Allow any image, sensation, or thought to occur. The image may be in black and white or in color, or it may be a bodily sensation or an emotion ... Whatever occurs, let it be ...

Now, let go of that image ... Allow an image to form that represents wholeness and health ...

Visualize a process by which healing and wholeness will occur, a process that transforms what you saw during the inspection into health and wholeness ... See and feel the healing process ... For the next few minutes, allow the healing process to continue ... Seeing, feeling, sensing a dynamic process that allows the problem to be transformed into healing ...

... Know that the healing process continues all the time; let it be become like a melody that occurs in the back of our minds all day long ... Feel the healing being carried through to completion ... Let a single image or symbol come to you that you can hold in your mind throughout the day ...

... Let go of the healing-process image and see, feel, sense as healthy and whole ... Experience a deep, gentle quietness ... Allow your breath to move

*easily in and out ... in and out. Imagine that as you inhale, a healing energy
comes into you like the rays of the sun, penetrating every cell with a shimmering
light, and as you exhale, the healing energy spreads outward like a blue cloud
or wave ... Allow this process to continue for a few minutes ... See yourself joy-
ously moving through your day, doing the things you love to do, enjoying just
being yourself, feeling free and content ...*

*... Each time you do the self-healing visualization, you are mobilizing your
self-healing potential ... Congratulate yourself for taking the time to care for
yourself and for supporting your healing process ... Allow the healing process
and healing imagery to continue to flow through you during the day ...*

*Now you choose whether to become more aware of the present environment
or to allow yourself to fall asleep ... If you want to get up, take a deep breath,
feeling relaxed yet alert, and then gently open your eyes while stretching your
arms. Whether asleep or awake, be aware that the healing process continues
all the time, and consciously evoke the healing process whenever you worry or
think of the disease or treatment.*

What did you notice? Many patients report that they feel better and
that they see themselves actively participating in mobilizing their own
health. The more they practiced, the easier it became, and the more
deeply they felt the imagery as an actual experience.

Evoking the Healing Process during the Day

Whenever you're tempted to worry, day or night, each time you begin
to think of the illness or the treatment, use that thought as a trigger to
evoke your healing imagery. Instead of letting worry run in the background of your mind, develop the habit of keeping thoughts or images
of healing running, and let them fill your mind. Each time a worry or
thought about the cancer occurs, redirect you attention and evoke the
healing process image again. For example, if you are receiving chemo

and dreading an upcoming appointment, you can work with your thoughts. The moment you are aware of such a thought or feeling, take a breath and exhale, and do your ritual to evoke your healing imagery. Or, when you're exhausted and the thoughts start racing, use that as a reminder to evoke healing imagery. Whenever you feel stressed, use that as a cue to evoke the healing image. Many patients report that years later, they can still evoke their healing images when the need arises.

The self-healing imagery can be done in anticipation of treatment. For example, a patient who was being driven to the hospital for her radiation treatment imagined all her cancer cells moving to her liver, which would get the radiation beam, and all the healthy cells vacating that area as much as possible. The ones that had to stay behind all received a silver radiation-resistant umbrella, which they put up to deflect the radiation. Every time she felt anxious or thought about the radiation treatment, she would use that as the trigger to evoke this self-healing imagery. This practice reduced her anxiety and made her feel in control. To her surprise, she experienced no side effects from the radiation. In addition, her husband recorded a long and short version of the self-healing script, which she played on her iPod. Each one began with the same music as she began her relaxation and self-healing imagery. In the short version, her husband's voice guided her quickly through the relaxation, by just reminding her of the key concepts: "Tighten your muscles and relax ... Breathe slowly ... Think of being at Nanna's house [her grandmother's house] ... exploring the problem ... See being whole and well ... the healing process, feeling whole ..." The long version also started with the same music and was adapted from the one described above. She practiced this before breakfast and most evenings before going to bed.

In summary, your thoughts and images form the blueprints of the future. As you become skilled at visualization, you will be able to transform negative thinking into positive thoughts and images. This is a strategy you will be able to apply in many areas of your life. You can use visualization to support you as an active participant in the healing process—and to mobilize your immune system and your self-healing processes.

Consider the following resources on healing visualization:

Norris, P., and G. Porter. *I Choose Life.* Walpole, NH: Stillpoint Publishing, 1985.

This book presents a detailed description of the use of imagery and biofeedback in an eleven-year-old boy's remarkable recovery from a life-threatening astrocytoma.

Peper, E., K. H. Gibney, and C. Holt. *Make Health Happen: Training Yourself to Create Wellness.* Dubuque, IA: Kendall-Hunt, 2002.

This is an outstanding, structured manual for learning and practicing relaxation and self-healing imagery.

Rossman, M. L. *Guided Imagery for Self-Healing.* New York: New World Library, 2000.

This book provides detailed instructions and case examples of using imagery for self-healing.

Samuels, M. *Healing with the Mind's Eye: How to Use Guided Imagery and Visions to Heal Body, Mind, and Spirit.* New York: Wiley, 2003.

This text presents outstanding background and descriptions of the use of healing with visualizations.

Simonton, O. C., S. Matthews-Simonton, and J. L. Creighton. *Getting Well Again.* New York: Bantam Books, 1992.

This is one of the first books to describe the successful use of imagery with cancer patients.

Chapter 15

THE ROLE OF HOPE

One of the doctors told me I have an 80 percent chance of dying. For me it's not 80 percent. It's either all or nothing—I will survive or not. The 80 percent is just a statistic, and I am one person, not a statistic.

A week after I got my cancer diagnosis, I contacted a cancer physician in Cologne, Dr. Robert Gorter. When I met with him, he stated clearly that he did not know if the treatment would specifically help me, although for some patients there was remission, and others were able to stabilize and have quality of life. That simple shift from the threat of dying to the possibility of living changed my perspective. Rather than preparing for death and saying goodbye, I began focusing on what I could do to mobilize my own healing.

This wasn't false hope. Dr. Gorter and I both knew that I could die. But now I saw every day as another opportunity to heal, to grow. I continued with the treatments recommended by my oncologist to destroy the cancer, but I also began the Gorter Model. For the first time since the diagnosis I felt hopeful.

HEINZ HAGEMEYER

The journey to healing is paved with both hope and disappointment—and also with acceptance, love, and a passion to live. Although we may not beat cancer by thinking good thoughts, we may be able to tip the balance in our favor by being conscious of the health factors that are within our control. We might otherwise overlook the influence of factors such as our personal beliefs and the subtle suggestions from those around us. These effects are usually described as *placebo* and *nocebo*.

The Placebo

A placebo[285] is a pill or procedure that evokes a healing response, while the nocebo is a pill or procedure that inhibits healing. A "placebo response" describes improvement in healing evoked by the patient's belief, rather than as a response to the treatment itself. A powerful example can be seen in the interaction of pain medication and placebo. When soldiers in battle believe that they are receiving a morphine injection, more than 50 percent can be injected with an inert solution that contains no medication, and their pain disappears. In a hospital setting, those given morphine by injection require 50 percent less medication than do those whose morphine is given in a continuous IV, because with the IV they are unaware of when they are actually receiving the painkiller.

If patients expect the medication to be more powerful because it is more expensive or because it is a trade name versus a generic, they usually feel better and experience more benefits, regardless of the actual efficacy of the medication. The placebo evokes the belief that the treatment will be effective and therefore establishes a sense of hope and safety in the patient. Symptoms are now interpreted as positive and sometimes even as a sign of healing. This assurance enables patients to shift out of a vigilant mode into a regeneration state, so energy can be expended on repair and healing rather than on self-protection.

The placebo effect also shows up in studies of skin allergies. Consider the series of poison oak studies conducted in Japan. Patients were told by their doctor that they were being exposed to poison oak, when in reality their skin was simply being stroked by a harmless leaf. Many of the patients developed reactions resembling poison oak. The study was also repeated in another variation. The doctor told patients that they were simply being stroked with a harmless leaf, when in reality they were being stroked with a poison oak leaf. Very few of the patients had reactions.

When we hold a belief or have a particular expectation, it influences the outcome. Words and images are the communicative language of the unconscious and the autonomic nervous system. They can create the blueprints for what will occur. An instruction or a procedure is not just a mechanical process—it is also a covert message that encourages hope or hopelessness. These messages communicate to the patient whether they should expect a procedure to be helpful or not. Patients with heart problems who were prescribed aspirin and warned about possible side effects were nearly three times as likely to develop ulcer symptoms and gastric bleeding—in contrast with those who were not warned about the side effects of repeated aspirin use.[286]

The Nocebo

A nocebo[287] response is the opposite of the placebo response—it triggers a nonhealing response instead of a healing response. It is probable that the nocebo evokes aspects of the flight/fight/freeze response, and often patients tend to be more fearful, more despairing, and less hopeful. Any sensations are interpreted as a signal that the disease process has worsened. Consider an account told by Bernie Segal, MD, of a patient who was told she was going to receive chemotherapy and was provided information on the side effects. Initially she was actually given an electrolyte injection (an inert solution that simply contained minerals, but no medication). Based on the belief that she had received chemo, all her hair fell out.

The nocebo signals the brain that a situation is dangerous or life threatening and thus mounts an alarm response in self-defense. When patients believe that there is no hope or that the treatment will not be effective, the immune system often shuts down, and their outcome tends to be much poorer. This is also true if they tend to have catastrophic thinking in which every event is interpreted pessimistically. In patients with pain, those who have a catastrophic pattern of thinking tend to have poorer clinical outcomes and suffer much more pain. Our mental habits frame the way we see and experience the world. For example, cardiac patients may experience tremendous fear and panic whenever they develop chest pain. However, following bypass surgery, chest pain is a reminder that they have survived and is therefore a sign of hope and healing. A chronic negative perspective can reduce the motivation for proactive self-care. Catastrophic thinking is often automatically triggered, yet we know from clinical experience that these habits of thinking can be improved with consistent effort.

Placebo and nocebo responses are part of *every* therapeutic interaction. The provider's expectations set in motion the placebo and nocebo reactions, which influence the outcome. This occurs covertly, usually without the awareness of either the physician or the patient. It is part and parcel of the therapeutic interaction, conveyed unconsciously at every step in the process.

The health care setting also triggers the placebo and nocebo responses. Messages of hope and healing are conveyed by the initial experience in the waiting room, the attitude of the receptionist, the intake process, the handshake with the doctor, the injection, the opportunity for the patient to tell his or her story (or not), the prognosis, and the treatment protocol recommended. These interactions all influence the beliefs of the patient. Namely, if the health provider expects that the patient will respond well to the treatment, this will increases the probability that the patient will experience improvement.[288] There are thousands of studies confirming the power of placebo—every example reflects the power of your unconscious mind to influence your body. The studies on pain and allergies also show the powerful effect of suggestion by the presence of an authority figure such as a physician—an expert with training, credentials, and the backing of a respected institution.

The Physician as a Source of Hope

Clear-eyed, hope gives us the courage to confront our circumstances and the capacity to surmount them.... During the course of an illness, then, hope can be imagined as a domino effect, a chain reaction in which each link makes improvement more likely. It changes us profoundly in spirit and in body.

JEROME GROOPMAN[289]

In medicine, authority figures such as physicians and surgeons influence the course of people's lives. A case of poison oak is a minor matter for most people. But when a patient is given a cancer diagnosis of only a few months to live and offered highly aggressive treatments, the power of authority can affect the patient's decision-making, their treatment options, the quality of their life, and even how long the patient lives.

To instill hope in the patient is the duty of all physicians.[290] This does not mean promising remission, which could be unethical and in specific cases unrealistic. However, it can include offering patients support in their quest for quality of life and supportive therapies such as nutrition, moderate exercise, stress management, and immune support, which often tends to be overlooked in conventional oncology treatment. This approach means keeping an open mind, and looking carefully and thoughtfully at treatment options.

Doctors can create an atmosphere of safety, a protective psychological cocoon that supports healing. When physicians provide this type of positive perspective—within the confines of what is realistically possible—patients can begin to hope, and their faith is nurtured. This supports the opportunity to heal as much as possible and to maximize quality of life.

To be met, supported, and understood by the physician allows anxiety to dissipate. To be accepted for who one is—and not just for the disease—initiates the first steps of healing to evoke wholeness. It implies emotional and spiritual wholeness, as well as physical recovery. In many cases the physical body cannot be healed. However, the person can still become whole and experience acceptance of death, thus allowing their transition to be peaceful.

On the other hand, physicians may also evoke a nocebo response, unconsciously discouraging to patients in their efforts to heal. If the attempts to explore other options are met with criticism or dismissal, patients may find themselves feeling frustrated and powerless. Often patients experience the diagnosis, prognosis, and treatment as the only options—the only legitimate approach. Frequently they are not aware that treatment recommendations are based on statistical results reflecting the aggregated results of thousands of treatments.

The system is not currently designed for individual differences or for the possibility that there may be additional viable options. In reality, disease progression and treatment protocol are based on pooled research data, averaged over hundreds or thousands of patients. The current approach, based on statistics, cannot take into account the specifics of the individual patient's genetics, lifestyle, support system, resources, or motivation level. Nor do the statistics explain the outlier who successfully survives and beats the statistical odds.

Critical life and death information about treatment and the probability of survival is conveyed through both verbal and nonverbal communication by the doctor. The words spoken—and unspoken messages conveyed through body language—influence the patient's mind-set for better or for worse. These messages may motivate the patient to be proactive or indirectly suggest to them that nothing more can be done.

The qualities of a health care provider that support healing are effective, in part, because they evoke the placebo response. (Those that inhibit healing are unconsciously evoking the nocebo response.) Table 15.1 shows the factors that were reported as promoting or reducing healing in a survey of hundreds of people.

Factors that promote healing as perceived by the patient

- Treated as a whole person
- Good listener
- Enough time to talk
- Provides information
- Expresses caring and compassion
- Spiritual inclusion
- Technically competent

Factors that reduce healing as perceived by the patient

- Treatment of body parts or of a diagnosis
- Subjective experiences not validated
- Lack of time, or being in a hurry
- No information
- Lack of personal contact
- Dismisses spiritual concerns
- Technically incompetent

Table 15.1. Peoples' descriptions of health care professionals' factors that promote or reduce their healing

The role of the physician as healer can also be to facilitate a peaceful transition to death. Death is not a failure of medicine. Death is an inherent aspect of the life cycle—a process that is beyond comprehension. Thus, supporting and nurturing the patient and his or her family and friends brings dignity and peace of mind. This perspective is most clearly expressed in the hospice movement.

Obviously, each patient needs to periodically ask the question, "At what point do I ask for additional aggressive treatment, and when do I let go?" Letting go is the acknowledgement that a patient is at the end of her life, and nothing more can really be done medically except to reduce discomfort and offer support.

The choices in this process are never easy—for the patient or the provider—but they can be facilitated by open communication with a compassionate physician. The challenge is to know when to make these decisions.

Hope and Healing

Getting better means different things to different people. For one, it's the ability to walk again, for another it's a reduction in pain, being able to live with the illness, or surviving long enough to see a daughter graduate. For many it is a desire to be as healthy as they were before the onset of the illness. Most patients want to get well—a state without disease or limitation—although they may have to settle for reduced suffering.

What does it mean to get better?

- To avoid death?
- To be cured?
- To have no pain?
- To be like before the illness?
- To reduce suffering?
- To feel safe?
- To be loved?
- To accept the illness and its consequences?
- To allow a peaceful death?
- To maintain good quality life?
- To be in complete remission?
- Not to be a burden to loved ones?
- To keep dignity and independence?

In some cases, the implied or explicit wish is, "Make me better. Make me well again." This means that the patient wants to be as he was before the illness struck—to lead the life he did before he got sick, and be able to do the things he did before.

You Can't Go Back

The paradox is that if we want to be as we were before the illness, then nothing has changed—we haven't really learned how to take care of ourselves, and we may become ill again. It's impossible to go back because that would imply negating all of the experiences we have gained through the illness. Our bodies and our minds are continually growing and changing—we are not the same as we were ten minutes ago, and definitely not the same as five years ago. Our awareness is continuously created, and present and future are influenced by the past. The cells in our bodies are continually being replaced in response to the demands on growth and repair. Similarly, our consciousness is continuously updated by the interaction between present and past experience. This is the process of attaining new wisdom. Mental health can be framed as the opportunity to find new meaning.

Wishing to be the same as before the illness means we prevent any growth or learning during the illness. Although this feeling is, in many ways, understandable, it blocks the ongoing flow of growth and personal development. Life has only one direction—a flow that cannot be reversed. To be truly healed is to be open to new experiences in the present, and to make the best of the situation at hand. For example, when chemotherapy prevents people from doing their normal exercise, it is a temptation to be angry and resentful. The other option is to acknowledge that at this moment, exertive physical activity is not possible, and instead patients can focus on things they can do that give them joy. For example, instead of cycling intensely for twenty miles, the person takes a gentle walk, practices yoga, or listens to music. The healing process includes ongoing growth and adapting—without resignation—to the present state of being, and at the same time continuing to maintain faith and hope.

Going through a disease process is like hastening our development, as if a major part of one's life had been intensely compressed. Once ill, patients have the choice to resign to the illness, to accept it, or to embrace it and all the unknown consequences that accompany it, good and bad.

Psychological studies of patients who have survived cancer consistently demonstrate that patients who are optimistic and play an active role in their medical decision making and their own healing often experience better quality of life and have longer survival rates than do other patients.[291] Patients who are proactive, putting their own life purpose and goals first, do much better than do those who comply simply to please their family and their physicians.

Embracing Illness and Health

Illness occurs to each of us—it is an inherent aspect of the human condition. Yet how we deal with it affects the outcome. When illness strikes, it is both a crisis and an opportunity. We have the choice of doing nothing or changing and growing. In fact, even the idea that "illness strikes" implies that we are victims who did nothing to contribute to its occurrence—and therefore we cannot possibly do anything about the outcome.

> It is remarkable—in the beginning, Els (my wife) had to bring me because I was very tired. So Els had to drive to the clinic and I was a wreck. After two or three hyperthermia sessions I said to Els, "I'm my old self-again."... You must always keep believing in your own recovery. Of course, you must try to break through the dogmas, and you need to be lucky. It's not all in your own hands, but there definitely is a future.
>
> RINUS GOEMAN, FIVE-YEAR SURVIVOR OF STAGE IV
> COLORECTAL CARCINOMA METASTASIZED TO LIVER AND LUNGS

From the authors' perspective, we believe that one can always do something about the outcome. Illness always creates opportunities for growth and change. Sometimes we can actively influence the course of the disease; at other times we can take control of our emotions and our energy level to mobilize potential health.

Acceptance or resignation. Recognizing and acknowledging that one has a severe illness are the first steps in the process of coping that leads to acceptance or resignation. Accepting the illness means taking a neutral stance from which to deal with the situation. Resigning to the illness implies a more negative stance, which evokes depression or a sense of helplessness. Remember that doing nothing is still making a choice.

Denial and fear. Denial is usually rooted in fear and flight from this fear. Fear is a negative force that can lead to various stages of paralysis, both physiologically (e.g., fatigue, constipation, cold hands and feet, or muscle tension in the neck, shoulders, or back) and mentally (e.g., mood swings, depression, apathy, panic reactions, insomnia, forgetfulness, loss of appetite, or weight loss). One could see fear as a force opposite to faith, love, and hope.

Opportunity for growth. Embracing the illness as an opportunity for growth is another option. By embracing illness, one experiences hope and an expansion of energy. It is this energy that mobilizes the immune system and the body's repair mechanisms. Embracing and accepting one's illness sounds strange at first, but it is a powerful force in the soul, with the potential to improve one's quality of life, life expectancy, and the healing process.

Dealing with a severe illness is always a matter of choice. A cancer diagnosis is a given fact. One has no choice that the illness exists. However, the way in which we deal with it is within our control. One way to increase control is to ask questions of your health care provider. The goal is to do no harm—or if harm must be done, then the benefits of the procedure must outweigh the possible harm. Explore some of the following questions with your provider:

- To what extend will the treatment improve my quality of life (and that includes the time during treatment)?
- Will my immediate reduction of symptoms improve my long-term health or ultimately have an adverse effect?
- How can the negative side effects of treatment be reduced?
- To what extent do the treatment strategies cause immune suppression?
- What can be done to empower my own immune system?
- How can I take my biography in my own hands?

Getting the answer to these questions can help us make more informed decisions. The questions we ask and how we use the information depend on the individuals and their health care provider. Ultimately these choices are different for each patient. The process of medical decision making can be challenging, and even tortuous. As uncomfortable as it is to ask questions and face hard decisions, we encourage patients to participate in their own care to the degree that they are comfortable. For some patients, this means entrusting decision making to family members or to their physician. For others, it means being an active participant at every phase of their care.

Patients who come to the Medical Center Cologne for treatment tend to be those who take a proactive approach to their cancer. Most have investigated this treatment carefully. They then made a calculated leap of faith, with the awareness that this nontoxic procedure supports quality of life. Stage IV patients who are struggling with the possibility of death often take the attitude that they have nothing left to lose. They might also come at the referral of a friend, so they know firsthand that the treatment can also prolong life.

The journey to healing is reflected in the stories throughout this book and is described in detail in inspiring video documentaries of patients at the Medical Center Cologne, which can be accessed at www.medical-center-cologne.com.

The factors that contribute to remission include the type of treatment chosen, the patients' psychological attitude, the physicians' skill, and many other unknowns. Psychological factors can also play a role in remission. For example, one survivor, whom we'll call Michael Burton, reported that before he was diagnosed with Stage II tongue cancer, his wife had a stillbirth, and she became extremely depressed. Instead of expressing his feelings, he worked obsessively in his study and only came down to eat. One wonders if the cancer was the result of not being able or willing to give voice to his feelings.

The effects of another such patient's mental and emotional perspectives are described in the case of Heinz Hagemeyer, a sixty-six-year-old high school teacher who was diagnosed with Stage IIIb metastasized prostate cancer in 2004. Now, after seven years, he is practically cancer-free (one persistent metastasis remains in one of his vertebrae) and is fully employed. Embedded within his story are psychological factors that are commonly observed in the patients who experience cancer remission.

One Patient's Journey

Before Heinz developed cancer, he reported being very dissatisfied with his work. For more than fifteen years each morning when he left home, he wished that it were his last day at his job. In addition, he had conflicts with his wife for many years.

Most cancer patients report some form of significant loss or long-term dissatisfaction in the years before the cancer diagnosis. For many people, life is experienced as being on a treadmill. Each day, they heroically wake up and get back on the treadmill. And they continue—day after day—without any hope that it will get better. It is not that patients complain of this fact, they just go on with their task. They seem to be living the myth of Sisyphus, the king in Greek mythology who was condemned to push an enormous rock uphill for all eternity. Just as the goal is in sight, the rock slips out of their grasp and rolls down the hill, and they have to push it up the hill again and again. (See figure 15.1.)

The immune system becomes less competent when we experience significant psychological stress. For example, this process is involved in the intense grief caused by the loss of a baby. For some it is the anger of hating the job in which people feel trapped but must keep working because they are responsible for their family income. For others the stress is caused by burning the candle at both ends—living a lifestyle without opportunities for regeneration. (Clearly sleep deprivation is an immune suppressant.) Stress in any form is usually intensified by feeling powerless to change the situation.

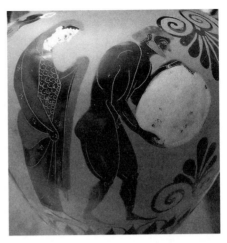

Figure 15.1. Persephone supervising Sisyphus while he pushes his rock in the underworld. Side A of an Attic black-figure amphora, ca. 530 BC. Staatliche Antiken-sammlungen (Inv.1494). Used with permission from: http://en.wikipedia.org/wiki/Sisyphus.

Clinical research shows that when patients take action, that tends to activate the body's defenses. The immune system becomes more competent when we acknowledge our situation and begin to improve it. For some patients, disease becomes an opportunity to bring about real change. However, many patients are so embedded in their lives that change appears impossible. These situations can be compared to the life of an abused woman who returns to live with the abuser because she feels that there is nothing else that she can do. Yet, when we begin to take action, change and health can be possible.

For Heinz, a turning point occurred soon after he received a terminal diagnosis. He began to look at his life situation differently, and the shift reflected that change. At the same time, he still had to deal with the diagnosis of his disease. As he said, "Why should I become depressed now? I decided to begin leading a smarter life. At that moment I jumped out of bed. I had just overcome the first obstacle on my path." When the doctors decided that an operation was not possible, Heinz requested a second opinion. The surgeon who examined him felt that prostate surgery would not help, although he recommended having all affected lymph nodes removed. Heinz notes,

> *A week later I underwent surgery, and the lymph nodes in my abdomen were removed. They were examined, and the pathology report showed that they had been affected. Thus from a medical point of view the prostate surgery was no longer necessary.*

His request for a second opinion indicated that he was not satisfied by simply complying with the treatment and following instructions without thought. He took the initiative to seek out information that would enable him to see the situation—and his diagnosis—from a different perspective. Patients who are assertive, who listen to their own heart, and who advocate for themselves usually have a better response to treatment and better outcomes. Implicitly, by taking charge, the patient's energy overcomes the sense of helplessness.

After the surgical removal of his abdominal lymph nodes, the oncologist prescribed hormone therapy with Zoladex injections and various oral medication—drugs that suppress testosterone production and make prostate cancer cells less responsive to the effects of testosterone. Unfortunately, all of these medications have significant side effects. In Heinz's words,

> *The hormone therapy has side effects that you don't want to know before you start. I won't elaborate on everything it does to you. Menopause pales in comparison. You sweat profusely. Get depressed. It does all the things you want to get rid of when you're sick.*

You feel absolutely horrible. You're constantly exhausted. I had never experienced anything like it. But I tried to handle it in a positive way. It also makes you impotent—that's obvious. My testosterone virtually dropped to zero. Nothing is going to happen then. That's how it is. It's a terrible burden.

Realizing that this therapy only postpones the cancer's progression—that's not a particularly pleasant insight. I thought it was worth it, because if I lived two or three more years, I'd be able to lead a decent life even with the burden of the side effects. I asked for help and went to a psychotherapist. So I felt a little bit better again.

Heinz describes his emotional and subjective experiences with a sense of humor—but not cynical humor. He has a willingness to describe the subjective experience without hiding his feelings behind a facade. This means that less energy is bound up in masking emotions and more energy is available for living. As a rule, patients who have humor and are able to communicate their experience do significantly better. In Heinz's case, despite his difficult diagnosis, he did not perceive himself as a victim. Even in his initial description of his diagnosis, he called it a "stupid diagnosis," implying that he was more powerful than the cancer. Patients who tend to describe their cancer as something that is powerless and can easily be overcome tend to have a significantly better prognosis. For example an eleven-year-old boy who experienced a total remission of life-threatening astrocytoma always described and pictured his tumor as dumb or looking like a hamburger that could easily be destroyed in his imagery by his white cells.[292]

Another factor is to communicate and look at possibilities. Again, Heinz can describe the discomfort and burden of side effects, but he does not feel sorry for himself or ask others to feel sorry for him. He has reframed his symptoms positively and accepts the side effects—and he feels that it was worthwhile if he can live a good life. He has taken over the rudder of his life and is less dependent on the winds of change. The disease has occurred, and now it is time not to find blame, but to focus on problem solving and on what can be done to optimize his health.

He has the courage, skill, support, and resources to initiate change. He is willing to ask for help. Asking for help is an indicator of the desire to take charge of certain aspects of his life. It also reflects the awareness that one cannot control everything. Asking for help shows a willingness to acknowledge that I am not perfect but am worthwhile and deserving of help from others. Heinz remembers,

One day I was watching television. One of the public networks had a program on alternative cancer therapies. At the end they introduced a Dutch patient who said that he been told he only had six more weeks to live.

But he said that those six weeks went by six years ago. He had prostate cancer, the same cancer I had. That's when I began listening attentively. I ran to my computer and sent an email to the station asking them the name of the hospital and the doctor who had treated this patient. The reply was that it was Dr. Gorter in Cologne. They also gave me the telephone number. I talked about it with my wife and called them the next day. I felt that this was something I needed to look into. I knew I could always make a decision later on.

Heinz visited the Medical Center Cologne. Dr. Gorter recommended that he do dendritic cell therapy with hyperthermia, while continuing with the hormone treatment (Zoladex to block the effects of testosterone and Zometa to slow down the progression of his bone metastases). Heinz discussed this with both his general practitioner and his urologist. This is another situation in which Heinz took charge by contacting Dr. Gorter and then by actively seeking the input of his physicians. Fewer than 20 percent of patients take steps to follow up on new possibilities. It is a giant step because you have to go outside your frame of comfort and familiarity. Heinz had to become less concerned with what other people thought about him and open to do what he needed to do for himself. Heinz continues,

I wanted a solid understanding of the treatment. As a layperson I can't judge whether this is a charlatan at work or not. After reading through the material, my family doctor spontaneously said, "If I had known this, it would have helped my brother." His brother had died of cancer. He said, "I would definitely give it a try." The pharmacist said the same thing. The urologist said, "I cannot give you an opinion, but if you want to do this, you have my support."

Heinz was very fortunate that neither his wife nor his doctors explicitly or implicitly opposed his treatment choices. Although he had a very serious disease, no doctor had given him a diagnosis with a timeline for his mortality. Instead, his physicians offered support. He received positive input from his own family doctor, who stated that he had wished his own brother-in-law could have received the treatment. This is a very powerful suggestion of hope and a statement that the proposed nontoxic therapy could potentially be useful. This kind of encouragement activates hope through the placebo effect, thus enhancing the self-healing process, which further supports the efficacy of the treatment.

In many cases, patients experience the opposite response from their health care providers. When they share with their general practitioner or oncologist that they would like to do something besides traditional orthodox treatment, they hear verbally (or sense nonverbally) that this would be a waste of time or that there are no controlled studies demonstrating efficacy. Such responses are powerful negative suggestions that trigger a nocebo response, which inhibits the self-healing process. In Heinz's case, his physicians increased his hope and motivation. Always remember that if no controlled studies have demonstrated clinical efficacy, it does not prove that it is not helpful. It only states that no controlled study has been done. Heinz recalls,

At the end of 2005, I started hyperthermia and dendritic cell injections. I went to Cologne for treatment periodically throughout that winter. Dr. Gorter recommended that I continue conventional treatment (in my case, hormone therapy) and await further examination.

After the initial treatment stage he said I should continue treatment and have one hyperthermia session every six months, which of course I did. After two years of treatment he said, "Alright, let's stop the hormone therapy and monitor your progress." All in all it took one year off the hormones before the tests showed normal levels again. My PSA level began to rise again slowly but only very little. This was nothing to worry about. My urologist gave me dark looks. He said, "An increase isn't good. I'd prefer things to be stable." I responded with a question: "Since I still have my prostate, couldn't this be a healthy sign? You said that every prostate produces PSA. Even a healthy one. So as long as it stays within certain limits, I'm OK with this."

Like many of the patients who undergo hyperthermia and dendritic cell treatment, the cancer progression had stopped. For Heinz, as for about 20 to 70 percent (depending on the kind of tumor) of the patients who receive hyperthermia, the disease process reverses and goes into partial or complete remission (unpublished data by Robert Gorter). Every aspect of treatment is working together—the psychological state is supporting the healing that is occurring within the body. Patients who tend to take charge and are seen as too assertive or independent have a significantly better prognosis. Assertiveness and independence are the opposite of powerlessness and helplessness.

In addition, Heinz has demonstrated a commitment to treatment. Once he agreed to start the treatment, he did it willingly, not because he "should." Nor did he passively follow the instructions of the physician. He made the choice consciously and actively wanted the treatment, so he willingly participates in the protocol:

The hardest, most strenuous part is full-body hyperthermia, perhaps because I have had hormone therapy and because I tend to be quite sensitive to heat. When you lie there, and they induce an artificial fever by applying heat, that takes its toll on you. For the four hours I was there, I didn't feel particularly well.

Local hyperthermia didn't bother me. That's when the tumor is heated locally. I could handle that, but for me, full-body hyperthermia was pretty tough. But at the same time you can take it. After the first time, you know that it will be over after those four hours. They slowly cool you down—otherwise it would be too hard. It's like a super sauna, except that after a sauna you can jump into the cold water, but your system wouldn't be able to handle that after this treatment. That's probably too dangerous. You slowly cool down until you've reached your normal temperature. It's bliss to take a shower at that point, and then you feel well. Even the week after you feel great. It makes you feel very fit.

As far as dendritic cells were concerned, in the first stage of treatment, I had six treatments in four weeks. Dr. Gorter had told me to bring somebody along the first time because you don't know how you will respond to it. After one to one and a half hours, I started getting a fever. Before I got home I would already have a fairly high fever. I would start trembling all over. I never took my temperature, but it had to be fairly high. It's not an unpleasant fever. It doesn't make you feel weak. Normally, a fever will wear you down. In this case, when I lie down and wrap myself in a blanket and close my eyes, I always fall asleep fairly quickly.

After the first two years of treatment, I get hyperthermia once every six months, along with an injection of dendritic cells. When I wake up the next day, it has already subsided a little. I always get mild headaches after that. One cannot take aspirin because that would be counterproductive. I don't, because the headaches are bearable, but I do take it easy that day. I go for a walk, get some fresh air, and in the evening it's gone. That's it. Those are the side effects.

Heinz realized that fever was not an illness but an indicator that his immune system was activated. So he agreed not to use medication to suppress the fever, and he was willing to live with the minor, short-term effects of the treatment. Hyperthermia is uncomfortable for about two to four hours. The symptoms of the dendritic cell therapy are limited to one day. After that, patients feel better and can do what they want. Thus, the treatment is not so exhausting, and because they are not exhausted, it is much easier to stay optimistic.

What a difference in quality of life there is with the nontoxic treatment as compared to the side effects of radiation or chemotherapy! Research shows that one person in five with cancer will become so traumatized by the treatment that they develop post-traumatic stress disorder. Many report experiencing a condition described as "chemo brain," a state in which cognition and memory are impaired for three months or longer. Other patients become exhausted, which may invoke depressive thoughts and feelings. It's a challenge to continue to be hopeful while feeling totally exhausted, nauseous, and hairless from the side effects.

There are none of these side effects with nontoxic treatment. Heinz began initially with six sessions of fever-range, total-body hyperthermia and dendritic cell injections for four weeks. After that he continued to come once every six months for follow-up treatments. The following year his body scans showed that his primary tumor was gone, and he has not undergone any other treatment besides Dr. Gorter's for more than five years by now. As Heinz says,

I had a primary tumor. It is no longer there. You can feel it when the primary tumor in the prostate is gone, and you can also see it on an ultrasound. It's gone. They can't feel anything. Nothing on the ultrasound. The PSA is in the normal range. Now my PSA is around 6.0. Not a single urologist will frown if somebody of my age has 6.0.

I have changed my life. I've changed my psyche. I've become friendlier, and I'm not as dissatisfied as I used to be. People around me confirm this. I hardly notice it, but people say that I've become a different person. If I push the boundaries, I could say that this disease has done me good. That's pushing it, of course. I'm not happy that I got sick. Let's not have any misunderstandings on this, but it has shown me the right way, that's true.

My health is much better, I feel healthy. I go for walks, swim, ride my bike, go on holidays, and go mountain climbing—ever since my own hormones are back. Of course, I've lost muscle tissue after the treatment. I need to work out, but that will take a while. The older you get, the harder it gets, but there are no other limitations.

Of course there's still some risk left, but the main thing in all of this is that you enjoy life. I have learned the important lesson that one cannot fight the disease. The disease is a part of me. A very smart woman told me that. You need to live with the disease—that's what matters. You can be happy.

Heinz Hagemeyer has changed. Instead of dreading each day, he looks forward to the day and what life may bring. He also is aware that the illness had beneficial components because it created an opportunity for him to change and grow (or pushed him in that direction, depending on how you look at it). He also realizes that cancer is now part of him. To some degree, illness is always an aspect of being alive. The body is continually seeking a dynamic balance between breakdown and growth. In Hagemeyer's case, the Gorter Model treatment stimulated his immune function so that it could eliminate the cancer, and his psychological choices also augmented his immune response. He freed his bound energy to support his own healing by changing his perspective, developing more autonomy, and remaining attuned to improvements that supported a realistic, yet positive outlook.

This book has described the Gorter Model, which addresses cancer by supporting the immune system through nontoxic treatment. The remarkable remission of some of the patients with cancer who have been treated with the Gorter Model strongly suggests that in many cases this nontoxic treatment is effective. That the Gorter Model has been successful with quite a few Stage IV cancers suggests that instead of waiting to do this approach combined with self-care after traditional treatment has failed, it should be done first as part of the initial treatment approaches.

As discussed in the earlier chapters, cancer is a complex disease. Health, healing, illness, and death are all part of the cycle of life and are not totally in our control. Yet often there are steps we can take to encourage the shift toward healing. Regardless of whether you use this approach or not, there are many things that you can do to nurture the possibility of a positive outcome and to improve your quality of life. Self-care can be overwhelming because it includes many aspects of our lives—but it is worth the effort because self-care is one of the foundations of healing. The process is unique to each individual. You can use the practices in this book to focus your efforts at self-care to improve your quality of life and support immune function, and mobilize your potential for health.

In 2009, the doctor told me that I had breast cancer with metastasis to the liver and that it was incurable—and that there was nothing that could be done. In terms of treatment, I took responsibility upon myself. It is my life, and I decide what I want to do with my life and my body. I decided to continue conventional treatment with Femara medication, an aromatase inhibitor used for the treatment of ER+ early breast cancer, with the Houtsmuller diet which consisted of large amounts of vitamins, minerals, antioxidants, vegetables, fruit, and very low sugar.

At the Medical Center Cologne, I received both whole-body and localized hyperthermia, and treatment with dendritic cells vaccine.

The local hyperthermia treatments were easy to take. They're not an ordeal at all. As for the total hyperthermia, the first time was very exciting. I didn't really mind. At the end it got very hot. For me it was very easy to take. I felt well in all respects—physically, emotionally, and especially mentally.

When I look at it now, one year later, I consider myself fortunate that everything went as well as it did. I'm happy again. I have a future again. My family and I can make plans again. That feeling is almost impossible to describe. That's how wonderful it is.

LIEN VOLDERS, SURVIVOR WITH TOTAL REMISSION
OF HORMONE-SENSITIVE BREAST CANCER METASTASIZED
TO THE LIVER, TREATED WITH THE GORTER MODEL

Appendix A
PROBLEM SOLVING

What do you do if you're faced with an important medical decision and there doesn't seem to be enough information? How can you make a decision if you're tying together a puzzle with missing pieces? What if there are too many choices, and then at some point there may not be enough choices? When that happens, it's a temptation to feel overwhelmed. This problem-solving approach can be used in a broad range of situations. The purpose is to get distance for a moment so you can reflect and make the best possible decisions.

Choices in healing can be very challenging. So often the knowledge is incomplete (see Appendix B for more information). It is challenging to know what the right answer is or even if a right answer exists. This is especially true with cancer—the answers are almost never clear-cut.[293] Are the side effects of the treatment worth the possibility of living longer? How do I know that I will live longer and not die of the side effects? It is even more difficult because these are often life-and-death decisions, so underneath we feel overwhelmed by emotion. At the same time, we want to make decisions rationally. There are no magic answers. Ultimately, we need to make the choices for ourselves.

Receiving the cancer diagnosis is usually a crisis. Nevertheless, remember that even though the cancer may be fulminant and aggressive, usually it has been present for eight years, ten years, or more. For most people, the risk is not increased by taking time to make a good decision—whether that means taking an extra day or even a week. Think carefully about what you really want to do. Agreement means to know that you have chosen this treatment approach, and this is different from passively complying with or resigning to the treatment.

A few guidelines are offered here to support your decision making.

- Stay centered. If you feel more than 20 percent angry, resentful, or depressed, stop and take the time to become calm again. Let the immediacy of your emotions wash through you and then ebb away like a wave. Even though the anger may mobilize you to action, make final decisions only when you have found your center again.
- For difficult decisions, "sleep on it." Make the decision, then wait a day and see if you still agree with your decision. At that point, you may find that you feel surer and are ready to act on it. If you're still unclear, that is actually a "no" or "probably not," which means going back into the decision-making process.
- You have the right to say "No." You have the right to tell anyone who is pushing you for a decision that you need time. You can take time out and become centered before deciding what to do—this is wisdom. Remind yourself again that cancer usually has been smoldering in the body for possibly ten years or more before it was detected. Also remember that you have an equal right to accept or reject any form of diagnostic procedure or treatment. You have the right to make your own decisions and choices. The health care professionals advising you will return to their own life, their home, family, and profession. You (and your partner or immediate family) will have to live with the consequences.
- Look at all the options. Consider your cancer from the perspective of another discipline. Get a second opinion, and a third. In short, explore other approaches and make a list of advantages and disadvantages for treatment and supportive care that you are considering
- Remind yourself that not making a choice is still a choice.
- Ask for advice from friends, relatives, health care providers, and others. However, remember that it is only advice. You have to make the choice because it is your life. Here again, remind yourself that you will be the one to live with the consequences.

In most cases, focus on what can be done and begin to initiate some action. Identifying possible solutions for problems takes creativity and out-of-the-box thinking. By taking an active approach to identify and resolve problems, quality of life may be improved and discomfort reduced. It may also be possible that there are no solutions, and the problem-solving process then focuses on acceptance and enhancing the quality of life.

You can use the following problem-solving strategy to identify the problem more clearly, generate possible solutions, and explore how you want to implement your action plan and how you want to follow up and assess the outcome. Nevertheless, the key to problem solving is to focus on an aspect of the problem that can be changed or solved. Thus, explore the problem-solving approach for challenges that have some possibility, however small, to be changed.

Some problems have a creative and achievable solution, even though it may not be obvious at first. It may require that we think "outside the box." The following six-step problem-solving process is useful in resolving most problems.

1. *Define the problem.* List all the issues associated with your situation, allowing them to flow freely onto the paper without editing them.[294] When you are done, identify the one issue you want to focus on *now.* Describe the major aspects of the issue in detail—for example, treatment side effects, distress in the family, worry about children, or financial concerns. You may want to prioritize the issues and explore the one on which you want to work first. Describe the how, when, how often, where, with whom, and what.

2. *Brainstorm possible solutions.* Write down every solution you can think of. Make a list of all of your generated solutions. Just write them down in any order. Do not *judge* or *criticize* the possible resolutions at this early stage. Allow a free flow of ideas. Allow a broad range of possible solution to occur. Postpone judgment during the

brainstorming stage; this is your chance to think outside the box. When critical thoughts arise, just acknowledge them and any self-critique and put them to the side. Then encourage other creative ideas to come forth.

3. *Pause and take a break.* After generating all possible solutions, take a break and see if other thoughts pop up. Expand the range of possible solutions by asking your friends, family members, or colleagues for additional ideas.

4. *Review and evaluate the possible solutions.* List all the pros (benefits) and cons (problems, difficulties) for each solution.

5. *Identify the best solution.* Review your assessments of the solutions, then rank them and select the best solution. Choose the solution that you can realistically use. If no solution appears viable, accept that you are still working on a resolution; write down the problem and schedule another brainstorming session at a later stage. Also, explore the risk benefits. How likely is it that the plan will work; what is the probability that the plan will not work? And is this worth the risk?

6. *Implement your solution and then follow up.* Keep notes of what happened when you carried out the action plan. Take time to review the outcome of the action plan. If successful, continue the implementation, or stop if your goal has been achieved. If less than successful, is there something that could be changed? Repeat the problem-solving process.

In summary, patients are surprised that initially they felt that there was nothing that could be changed. Yet when they started applying the problem-solving steps, they found there were some factors that they could influence and enhance their quality of life.

For more on problem solving, explore the following books:

Lerner, M. *Choices in Healing.* Cambridge: MIT Press, 1994.
This book explores in detail the dilemmas in decision making that face a patient with cancer—the choices between treatment or no treatment are not simple. This book is available at www.common-weal.org/pubs/choices-healing.html.

Taleb, N. N. *The Black Swan: The Impact of the Highly Improbable* (2nd ed.). New York: Random House, 2010.
This remarkably easy-to-read book points out that the world is not predictable but is more random and unknowable. It offers a foundation to think differently.

Watanabe, B. *Problem Solving 101: A Simple Book for Smart People.* New York: Portfolio, 2009.
This fun and easy guide to problem solving and decision making was initially developed for Japanese students to think like problem solvers and take a proactive role in their own education.

Appendix B
WEB RESOURCES

This appendix lists a number of internet resources and includes websites that provide specific types of information on cancer therapy and immune support.

The web is a fountain of information. For some people, having more information is empowering and increases their sense of control. For others, it may feel overwhelming. Some find community on the web, and others simply feel more isolated. If you feel overwhelmed by the information, stop and take a walk or talk to someone to whom you feel close.

Surfing from one site to another, from one link to the next, can take hours of time. What are my options? What information is useful, what is not, and what is harmful? Should I do conventional treatment or complementary therapies in combination with conventional treatment?

We recommend that you look at all the information with an open-minded skepticism—since many of the claims, even those on superbly constructed websites—represent the beliefs and biases of the site sponsors. Remember that the information on websites is not vetted for accuracy. In addition, many nonprofit websites have actually been created as marketing outlets for commercial interests.

If possible, find someone who shares your values with whom you can discuss the information you are finding and the questions it raises. You also want someone who is a compassionate listener.

Specific Resources on the Web

Video Documentaries of Patients from the Medical Center Cologne

www.medical-center-cologne.com

You can view documentaries of patients who have experienced cancer remission using the Gorter Model, including their experiences and how they dealt with cancer.

Audio Files on Imagery and Relaxation

www.medical-center-cologne.com or www.biofeedbackhealth.org

Audio files of the imagery scripts, relaxation practices, and exercises from this book can be downloaded for personal use.

Search Engines and Websites

The most common source of information is the keyword searches performed by search engines such as Google. Just enter a keyword or multiple words, and hyperlinked citations are displayed almost instantaneously. The following websites may useful in finding relevant information. We do not endorse or vouch for the content or accuracy of the information on any website.

www.google.com/

This search engine can literally scan databases that include millions of websites in a matter of seconds to locate sites and information based on keyword searches.

http://scholar.google.com/

This section of Google searches the web for scientific literature related to the keywords entered. Citations may include abstracts and/or full-length articles.

www.ncbi.nlm.nih.gov/sites/entrez

PubMed, U.S. National Library of Medicine, National Institutes of Health, offers keyword searches of the biomedical literature comprising more than nineteen million citations from the MEDLINE database.

www.cancerguide.org

This page provides information on how patients can research cancer information.

Complementary Medicine/Integrative and Functional Medicine

www.acamnet.org

American College for the Advancement of Medicine provides referrals to integrative physicians through the largest professional group of integrative providers in the United States. It is important to inquire how long the physician has been involved in cancer care, what types of cancers they treat, and the primary approaches they use.

www.functionalmedicine.org

The Institute for Functional Medicine provides referrals to physicians who practice functional medicine, a form of integrative practice that focuses on body chemistry. It is important to know how long physicians have been actively practicing functional medicine and how extensively they are involved in cancer care.

Mainstream Integrative Medicine

www.blockmd.com

The Block Center for Integrative Cancer Care in Evanston, Illinois, is a cancer center that includes nutrition, immunotherapy, and European approaches to chemotherapy.

www.mskcc.org/mskcc/html/1979.cfm
Memorial Sloan-Kettering Cancer Center in New York provides mainstream cancer treatment in combination with adjunctive complementary therapies.

http://nccam.nih.gov/
The National Center for Complementary and Alternative Medicine
(NCCAM), at the National Institutes of Health, sponsors research on
complementary medicine, including cancer therapies.

www.dendritic-cells.org/EN/index.html
This website from the Medical Center Cologne provides information
on dendritic cells and their applications in oncologic treatment. It
includes selected information from scientific sources, patients' tes-
timonies (in writing and through video clips), and documentation
from clinicians and medical centers throughout the world with extensive experience in cancer therapies.

Nutrition and Diet

http://crazysexylife.com/
This is Kris Carr's website and network of blogs and brief inspirational
videos on vegetarian and raw-food approaches to nutrition and other
aspects of healthy lifestyle for cancer support.

www.eatingwell.com/
This is *Eating Well* magazine's online version—another site with a broad
emphasis on good nutrition. Recipes, videos, and nutritional information on the Mediterranean diet and other healthy approaches to
delicious food are provided.

www.livestrong.org/
The Lance Armstrong Foundation website provides extensive resources
on diet and exercise, primarily focused on weight loss.

www.vrg.org/

The Vegetarian Resource Group has a broadly focused website on vegetarian food, diet, recipes, and restaurants.

Minimizing Toxic Exposures

www.appetiteforprofit.com/

This nonprofit group's website educates people about plant-based eating and the problems associated with Big Food and agribusiness.

www.cspinet.org/

This website from Center for Science in the Public Interest provides excellent data on food additives and what to avoid.

www.ewg.org/

The Environmental Working Group offers accessible information and research on minimizing toxic exposure in food and water, consumer products, and cosmetics and on finding kid-safe products.

www.FoodIncMovie.com/

This site updates the issues raised in Eric Schlosser's movie *Food Inc.*, which provides a behind-the-scenes look at factory farming in the United States today.

Personal Care Products

www.cosmeticsdatabase.com/

Skin Deep, the cosmetic safety database of the Environmental Working Group, lists products, especially cosmetics, that contain hormone disruptors and other toxins.

www.healthystuff.org

Healthy Stuff, a site sponsored by the Ecology Center, lists harmful ingredients in common household items and children's products.

Resource for Caregivers

http://cancer.ucsf.edu/_docs/crc/Caregiver_GEN.pdf

The Osher Center for Integrative Medicine and the Caregivers Project provides a downloadable sixty-five-page handbook for family caregivers helping to care for loved ones with serious illness.

Mainstream Resources: Government and Conventional Medical Resources

www.aicr.org/

The American Institute for Cancer Research provides cancer information.

www.cancer.gov/

This website of the National Cancer Institute at the NIH, the U.S. government agency for cancer research, gives information on specific types of cancer and clinical trials.

www.cancer.net

This site is sponsored by the American Society for Clinical Oncology.

www.cancer.org/

The American Cancer Society's website provides information on conventional medical approaches to cancer treatment, medications, and services.

http://cancer.ucsf.edu/cancerinfo/

This is the website of the University of California–San Francisco Cancer Center.

www.healthfinder.gov/

This is a resource from the U.S. Department of Health and Human Services for finding government and nonprofit health and human services information on the internet.

www.webmd.com/

WebMD is a corporate, for-profit site that provides comprehensive health information from the perspective of mainstream medicine.

Support

www.acor.org/

The Association of Cancer Online Resources provides mainstream cancer resources such as special interest groups, support groups, and links to cancer clinical trials.

www.blochcancer.org/

The Bloch Cancer Foundation provides support for cancer patients from a mainstream perspective, including a step-by-step guide and a hotline.

www.cancersupportivecare.com/Survivor/index.html

The Cancer Supportive Care website provides access to information and books on cancer survivorship.

www.vitaloptions.org/

This support website provides conventional options through media such as a weekly talk show in conjunction with the National Cancer Institute and the American Society of Clinical Oncology.

Drug, Herb, and Supplement Information

http://dietarysupplements.nlm.nih.gov/dietary/

The National Library of Medicine's dietary supplements labels database gives information on ingredients in dietary supplements and on the health claims by manufacturers.

www.doublecheckmd.com/

This commercial website allows users to check their prescription medications for potential interactions and gives information on side effects.

www.fda.gov/Drugs/default.htm

This website from the U.S. Food and Drug Administration provides information on medication labeling and indications for use, which can be searched by disease condition.

www.mskcc.org/mskcc/html/11570.cfm

On this website, Memorial Sloan-Kettering provides analysis of herbs and possible harmful herb interactions for cancer patients.

Appendix C
GLOSSARY

absolute risk: The actual risk of an occurrence, expressed as a percentage—one chance in one hundred would be 1 percent; ten in one hundred would be 10 percent.

anabolism: The constructive/regenerative phase of metabolism when growth and repair occur. An anabolic (growth) state is the opposite of the catabolic (breakdown) state. *See also* catabolism.

antioxidants: Molecules derived from food that prevent or slow the oxidation of other molecules—oxidation can be compared to rusting. Antioxidants prevent damage caused by free radicals, which are highly reactive. In the human body various nutrients such as vitamin E, vitamin C, and beta-carotene and minerals such as selenium act as antioxidants.

anthroposophy: A spiritual philosophy and method that states that the spiritual world is directly accessible through exercise and discipline, which leads to inner experience and sensory experience and which integrates spirituality with a scientific perspective. It was founded by Rudolf Steiner (1861–1924).

autonomic nervous system (ANS): The branch of the central nervous system that controls most automatic functions such as heart rate, digestion, salivation, perspiration, pupil dilation, and respiration. Most of these functions are typically not under voluntary control (breathing is a notable exception). The ANS divides into the sympathetic nervous system (SNS), which prepares the body for the fight/flight/freeze response, and the parasympathetic nervous system (PNS), which promotes relaxation and regeneration.

Some definitions have been adapted from Wikipedia (http://en.wikipedia.org/wiki/Main_Page)

biphenol A (BPA): A commonly used chemical found in plastics such as polycarbonate plastics and epoxy resins. BPA acts as a hormone disregulator and appears to contribute to cancer growth or interfere with healing.

bracing: The tensing of muscles, usually related to stress or expectation of pain—but not necessary for the performance of a task.

catabolism: The destructive phase of metabolism when breakdown occurs. It is the result of excessive and prolonged activity and/or arousal (e.g., frequent activation of the fight/flight/freeze response) without regenerative breaks. It is the opposite of the anabolic state.

cellular immunity: One component of the immune system that defends the body from cancerous cells and viruses lodged within our bodies' own cells or produced by the body itself. Cellular immunity includes white blood cells such as T cells and other infection fighters. When cellular immunity is compromised or shut down, the body becomes vulnerable to cancer. *See also* humoral immunity.

cholangiocarcinoma: Bile duct cancer.

circadian rhythm: An approximately twenty-four-hour cycle of physiological, biochemical, or behavioral processes that occurs in living organisms.

diaphragm: The major muscle involved in active breathing that is located beneath the ribs and above the stomach. It is a broad, flat panel of muscle below the lungs that can be compared to the bottom of a drum. The diaphragm contracts (flattens and drops) during inhalation and relaxes and moves upward, compressing the lungs, during exhalation.

diaphragmatic breathing: A breathing pattern in which the major movement is initiated with the diaphragm. During inhalation, the abdomen increases in circumference, and during exhalation the abdomen decreases in circumference. A slight chest expansion may occur near the end of inhalation to increase inhalation volume. It is usually associated with an effortless, slower breathing rate, followed by a postexhalation pause and lower arousal. This breathing pattern, if done effortlessly, promotes an anabolic regenerative state.

diurnal rhythm: *See* circadian rhythm.

dysponesis: A term referring to misplaced efforts, muscle contractions, or energy expenditures during an activity, which are not required for the performance of that activity. From the Greek *dys* (bad) and *ponos or ponesis* (effort, work, or energy).

edema: Swelling of the body or a body part due to excessive accumulation of fluid in the tissue.

eurhythmy: An art expression that synthesizes movement, music, and speech in which the body is an instrument for physical, emotional, and spiritual expression. It is based on Rudolf Steiner's anthroposophy. Eurhythmy can be applied therapeutically to support the healing efforts of the body.

fever-range, total-body hyperthermia: A form of treatment involving induced fever, through the slow heating of the patient's core body temperature to about 102.2°F (39°C) and sometimes to 104°F (40.0°C), to activate the patient's immune system. *See also* local or localized hyperthermia.

fight/flight/freeze response: An automatic physiological reaction to stressful stimuli that prepares the body for action by shifting blood away from the periphery and gastrointestinal tract toward the muscles. This response can occur at different levels of intensity, so it is also referred to as the stress response, an alarm reaction, or a startle response.

glioblastoma multiforme: A primary brain tumor in humans that is most common and aggressive and involves the glial cells. It is the cause of 52 percent of all parenchymal brain tumor cases and 20 percent of all intracranial tumors.

glycemic index: A simple measure of how quickly various carbohydrates raise the level of glucose in the blood. Foods that contain refined carbohydrates such as sucrose/sugar are broken down the most rapidly into simple sugars. These fast-metabolizing foods have the highest rating.

hormone disregulators: A group of substances (environmental toxins such as BPA) that mimic naturally produced hormones of the body and may cause developmental pathology or increase the risk of cancer.

humoral immunity: The component of the immune system that produces antibodies (microscopic protein fragments used by the immune system as artillery). Antibodies are produced by mature B cells to defend the body against pathogens and allergens. *See also* cellular immunity.

hyperthermia: Fever induced for therapeutic purposes. Localized hyperthermia involves focused heating of a small area of tissue in the body—in cancer treatment it involves specifically heating tumor cells to destroy them. The fever-range, total-body hyperthermia is a form of induced fever in which the entire body is heated to a low- to midrange fever temperature in order to stimulate immune activity.

hyperventilation: A term referring to rapid overbreathing, which causes abnormally low levels of carbon dioxide in the blood. Hyperventilation can cause dizziness, increases in muscle spasms, and a sense of anxiety or panic.

hypervigilance: Increased arousal and responsiveness to stimuli, usually in response to the threat of danger or compromise of well-being.

immunity: *See* cellular immunity; humoral immunity.

local or localized hyperthermia: Selective heating of a specific area within the body for therapeutic purposes. The temperature in the tissue is increased to 107.6°F (42°C). In cancer treatment, this causes the malignant cell to increase its metabolism. As a result, lactic acid production increases, which causes the cancer cells to become highly acidic (pH declines) to the degree that these cells die (necrosis). This process does not affect neighboring healthy cells, which remain at normal body temperature. *See also* fever-range, total-body hyperthermia.

melanoma: A malignant cancer of the skin.

mindfulness: An attitude of remaining present, watchful, and aware of what is happening without becoming involved or captured by mental

images or feelings. Being truly present implies the absence of anticipating, ruminating, or letting the mind wander.

mistletoe: A plant *(Viscum album)* that has medicinal properties shown
to have anticancer activities.

natural killer (NK) cell: A type of white blood cell that activates or
inhibits part of an immune response. It destroys tumor cells and cells
infected by viruses or minute bacteria that behave like viruses.

natural killer (NK) T cell: A subset of T cells that have an important
immune function to activate or suppress immune responses through
their rapid release of messenger chemicals (cytokines). *See also* natural
killer (NK) cell.

Newcastle disease virus: A bird pest virus that has properties destructive selectively to cancer cells (oncolytic effects). The virus is otherwise
benign in human beings and mammals and is used as a treatment strategy to kill cancer cells.

nocebo: A pill or procedure that in itself has no pharmacological activity
or medical effects but that evokes a nonhealing response and increases
the symptoms or illness. From the Latin, "I will harm."

nonsteroidal anti-inflammatory drugs (NSAIDs): Over-the-counter
analgesic (pain reliever) and antipyretic (fever reducer) medication
such as aspirin, ibuprofen, and Tylenol (acetaminophen) or prescription
drug such as celecoxib and indomethacin. Possible negative side effects
include gastrointestinal ulcers and stomach bleeding.

parasympathetic nervous system (PNS): The branch of the autonomic nervous system that promotes relaxation and regeneration by
shifting the blood from the muscles back to the digestive system while
slowing down the heart rate, thus decreasing arousal. *See also* autonomic
nervous system (ANS).

phagocytosis: A process in which large white blood cells engulf and
ingest harmful foreign particles, bacteria, and dead or dying cells as part
of the immune response.

placebo: A pill or procedure that in itself has no pharmacological activity or medical effects but that evokes a healing response. From the Latin, "I will please."

prostate specific antigen (PSA): A protein manufactured by the prostate gland. High levels of PSA circulating in the blood are often an indicator of prostate cancer or other prostate diseases.

relative risk: The percentage change of one risk as compared with a second risk. This expression of risk can skew the impression of safety or risk. A more realistic estimate is obtained by looking at absolute risk.

REM sleep: State of sleep during which dreaming usually occurs, characterized by rapidly shifting eye movements and mild, involuntary muscle movements.

self-talk: The internal/private dialogue within a person's own mind. Self-talk can positively or negatively affect health and/or performance. Positive self-talk that is supportive and caring leads to feelings of self-efficacy and higher self-esteem, whereas negative self-talk that is non-caring and critical leads to negative feelings of embarrassment or shame.

SNS: *See* sympathetic nervous system (SNS).

Stage IV cancer: The most severe stage in the rating of cancer, with Stage I being the least severe. A Stage IV condition suggests that the tumor has penetrated other tissue and has metastasized and spread to distant organs. The staging of cancer is often a predictor of survival (though not always) and influences treatment strategies.

Steiner, Rudolf: An Austrian philosopher and scientist (1861–1925) who founded anthroposophy, which synthesizes science and spiritual perspectives. His philosophy forms the basis of Waldorf education, biodynamic agriculture, eurythmia (a natural form of dance), and anthroposophical medicine.

sympathetic arousal (flight/fight/freeze): A term referring to the activation of the sympathetic branch of the autonomic (automatic) nervous system. This reaction, which prepares the body for vigorous action, results in an increase in arterial blood pressure, increased cardiac output, increased blood flow to muscles, decreased blood flow to the organs (since that is not needed for rapid physical activity), increased cellular metabolism through the body, increased muscle strength, and increased mental alertness and hypervigilance. Prolonged or chronically high stress and sympathetic arousal shifts the body to a catabolic state depleting physical resources.

sympathetic nervous system (SNS): The branch of the autonomic nervous system that prepares the body for the fight/flight/freeze response by shifting the blood from the gastrointestinal tract and periphery to the muscles. *See also* autonomic nervous system (ANS).

T cell: *See* natural killer (NK) T cell.

thoracic breathing: A dysfunctional and strained breathing pattern in which the major movement is initiated by lifting the chest and that is usually associated with a faster breathing rate, rapid shallow inhalation, and increased arousal. In most cases there is minimal diaphragmatic breathing, evidenced by less abdominal movement.

total-body hyperthermia: *See* fever-range, total-body hyperthermia.

Viscum album. *See* mistletoe.

Notes

Prologue

1. E. Simpson, "The Perfection of Hope," *The Globe and Mail* (Toronto), March 16, 1996, D5.

Chapter 1

2. H. Wagenmakers, *Artsen uit de Wereld van het Licht-Over wonderbaarlijke genezingen* (Deventer, Netherlands: Ankh-Hermes B.V., 2007). In this book, Harmen describes his remarkable recovery from end-stage bile-duct cancer.

3. C. Hirschberg and M. Barasch, *Remarkable Recovery: What Extraordinary Healings Tell Us about Getting Well and Staying Well* (New York: Riverhead Trade, 1996). L. LeShan, *Cancer as a Turning Point* (New York: Plume, 1999). E. F. Lewison, "Spontaneous Regression of Breast Cancer," *Journal of the National Cancer Institute Monographs*, 44 (1976): 23–26. R. Van Overbruggen, *Healing Psyche: Patterns and Structure of Complementary Psychological Cancer Treatment (CPCT)* (Charleston, SC: BookSurge, 2006).

4. R. Gorter and E. Peper, "Treating Prostate Cancer with Immune Therapy Using the Gorter Model," *Townsend Letter—The Examiner of Alternative Medicine* 329 (2010): 44–49.

5. D. Krex, B. Klink, C. Hartmann, et al., "Long-term Survival with Glioblastoma Multiforme," *Brain* 130, no. 10 (2007): 2596–2606. E. G. Shawl, W. Seiferheld, C. Scott, et al., "Re-examining the Radiation Therapy Oncology Group (RTOG) Recursive Partitioning Analysis (RPA) for Glioblastoma Multiforme (GBM) Patients," *International Journal of Radiation Oncology, Biology, Physics* 57, no. 2 (2003): S135–136.

6. G. Kolata, "Advances Elusive in the Drive to Cure Cancer," *New York Times*, April 24, 2009. Data adapted from CDC/NCHS, National Vital Statistics System, Health, United States, 2009, Figure 18.

7. Data adapted from CDC/NCHS, National Vital Statistics System, Health, United States, 2009, Figure 18.

8. Heidi D. Nelson, K. Tyne, A. Naik, C. Bougatsos, B. K. Chan, and L. Humphrey, "Screening for Breast Cancer: An Update for the U.S. Preventive Services Task Force," *Annals of Internal Medicine* 17, no. 151 (2009); 727–737. P. Zahl, J. Maehlen, and H. G. Welch, "The Natural History of Invasive Breast Cancers

Detected by Screening Mammography," *Archives of Internal Medicine* 168, no. 21 (2008): 2311–2316.

9. In 2006, the latest year for which statistics are available from USCS, 191,410 women were diagnosed with breast cancer, and 40,820 women died from the disease, Data from the Centers for Disease Control and Prevention, www.cdc.gov/cancer/breast/.

10. N. N. Taleb, *The Black Swan: The Impact of the Highly Improbable* (New York: Penguin Books, 2007).

11. J. P. Van Netten and C. van Netten, "Dr. William Coley and Tumour Regression: A Place in History or in the Future," *Journal of Postgraduate Medicine* 799, no. 38 (2003): 672–680. U. Hobohm, "Fever and Cancer in Perspective," *Cancer Immunology Immunotherapy* 50 (2001): 391–396. H. Coley-Nauts, W. E. Swift, and B. L. Coley, "The Treatment of Malignant Tumors by Bacterial Toxins as Developed by the Late William B. Coley, MM, Reviewed in the Light of Modern Research," *Cancer Research* (1946): 205–216. R. Kleef and D. Hager, "Incidence of Malignancies and Missing History of Fever," in *Hyperthermia in Cancer Treatment: A Primer*, ed. G. F. Baronzio and E. Hager (New York: Springer, 2006), 276–337.

12. Japanese Society for Thermal Medicine, *Hyperthermia* (Kobe, Japan: Shinkyobuko, 2008). T. Yoshikawa and S. Kokura, *Hyperthermic Immunology for Cancer* (Tokyo: Sindan To Chiryo Sha, 2008). U.S. Department of Health and Human Services, National Institutes of Health, "FactSheet: Hyperthermia," in Cancer Treatment: Questions and Answers (2004), available at www.cancer.gov.

13. D. Ornish, *Dr. Dean Ornish's Program for Reversing Heart Disease* (New York: Ballantine Books, 1992).

Chapter 2

14. J. K. Kiecolt-Glaser, L. McGuire, T. F. Robles, and R. Glaser, "Emotions, Morbidity, and Mortality: New Perspectives from Psychoneuroimmunology," *Annual Review of Psychology* 53 (2002): 83–107.

15. S. W. Porges, "The Polyvagal Perspective," *Biological Psychology* 74 (2007): 116–143.

16. The diagnosis and especially cancer treatment can cause posttraumatic stress disorder in patients. L. J. Kwekeboom and S. J. Seng, "Recognizing and Responding to Post-traumatic Stress Disorder in People with Cancer," *Oncology Nursing Forum* 29, no. 4 (2002): 643–649. Post-traumatic Stress Disorder (PDQ®), National Cancer Institute, U.S. National Institutes of Health, available at www.cancer.gov/cancertopics/pdq/supportivecare/post-traumatic-stress/

Patient/page2. M. Y. Smith, W. H. Redd, C. Peyser, and D. Vogl, "Post-traumatic Stress Disorder in Cancer: A Review," *Psycho-Oncology* 8, no. 6 (1999): 521–537.

17. This is a movement art expression developed by Rudolph Steiner that is taught in the anthroposophy-based Waldorf Schools. It synthesizes movement, music, and speech.

18. S. Greer, T. Morris, and K. Pettingale, "Psychological Response to Breast Cancer: Effect on Outcome," *Lancet* 335 (1979): 49–50. R. Van Overbruggen, *Healing Psyche* (Charleston, SC: BookSurge, 2006). S. Seeman and S. Lewis, "Powerlessness, Health, and Mortality: A Longitudinal Study of Older Men and Mature Women," *Social Science and Medicine* 41, no. 4 (1995): 517–525. J. K. Kiecolt-Glaser, L. McGuire, T. F. Robles, and R. Glaser, "Emotions, Morbidity, and Mortality: New Perspectives from Psychoneuroimmunology," *Annual Review of Psychology,* 53 (2002): 83–107.

19. L. Payer, *Medicine and Culture* (New York: Henry Holt, 1988).

20. P. Zahl, J. Mæhlen, and H. G. Welch, "The Natural History of Invasive Breast Cancers Detected by Screening Mammography," *Archives of Internal Medicine* 168, no. 21 (2008): 2311–2316.

21. U.S. Preventive Services Task Force, "Screening for Breast Cancer: U.S. Preventive Services Task Force Recommendation Statement," *Annals of Internal Medicine* 15, no. 10 (2009): 716–726. U.S. Preventive Services Task Force, www.ahrq.gov/clinic/uspstfab.htm (Rockville, MD: Agency for Healthcare Research and Quality, June 2010).

22. National Cancer Institute (NCI) and the National Institute of Environmental Health Sciences (NIEHS), *Cancer and the Environment: What You Need to Know; What You Can Do,* NIH Publication No. 03–2039 (2003).

23. D. Ornish, M. J. Magbanua, G. Weidner, et al., "Intensive Lifestyle Changes May Affect the Progression of Prostate Cancer," *Journal of Urology* 174, no. 3 (2005): 1065–69 (discussion 9–70). See also D. Servan-Schreiber, *Anticancer: A New Way of Life* (New York: Viking Press, 2008).

24. H. G. Welch, *Should I Be Tested for Cancer?* (Berkeley: University of California Press, 2004).

25. E. D. Robin, *Matters of Life and Death: Risks versus Benefits of Medical Care* (New York: Freeman, 1984).

26. W. Bogdanich, "Radiation Boom: Radiation Offers New Cures, and Ways to Do Harm," *New York Times,* January 24, 2010. B. M. Kuehn, "FDA Warning: CT Scans Exceeded Proper Doses," *JAMA* 303, no. 2 (2010): 124.

27. S. Ben-Eliyahu, "The Promotion of Tumor Metastasis by Surgery and Stress: Immunological Basis and Implications for Psychoneuroimmunology. *Brain, Behavior, and Immunity* 17, no. 1, suppl. 1 (2003): 27–36.

28. H. G. Welch, *Should I Be Tested For Cancer?* (Berkeley: University of California Press, 2004).

Chapter 3

29. P. Lichtenstein, N. V. Holm, P. K. Verkasalo, A. Iliadou, J. Kaprio, M. Koskenvuo, E. Pukkala, A. Skythe, and K. Hemminki, "Environmental and Heritable Factors in the Causation of Cancer: Analyses of Cohorts of Twins from Sweden, Denmark, and Finland," *New England Journal of Medicine* 343, no. 2 (2000): 78–85.

30. Colborn, T., D. Dumanoski, and J. P. Myers, *Our Stolen Future* (New York: Dutton, 1996). J. Rizzo, "BPA and Breast Cancer," *Strong Voices*, 14 (2009): 1–7 (available at www.breastcancerfund.org). National Cancer Institute (NCI) and the National Institute of Environmental Health Sciences (NIEHS), *Cancer and the Environment What You Need to Know What You Can Do*, NIH Publication No. 03-2039 (2003). S. Steingraber, *Living Downstream* (New York: Vintage Books, 1998). The President's Cancer Panel, "Reducing Environmental Cancer Risk: What We Can Do Now," National Cancer Institute, National Institutes of Health, U.S. Department of Health and Human Services, April 2010.

31. J. R. Satin, W. Linden, and M. J. Phillips, "Depression as a Predictor of Disease Progression and Mortality in Cancer Patients: A Meta-Analysis," *Cancer* 115, no. 22 (2010): 5349–5361. R. Van Overbruggen, *Healing Psyche* (Charleston, SC: BookSurge, 2006).

Chapter 4

32. The President's Cancer Panel, "Reducing Environmental Cancer Risk: What We Can Do Now," National Cancer Institute, National Institutes of Health, U.S. Department of Health and Human Services, April 2010.

33. R. Kleef and D. Hager, "Incidence of Malignancies and Missing History of Fever," in *Hyperthermia in Cancer Treatment: A Primer*, ed. G. F. Baronzio and E. Hager (New York: Springer, 2006), 276–337.

34. R. K. Beasley, T. Clayton, J. Crane, J. von Mutius, C. K. Lai, S. Montefort, A. Stewart, and Phase Three Study Group, "Association between Paracetamol Use in Infancy and Childhood, and Risk of Asthma, Rhinoconjunctivitis, and Eczema in Children Aged 6–7 Years: Analysis from Phase Three of the ISAAC Programme," *Lancet* 20, no. 372 (2008): 1039–1048.

Chapter 5

35. E. M. Sternberg, *Healing Spaces: The Science of Place and Well-Being* (Cambridge, MA: Harvard University Press, 2009).

Chapter 6

36. R. Kleef and D. Hager, "Incidence of Malignancies and Missing History of Fever" in *Hyperthermia in Cancer Treatment: A Primer*, ed. G. F. Baronzio and E. Hager (New York: Springer, 2006).

37. G. F. Baronzio and E. Hager, *Hyperthermia in Cancer Treatment: A Primer* (New York: Springer, 2006), 276–337. Japanese Society for Thermal Medicine, *Hyperthermia* (Kobe, Japan: Shinkyobuko, 2008). T. Yoshikawa and S. Kokura, *Hyperthermic Immunology for Cancer* (Tokyo: Sindan To Chiryo Sha, Inc., 2008).

38. J. F. Duffy, D. J. Dijk, E. G. Klerman, and C. A. Czeisler, "Later Endogenous Circadian Temperature Nadir Relative to an Earlier Wake Time in Older People," *Am J Physiol Regul Integr Comp Physiol* 8 (1998): 275.

39. Use of paracetamol in the first year of life and in later childhood is associated with risk of asthma, rhinoconjunctivitis, and eczema at age 6 to 7 years. R. K. Beasley, T. Clayton, J. Crane, J. von Mutius, C. K. Lai, S. Montefort, A. Stewart, and Phase Three Study Group, "Association between Paracetamol Use in Infancy and Childhood, and Risk of Asthma, Rhinoconjunctivitis, and Eczema in Children Aged 6–7 Years: Analysis from Phase Three of the ISAAC Programme," *Lancet* 20, no. 372 (2008): 1039–1048.

40. Teun van Vliet's remarkable recovery from end-stage primary brain cancer has been written up in the following book: G. Bindels, *Teun van Vliet-Drank, Vrouwen, de Koers en de Dood* (Leeuwarden, Netherlands: Elikser, 2010).

41. J. Overgaard, "Effect of Hyperthermia on Malignant Cells *In Vivo:* A Review and a Hypothesis," *Cancer* 39, no. 6 (2006): 2637–2646.

42. The electro-hyperthermia equipment used in this protocol was developed by the German company Celsius 42.

43. F. Dietzel, "Basic Principles in Hyperthermic Tumor Therapy," *Recent Respite Cancer Res* 86 (1983): 177–190. T. Kerner et al., "Whole Body Hyperthermia: A Secure Procedure for Patients with Various Malignancies?" *Intensive Care Med* 25, no. 9 (1999): 959–965. W. G. Kraybill et al., "A Phase I Study of Fever-Range Whole Body Hyperthermia (FR-WBH) in Patients with Advanced Solid Tumours: Correlation with Mouse Models," *Int J Hyperthermia* 18, no. 3 (2002): 253–266.

44. D. Atanackovic et al., "Patients with Solid Tumors Treated with High-

Temperature Whole Body Hyperthermia Show a Redistribution of Naïve/Memory T-Cell Subtypes," *Am J Physiol Regul Integr Comp Physiol* 290, no. 3 (2006): R585–594.

45. H. Wehner, A. von Arden, and S. Kaltofen, "Whole-Body Hyperthermia with Water-Filtered Infrared Radiation: Technical-Physical Aspects and Clinical Experiences," *Int J Hyperthermia* 17, no. 1 (2001): 19–30.

46. T. J. Doering et al., "Cerebral Autoregulation during Whole-Body Hyperthermia and Hyperthermia Stimulus," *Am J Phys Med Rehabil* 78, no. 1 (1999): 33–38.

47. I. Bedrosian et al., "Intranodal Administration of Peptide-Pulsed Mature Dendritic Cell Vaccines Results in Superior CD8+ T-Cell Function in Melanoma Patients," *J Clin Oncol* 21, no. 20 (2003): 3826–3835.

48. M. Franckena et al., "Radiotherapy and Hyperthermia for Treatment of Primary Locally Advanced Cervix Cancer: Results in 378 Patients," *Int J Radiat Oncol Biol Phys* 73, no. 1 (2009): 242–255.

49. J. M. Bull et al., "Fever-Range Whole-Body Thermal Therapy Combined with Cisplatin, Gemcitabine, and Daily Interferon-Alpha: Description of a Phase I–II Protocol," *Int J Hyperthermia* 24, no. 8 (2008): 649–662.

50. M. Kappel et al., "Somatostatin Attenuates the Hyperthermia Induced Increase in Neurtrophil Concentration," *Euro J Appl Physiol Occup Physiol* 77, no. 1–2 (1998): 149–56.

51. Dietzel, "Basic Principles." Kerner et al., "Whole Body Hyperthermia."

52. M. Kappel, T. D. Poulsen, H. Galbo, and B. K. Pedersen, "Influence of Minor Increases in Plasma Catecholamines on Natural Killer Cell Activity," *Horm Res* 49, no. 1 (1998): 22–26.

53. P. Wust et al., "Feasibility and Analysis of Thermal Parameters for the Whole-Body-Hyperthermia System IRATHERM-2000," *Int J Hyperthermia* 16, no. 4 (2000): 325–339.

54. Dietzel, "Basic Principles." Kerner et al., "Whole Body Hyperthermia."

55. M. Zellner et al., "Human Monocyte Stimulation by Experimental Whole Body Hyperthermia," *Wien Klin Wochenschr* 114, no. 3 (2002): 102–107.

56. Doering et al., "Cerebral Autoregulation."

57. H. I. Robins et al., "Phase I Clinical Trial Of Melphalan and 41.8 Degrees C Whole-Body Hyperthermia in Cancer Patients," *Clin Oncol* 15, no. 1 (1997): 158–164.

58. R. Oehler et al., "Cell Type-Specific Variations in the Induction of hsp70

in Human Leukocytes by Feverlike Whole Body Hyperthermia," *Cell Stress Chaperones* 6, no. 4 (2001): 306–315.

59. Atanackovic et al., "Patients with Solid Tumors."

60. T. Brockow, A. Wagner, A. Franke, M. Offenbacher, and K. L. Resch, "A Randomized Controlled Trial on the Effectiveness of Mild Water-Filtered Near Infrared Whole-Body Hyperthermia as an Adjunct to a Standard Multimodal Rehabilitation in the Treatment of Fibromyalgia," *Clin J Pain* 23, no. 1 (2007): 67–75.

61. Kraybill et al., "A Phase I Study."

62. Franckena et al., "Radiotherapy and Hyperthermia."

63. Bull et al., "Fever-Range Whole-Body Thermal Therapy."

64. Wust et al., "Feasibility and Analysis."

65. Brockow et al. "A Randomized Controlled Trial."

66. Bedrosian et al., "Intranodal Administration."

67. Bull et al., "Fever-Range Whole-Body Thermal Therapy."

68. M. J. Kluger, "Fever: Role of Pyrogens and Cryogens," *Physiol Rev* 71, no. 1 (1991): 93–127. N. J. Roberts Jr., "The Immunological Consequences of Fever," in *Fever: Basic Mechanisms and Management,* ed. P. A. Mackowiak (New York: Raven, 1991), 125. N. J. Roberts Jr., "Impact of Temperature Elevation on Immunologic Defenses," *Rev Infect Dis* 13, no. 3 (1991): 462–72.

69. National Library of Medicine, MeSH Database, available at www.ncbi .nlm.nih.gov/sites/mesh (accessed July 20, 2010).

70. R. Kleef, W. B. Jonas, W. Knogler, and W. Stenzinger, "Fever, Cancer Incidence and Spontaneous Remissions," *Neuroimmunomodulation* 9, no. 2 (2001): 55–64. Kleef and Hager, "Incidence of Malignancies."

71. J. Z. Laurence, "The Diagnosis of Surgical Cancer (Liston Prize Essay for 1854)," (London: Churchill, 1854), 56.

72. R. Kleef and E. Dieter Hager, "Fever, Pyrogens and Cancer," available at www.ncbi.nlm.nih.gov/bookshelf/br.fcgi?book=eurekah&part=A59581 (accessed July 14, 2010).

73. W. Remy, K. Hammerschmidt, K. S. Zänker, et al., "Tumorträger haben selten Infekte in der Anamnese" *Med Klinik* 78 (1983): 95–98.

74. K. Kölmel, O. Gefeller, and B. Haverkamp, "Febrile Infections and Malignant Melanoma: Results of a Case-Control Study," *Melanoma Res* 2 (1992): 207–211.

75. B. Schlehofer, M. Blettner, N. Becker, et al., "Medical Risk Factors and Development of Brain Tumors," *Cancer* 69 (1992): 2541–2547.

76. C. A. Dinarello, "Endogenous Pyrogens," in *Fever: Basic Mechanisms and Management*, ed. P. A. Mackowiak (New York: Raven, 1991): 23. C. A. Dinarello, "Thermoregulation and the Pathogenesis of Fever," *Infect Dis Clin North Am* 10, no. 2 (1996): 433–49.

77. R. H. Burdon, "The Heat Shock Proteins," *Endeavour* 12, no. 3 (1988): 133–138. R. Dressel, L. Heine, L. Elsner, et al., "Induction of Heat Shock Protein 70 Genes in Human Lymphocytes during Fever Therapy," *Eur J Clin Invest* 26, no. 6 (1996): 499–505.

78. Roberts Jr., "The Immunological Consequences." Roberts Jr., "Impact of Temperature Elevation."

79. Kluger, "Fever." Roberts Jr., "The Immunological Consequences." Roberts Jr., "Impact of Temperature Elevation."

80. M. L. Newhouse, R. M. Pearson, J. M. Fullerton, et al., "A Case Control Study of Carcinoma of the Ovary," *Brit J Preventive Social Med* 31 (1977): 148–153.

81. T. Rønne, "Measles Virus Infection without Rash in Children Is Related to Disease in Adult Life," *Lancet* 8419 (1985): 1–5.

82. H. A. van Steensel-Moll, H. A. Valkenburg, and G. E. van Zanen, "Childhood Leukemia and Infectious Diseases in the First Year of Life: A Register Based Case-Control Study," *Am J Epidemiol* 124 (1986): 590–594.

83. H. Flöistrup, J. Swartz, A. Bergström, J. S. Alm, A. Scheynius, M. van Hage, M. Waser, C. Braun-Fahrländer, D. Schram-Bijkerk, M. Huber, A. Zutavern, E. von Mutius, E. Ublagger, J. Riedler, K. B. Michaels, G. Pershagen, and the Parsifal Study Group, "Allergic Disease and Sensitization in Steiner School Children," *J Allergy Clin Immunol* 117, no. 1 (2006): 59–66.

84. R. Gorter, unpublished clinical data, Medical Center Cologne (Cologne, Germany), 2010.

85. R. Gorter, unpublished data, Medical Center Cologne (Cologne, Germany), 2010.

86. R. Ader and N. Cohen, "Behaviorally Conditioned Immunosuppression," *Psychosomatic Medicine* 37, no. 4 (1975): 333–340. R. Ader, "Conditioned Immunomodulation: Research Needs and Directions," *Brain Behav Immun* 17, suppl. 1 (2003): S51–57. M. U. Goebel, A. E. Trebst, J. Steiner, Y. F. Xie, M. S. Exton, S. Frede, A. Canbay, M. C. Michel, U. Heeman, and M. Schedlowski, "Behavioral Conditioning of Immunosuppression Is Possible in Humans," *FASEB Journal* 16 (2002): 1869–1873. R. Hiramoto, C. Rogers, S. Demissie, C. M. Hsueh, N. Hiramoto, J. Lorden, and V. Ghanta, "The Use of Conditioning to Probe for CNS

Pathways That Regulate Fever and NK Cell Activity," *Int J Neurosci* 84, no. 1–4 (1996): 229–45.

87. D. Sevan-Schreiber, *Anticancer: A New Way of Life* (New York: Viking, 2008), 1.

88. A. Hildesheim, C. L. Han, L. A. Brinton, R. J. Kurman, and J. T. Schiller, "Human Papillomavirus Type 16 and Risk of Preinvasive and Invasive Vulvar Cancer: Results from a Seroepidemiological Case-Control Study," *Obstet Gynecol* 90, no. 5 (1997): 748–54.

89. Y. Zhu, Y. Jin, X. Guo, X. Bai, T. Chen, J. Wang, G. Qian, J. D. Groopman, J. Gu, J. Li, and H. Tu, "Comparison Study of Complete Sequences of Hepatitis B Virus Identifies New Mutations in Core Gene Associated with Hepatocellular Carcinoma," *Cancer Epidemiol Biomarkers Prev* (August 10, 2010; forthcoming).

90. P. M. Webb, K. J. Hengels, H. Møller, D. G. Newell, D. Palli, J. B. Elder, M. P. Coleman, G. De Backer, and D. Forman, "The Epidemiology of Low Serum Pepsinogen A Levels and an International Association with Gastric Cancer Rates: EUROGAST Study Group," *Gastroenterology* 107, no. 5 (1994): 1335–44.

91. Flöistrup et al., "Allergic Disease."

92. R. K. Beasley, T. Clayton, J. Crane, J. von Mutius, C. K. Lai, S. Montefort, A. Stewart, and Phase Three Study Group, "Association between Paracetamol Use in Infancy and Childhood, and Risk of Asthma, Rhinoconjunctivitis, and Eczema in Children Aged 6–7 Years: Analysis from Phase Three of the ISAAC Programme," *Lancet* 20, no. 372 (2008): 1039–1048.

93. Beasley et al., "Association between Paracetamol Use."

94. Available at www.healthsentinel.com (accessed July 14, 2010).

95. T. McKeown, *The Role of Medicine: Dream, Mirage, or Nemesis?* (Princeton, NJ: Princeton University Press, 1979).

96. M. von Ardenne, "Spontaneous Remission of Tumors following Hyperthermia: A Feedback Process?" *Naturwissenschaften* 52, no. 23 (1965): 645. M. von Ardenne, R. A. Chaplain, and P. G. Reitnauer, "In Vivo Studies on Cancer Multiple-Step Therapy Using the Attack Combination of Optimum Tumor Overacidification, Hyperthermia and Weak X-Irradiation," *Dtsch Gesundheitsw* 24, no. 20 (1969): 924–35. M. von Ardenne and P. G. Reitnauer, "Measurements on Selective Damage to Cancer Cells in Vitro by Attack-Combination with Hyperacidification Plus 40 Degree C Hyperthermia and Various Bile Acids with Favorable pH," *Arzneimittelforschung* 20, no. 3 (1970): 323–9. M. von Ardenne and F. Rieger, "On the Present State of Extreme Total-Body Hyperthermia as

Element in the Cancer Therapy," *Krebsforsch Klin Onkol Cancer Res Clin Oncol* (1967): 4341–4. M. von Ardenne, "Synergic Therapeutic Effect of Selective Local Hyperthermia and Selective Optimized Hyperacidity against Tumors: Theoretical and Experimental Bases," *Ther Ggw* 116, no. 7 (1977): 1299–316. S. R. Ash, C. R. Steinhart, M. F. Curfman, C. H. Gingrich, D. A. Sapir, E. L. Ash, J. M. Fausset, and M. B. Yatvin, "Extracorporeal Whole Body Hyperthermia Treatments for HIV Infection and AIDS," *ASAIO J* 43, no. 5 (1997): M830–8. A. Atmaca, S. E. Al-Batran, A. Neumann, Y. Kolassa, D. Jäger, A. Knuth, and E. Jäger, "Whole-Body Hyperthermia (WBH) in Combination with Carboplatin in Patients with Recurrent Ovarian Cancer: A Phase II Study," *Gynecol Oncol* 112, no. 2 (2009): 384–8. A. Bakhshandeh, I. Bruns, K. Eberhardt, and G. J. Wiedemann, "Chemotherapy in Combination with Whole-Body Hyperthermia in Advanced Malignant Pleural Mesothelioma [article in German]," *Dtsch Med Wochenschr* 125, no. 11 (2000): 317–9. A. Bakhshandeh, I. Bruns, A. Traynor, H. I. Robins, K. Eberhardt, A. Demedts, E. Kaukel, G. Koschel, U. Gatzemeier, T. Kohlmann, K. Dalhoff, E. M. Ehlers, Y. Gruber, R. Zumschlinge, S. Hegewisch-Becker, S. O. Peters, and G. J. Wiedemann, "Ifosfamide, Carboplatin and Etoposide Combined with 41.8 Degrees C Whole Body Hyperthermia for Malignant Pleural Mesothelioma," *Lung Cancer* 39, no. 3 (2003): 339–45. D. Blake, P. Bessey, I. Karl, et al., "Hyperthermia Induces IL-1 Alpha but Does Not Decrease Release of IL-1 Alpha or TNF-Alpha After Endotoxin," *Lymphokine Cytokine Res* 13, no. 5 (1994): 271–5. J. M. Bull, L. H. Cronau, B. M. Newman, K. Jabboury, S. J. Allen, S. Ohno, T. Smith, and A. S. Tonnesen, "Chemotherapy Resistant Sarcoma Treated with Whole Body Hyperthermia (WBH) Combined with 1-3-bis(2-chloroethyl)-1-nitrosourea (BCNU)," *Int J Hyperthermia* 8, no. 3 (1992): 297–304. R. Burd, T. S. Dziedzic, X. Yan, et al., "Tumor Cell Apoptosis, Lymphocyte Recruitment and Tumor Vascular Changes Are Induced by Low Temperature, Long Duration (Fever-Like) Whole Body Hyperthermia," *J Cell Physiol* 177 (1998): 137–147. I. Bruns, T. Kohlmann, G. J. Wiedemann, and A. Bakhshandeh, "Evaluation of the Therapeutic Benefit of 41.8 Degrees C Whole Body Hyperthermia Plus Ifosfamide, Carboplatin and Etoposide (ICE) for Patients with Malignant Pleural Mesothelioma Using the Modified Brunner-Score (MBS) [article in German]," *Pneumologie* 58, no. 4 (2004): 210–6. J. E. Ensor, S. M. Wiener, and K. A. McCrea, et al., "Differential Effects of Hyperthermia on Macrophage Interleukin-6 and Tumor Necrosis Factor-Alpha Expression," *Am J Physiol* 266, no. 4, pt. 1 (1994): C967–74. M. Deja, B. Hildebrandt, O. Ahlers, H. Riess, P. Wust,

H. Gerlach, and T. Kerner, "Goal-Directed Therapy of Cardiac Preload in Induced Whole-Body Hyperthermia," *Chest* 128, no. 2 (2005): 580–6. R. Engelhardt, U. Müller, R. Weth-Simon, H. A. Neumann, and G. W. Löhr, "Treatment of Disseminated Malignant Melanoma with Cisplatin in Combination with Whole-Body Hyperthermia and Doxorubicin," *Int J Hyperthermia* 6, no. 3 (1990): 511–5. A. Fippel, A. Von Sandersleben, K. Bangert, J. Horn, A. Nierhaus, and F. Wappler, "Monitoring of Whole-Body Hyperthermia with Transesophageal Echocardiography (TEE)," *Int J Hyperthermia* 23, no. 5 (2007): 457–66. P. A. Hancock and G. R. Dirkin, "Central and Peripheral Visual Choice-Reaction Time under Conditions of Induced Cortical Hyperthermia," *Percept Mot Skills* 54, no. 2 (1982): 395–402. K. Haranaka, A. Sakurai, and N. Satomi, "Antitumor Activity of Recombinant Human Tumor Necrosis Factor in Combination with Hyperthermia, Chemotherapy, or Immunotherapy," *J Biol Response Mod* 6 (1987): 379–391. K. Haranaka, N. Satomi, A. Sakurai, et al., "Antitumour Effects of Tumour Necrosis Factor: Cytotoxic or Necrotizing Activity and Its Mechanism," *Ciba Found Symp* 131 (1987): 140–53. S. Hegewisch-Becker, Y. Gruber, A. Corovic, U. Pichlmeier, D. Atanackovic, A. Nierhaus, and D. K. Hossfeld, "Whole-Body Hyperthermia (41.8 Degrees C) Combined with Bimonthly Oxaliplatin, High-Dose Leucovorin and 5-Fluorouracil 48-Hour Continuous Infusion in pretreated Metastatic Colorectal Cancer: A Phase II Study," *Ann Oncol* 13, no. 8 (2002): 1197–204. B. Hildebrandt, J. Dräger, T. Kerner, M. Deja, J. Löffel, C. Stroszczynski, O. Ahlers, R. Felix, H. Riess, and P. Wust, "Whole-Body Hyperthermia in the Scope of von Ardenne's Systemic Cancer Multistep Therapy (sCMT) Combined with Chemotherapy in Patients with Metastatic Colorectal Cancer: A Phase I/II Study," *Int J Hyperthermia* 20, no. 3 (2004): 317–33. R. S. Ismail-Zade, "Whole Body Hyperthermia Supplemented with Urotropin in the Treatment of Malignant Tumors," *Exp Oncol* 27, no. 1 (2005): 61–4. Y. Iwashita, S. Goto, M. Tominaga, A. Sasaki, N. Ohmori, T. Goto, S. Sato, M. Ohta, and S. Kitano, "Dendritic Cell Immunotherapy with Poly(D,L-2,4-Diaminobutyric Acid)-Mediated Intratumoral Delivery of the Interleukin-12 Gene Suppresses Tumor Growth Significantly," *Cancer Sci* 96, no. 5 (2005): 303–7. C. Jimenez, B. Melin, G. Savourey, J. C. Launay, A. Alonso, and J. Mathieu, "Effects of Passive Hyperthermia versus Exercise-Induced Hyperthermia on Immune Responses: Hormonal Implications," *Eur Cytokine Netw* 18, no. 3 (2007): 154–61. J. A. Kalapurakal, M. Pierce, A. Chen, and V. Sathiaseelan, "Efficacy of Irradiation and External Hyperthermia in Locally Advanced, Hormone-Refractory or Radiation Recurrent Prostate Cancer: A Preliminary Report," *Int J Radiat Oncol Biol Phys* 57, no. 3 (2003): 654–64. N. Kan, S. Yamasaki, T. Harada, K. Satoh, Y. Ichinose, Y. Moriguchi, H. Kodama, and K. Ohgaki, "Augmentation of Therapeutic Effect of Adoptive Immunotherapy through a Synergy between Transferred Killer Cells and Host's Fresh Lymphocytes [article in Japanese]," *Hum Cell* 5, no. 3 (1992): 236–42. M. Kappel, N. Tvede, M. B. Hansen, et al., "Cytokine Production Ex Vivo: Effect of Raised Body Temperature," *Int J Hyperthermia* 11, no. 3 (1995): 329–35. D. M. Katschinski, R. Benndorf, G. J. Wiedemann, D. L. Mulkerin, R. Touhidi, and H. I. Robins, "Heat Shock Protein Antibodies in Sarcoma Patients Undergoing 41.8 Degrees C Whole Body Hyperthermia," *J Immunother* 22, no. 1 (1999): 67–70. D. M. Katschinski, G. J. Wiedemann, M. Mentzel, D. L. Mulkerin, R. Touhidi, and H. I. Robins, "Optimization of Chemotherapy Administration for Clinical 41.8 Degrees C Whole Body Hyperthermia," *Cancer Lett* 115, no. 2 (1997): 195–9. T. Kerner, M. Deja, O. Ahlers, B. Hildebrandt, A. Dieing, H. Riess, P. Wust, and H. Gerlach, "Monitoring Arterial Blood Pressure during Whole Body Hyperthermia," *Acta Anaesthesiol Scand* 46, no. 5 (2002): 561–6. T. Kerner, B. Hildebrandt, O. Ahlers, M. Deja, H. Riess, J. Draeger, P. Wust, and H. Gerlach, "Anaesthesiological Experiences with Whole Body Hyperthermia," *Int J Hyperthermia* 19, no. 1 (2003): 1–12. R. Kirsch, D. Schmidt, J. Fichler, et al., "Problems of Multiple Step-Therapy of Carcinoma: II. Effect of Hyperthermia on Cancer Tissue," *Dtsch Gesundheitsw* 22, no. 16 (1967): 732–5. R. Kirsch, D. Schmidt, and H. Schmidt, "Problems of Multiple Step-Therapy of Carcinoma. I. On the History of Hyperthermic Treatment," *Dtsch Gesundheitsw* 22 (1967): 15678–81. M. Kosaka, T. Suguhara, K. L. Schmidt, and E. Simon, eds., *Thermotherapy for Neoplasia Inflammation and Pain* (Tokyo: Springer, 2001). F. Lohr, K. Hu, Q. Huang, L. Zhang, T. V. Samulski, M. W. Dewhirst, and C. Y. Li, "Enhancement of Radiotherapy by Hyperthermia-Regulated Gene Therapy," *Int J Radiat Oncol Biol Phys* 48, no. 5 (2000): 1513–8. M. Maeta, S. Koga, J. Wada, M. Yokoyama, N. Kato, H. Kawahara, T. Sakai, M. Hino, T. Ono, and K. Yuasa, "Clinical Evaluation of Total-Body Hyperthermia Combined with Anticancer Chemotherapy for Far-Advanced Miscellaneous Cancer in Japan," *Cancer* 59, no. 6 (1987): 1101–6. M. F. McCarty and K. Kondo, "Integration of Allogeneic Lymphocyte Immunotherapy with Short-Course Chemotherapy and Hypoenergic Hyperthermia: A 'Triple-Threat' Treatment for Disseminated Cancer," *Med Hypotheses* 16, no. 1 (1985): 39–60. P. G. Martin, F. E. Marino, J. Rattey, D. Kay, and J. Cannon, "Reduced Voluntary Activation of Human Skeletal Muscle during Shortening and Lengthening Con-

tractions in Whole Body Hyperthermia," *Exp Physiol* 90, no. 2 (2005): 225–36.
T. Matsuda, Y. Tanaka, N. Takeshita, J. Ishiwata, and Y. Awane, "Clinical Significance of the Combined Use of Radiation Therapy and Hyperthermia [article in Japanese]," *Gan To Kagaku Ryoho* 14, no. 5, pt. 2 (1987): 1508–14. A. Michalsen, D. Löer, D. Melchart, and G. Dobos, "Changes of Short-Time Heart Rate Variability during Hyperthermia Treatment with Infrared A Whole Body Irradiation [article in German]," *Forsch Komplementarmed* 6, no. 4 (1999): 212–5. G. P. Midis, D. F. Fabian, and A. T Lefor, "Lymphocyte Migration to Tumors after Hyperthermia and Immunotherapy," *J Surg Res* 52, no. 5 (1992): 530–6. B. B. Mittal, M. A. Zimmer, V. Sathiaseelan, A. B. Benson III, R. R. Mittal, S. Dutta, S. T. Rosen, S. M. Spies, J. M. Mettler, and M. W. Groch, "Phase I/II Trial of Combined 131I Anti-CEA Monoclonal Antibody and Hyperthermia in Patients with Advanced Colorectal Adenocarcinoma," *Cancer* 78, no. 9 (1996): 1861–70. G. Myhr, "Multimodal Cancer Treatment: Real Time Monitoring, Optimization, and Synergistic Effects," *Technol Cancer Res Treat* 7, no. 5 (2008): 409–14. R. Oehler, E. Pusch, M. Zellner, P. Dungel, N. Hergovics, M. Homoncik, M. M. Eliasen, M. Brabec, and E. Roth, "Cell Type-Specific Variations in the Induction of Hsp70 in Human Leukocytes by Feverlike Whole Body Hyperthermia," *Cell Stress Chaperones* 6, no. 4 (2001): 306–15. M. M. Park, N. B. Hornback, S. Endres, et al., "The Effect of Whole Body Hyperthermia on the Immune Cell Activity of Cancer Patients," *Lymphokine Res* 9, no. 2 (1990): 213–23. G. Parmiani, M. L. Sensi, A. Balsari, M. P. Colombo, C. Gambacorti-Passerini, L. Grazioli, M. Rodolfo, N. Cascinelli, and G. Fossati, "Adoptive Immunotherapy of Cancer with Immune and Activated Lymphocytes: Experimental and Clinical Studies," *Ric Clin Lab* 16, no. 1 (1986): 1–20. R. T. Pettigrew, J. M. Galt, C. M. Ludgate, and A. N. Smith, "Clinical Effects of Whole-Body Hyperthermia in Advanced Malignancy," *Br Med J* 4, no. 5946 (1974): 679–82. M. T. Pritchard, J. R. Ostberg, S. S. Evans, et al., "Protocols for Simulating the Thermal Component of Fever: Preclinical and Clinical Experience," *Methods* 32, no. 1 (2004): 54–62. O. Richel, P. J. Zum Vörde Sive Vörding, R. Rietbroek, J. Van der Velden, J. D. Van Dijk, M. W. Schilthuis, and A. M. Westermann, "Phase II Study of Carboplatin and Whole Body Hyperthermia (WBH) in Recurrent and Metastatic Cervical Cancer," *Gynecol Oncol* 95, no. 3 (2004): 680–5. H. I. Robins, J. D. Cohen, C. L. Schmitt, K. D. Tutsch, C. Feierabend, R. Z. Arzoomanian, D. Alberti, F. d'Oleire, W. Longo, and C. Heiss, et al., "Phase I Clinical Trial of Carboplatin and 41.8 Degrees C Whole-Body Hyperthermia in Cancer Patients," *J Clin Oncol* 11, no. 9 (1993):

1787–94. H. I. Robins, E. Grosen, D. M. Katschinski, W. Longo, C. L. Tiggelaar, M. Kutz, J. Winawer, F. Graziano, "Whole Body Hyperthermia Induction of Soluble Tumor Necrosis Factor Receptors: Implications for Rheumatoid Diseases," *J Rheumatol* 26, no. 12 (1999): 2513–6. H. I. Robins, M. Kutz, G. J. Wiedemann, et al., "Cytokine Induction by 41.8 Degrees C Whole Body Hyperthermia," *Cancer Lett* 97, no. 2 (1995): 195–201. H. I. Robins, W. L. Longo, R. A. Steeves, J. D. Cohen, C. L. Schmitt, A. J. Neville, S. O'Keefe, R. Lagoni, and C. Riggs, "Adjunctive Therapy (Whole Body Hyperthermia versus Lonidamine) to Total Body Irradiation for the Treatment of Favorable B-Cell Neoplasms: A Report of Two Pilot Clinical Trials and Laboratory Investigations," *Int J Radiat Oncol Biol Phys* 18, no. 4 (1990): 909–20. H. I. Robins, K. M. Sielaff, B. Storer, M. J. Hawkins, and E. C. Borden, "Phase I Trial of Human Lymphoblastoid Interferon with Whole Body Hyperthermia in Advanced Cancer," *Cancer Res* 49, no. 6 (1989): 1609–15. R. N. Shen, L. Lu, P. Young, et al., "Influence of Elevated Temperature on Natural Killer Cell Activity, Lymphokine-Activated Killer Cell Activity and Lectin-Dependent Cytotoxicity of Human Umbilical Cord Blood and Adult Blood Cells," *Int J Radiat Oncol Biol Phys* 29, no. 4 (1994): 821–6. E. D. Strauch, D. F. Fabian, J. Turner, et al., "Combined Hyperthermia and Immunotherapy Treatment of Multiple Pulmonary Metastases in Mice," *Surg Oncol* 3, no. 1 (1994): 45–52. D. Steinhausen, W. K. Mayer and M. von Ardenne, "Evaluation of Systemic Tolerance of 42.0 Degrees C Infrared-A Whole-Body Hyperthermia in Combination with Hyperglycemia and Hyperoxemia, "A Phase-I Study," *Strahlenther Onkol* 170, no. 6 (1994): 322–34. R. Smith, J. M. Bull, D. E. Lees, and W. H. Schuette, "Whole Body Hyperthermia: Nursing Management and Intervention," *Cancer Nurs* 3, no. 3 (1980): 185–8. C. R. Steinhart, S. R. Ash, C. Gingrich, D. Sapir, G. N. Keeling, and M. B. Yatvin, "Effect of Whole-Body Hyperthermia on AIDS Patients with Kaposi's Sarcoma: A Pilot Study," *J Acquir Immune Defic Syndr Hum Retrovirol* 11, no. 3 (1996): 271–81. D. Steinhausen, W. K. Mayer, and M. von Ardenne, "Evaluation of Systemic Tolerance of 42.0 Degrees C Infrared-A Whole-Body Hyperthermia in Combination with Hyperglycemia and Hyperoxemia: A Phase-I Study," *Strahlenther Onkol* 170, no. 6 (1995): 322–34. T. Takeda, X. Dong, H. Takeda, A. Haba, and Y. Takeda, "Successful Immunotherapy Combined with Hyperthermia Therapy for Cancer Patients [article in Japanese]," *Gan To Kagaku Ryoho* 33, no. 12 (2006): 1739–41. T. Takeda, K. Fukunaga, K. Miyazawa, T. Takahashi, H. Takeda, Y. Takeda, K. Tanigawa, T. Morisaki, I. Yamamoto, and T. Hasegawa, "Hyperthermic Immuno-

Cellular Therapy: Basic and Clinical Study [article in Japanese]," *Gan To Kagaku Ryoho* 35, no. 12 (2008): 2244–6. R. A. Vertrees, J. B. Zwischenberger, L. C. Woodson, E. A. Bedell, D. J. Deyo, and J. M. Chernin, "Veno-Venous Perfusion-Induced Systemic Hyperthermia: Case Report with Perfusion Considerations," *Perfusion* 16, no. 3 (2001): 243–8. H. Wehner, A. von Ardenne, and S. Kaltofen, "Whole-Body Hyperthermia with Water-Filtered Infrared Radiation: Technical-Physical Aspects and Clinical Experiences," *Int J Hyperthermia* 17, no. 1 (2001): 19–30. A. M. Westermann, G. J. Wiedemann, E. Jager, D. Jager, D. M. Katschinski, A. Knuth, P. Z. Vörde Sive Vörding, J. D. Van Dijk, J. Finet, A. Neumann, W. Longo, A Bakhshandeh, C. L. Tiggelaar, W. Gillis, H. Bailey, S. O. Peters, H. I. Robins, and the Systemic Hyperthermia Oncologic Working Group, "A Systemic Hyperthermia Oncologic Working Group Trial: Ifosfamide, Carboplatin, and Etoposide Combined with 41.8 Degrees C Whole-Body Hyperthermia for Metastatic Soft Tissue Sarcoma," 64, no. 4 (2003): 312–21. G. J. Wiedemann, H. I. Robins, S. Gutsche, M. Mentzel, M. Deeken, D. M. Katschinski, S. Eleftheriadis, R. Crahé, C. Weiss, B. Storer, and T. Wagner, "Ifosfamide, Carboplatin and Etoposide (ICE) Combined with 41.8 Degrees C Whole Body Hyperthermia in Patients with Refractory Sarcoma," *Eur J Cancer* 32A, no. 5 (1996): 888–92. M. Zellner, N. Hergovics, E. Roth, B. Jilma, A. Spittler, and R. Oehler, "Human Monocyte Stimulation by Experimental Whole Body Hyperthermia," *Wien Klin Wochenschr* 114, no. 3 (2002): 102–7. T. Takeda, X. Dong, H. Takeda, A. Haba, and Y. Takeda, "Effects of Intratumoral Injection Therapy of Dendritic Cells Combined with Hyperthermia for Cancer Patients [article in Japanese]," *Gan To Kagaku Ryoho* 34, no. 12 (2007): 1905–7. J. van der Zee, G. J. van den Aardweg, and G. C. van Rhoon, "Thermal Enhancement of Both Tumour Necrosis Factor Alpha-Induced Systemic Toxicity and Tumour Cure in Rats," *Br J Cancer* 71, no. 6 (1995): 1158–62. M. Yonezawa, T. Otsuka, N. Matsui, et al., "Hyperthermia Induces Apoptosis in Malignant Fibrous Histiocytoma Cells in Vitro," *Int J Cancer* 66, no. 3 (1996): 347–51. K. S. Zanker and J. Lange, "Whole Body Hyperthermia and Natural Killer Cell Activity (Letter)," *Lancet* 1, no. 8280 (1982): 1079–80.

Chapter 7

97. K. Mashino, N. Sadanaga, F. Tanaka, M. Ohta, H. Yamaguchi, and M. Mori, "Effective Strategy of Dendritic Cell-Based Immunotherapy for Advanced Tumor-Bearing Hosts: The Critical Role of Th1-Dominant Immunity," *Mol Cancer Ther* 1, no. 10 (2002): 785–94.

98. E. Gilboa, S. K. Nair, and H. K. Lyerly, "Immunotherapy of Cancer with Dendritic-Cell-Based Vaccines," *Cancer Immunol Immunother* 46 (1998): 82–87.

99. F. M. Lemoine, M. Cherai, C. Giverne, D. Dimitri, M. Rosenzwajg, H. Trebeden-Negre, N. Chaput, B. Barrou, N. Thioun, B. Gattegnio, F. Selles, A. Six, N. Azar, J. P. Lotz, A. Buzyn, M. Sibony, A. Delcourt, O. Boyer, S. Herson, D. Klatzmann, and R. Lacave, "Massive Expansion of Regulatory T-Cells Following Interleukin 2 Treatment during a Phase I–II Dendritic Cell-Based Immunotherapy of Metastatic Renal Cancer," *Int J Oncol* 35, no. 3 (2009): 569–81. T. Bachleitner-Hofmann, J. Friedl, M. Hassler, H. Hayden, P. Dubsky, M. Sachet, E. Rieder, R. Pfragner, C. Brostjan, S. Riss, B. Niederle, M. Gnant, and A. Stift, "Pilot Trial of Autologous Dendritic Cells Loaded with Tumor Lysate(s) from Allogeneic Tumor Cell Lines in Patients with Metastatic Medullary Thyroid Carcinoma," *Oncol Rep* 21, no. 6 (2009): 1585–92. D. H. Palmer, R. S. Midgley, N. Mirza, E. E. Torr, F. Ahmed, J. C. Steele, N. M. Steven, D. J. Kerr, L. S. Young, D. H. Adams, "A Phase II Study of Adoptive Immunotherapy Using Dendritic Cells Pulsed with Tumor Lysate in Patients with Hepatocellular Carcinoma," *Hepatology* 49, no. 1 (2009): 124–32.

100. Lemoine et al., "Massive Expansion of Regulatory T-Cells." F. Tanaka, N. Haraguchi, K. Isikawa, H. Inoue, and M. Mori, "Potential Role of Dendritic Cell Vaccination with MAGE Peptides in Gastrointestinal Carcinomas," *Oncol Rep* 20, no. 5 (2008): 1111–1116. H. Kimura, T. Iizasa, A. Ishikawa, M. Shingyouji, M. Yoshino, M. Kimura, Y. Inada, and K. Matsubayashi, "Prospective Phase II Study of Post-Surgical Adjuvant Chemo-Immunotherapy Using Autologous Dendritic Cells and Activated Killer Cells from Tissue Culture of Tumor-Draining Lymph Nodes in Primary Lung Cancer Patients," *Anticancer Res* 28, no. 2B (2008): 1229–38.

101. B. G. Redman, A. E. Chang, J. Whitfield, P. Esper, G. Jiang, T. Braun, B. Roessler, and J. J. Mulé, "Phase Ib Trial Assessing Autologous, Tumor-Pulsed Dendritic Cells as a Vaccine Administered with or without IL-2 in Patients with Metastatic Melanoma," *J Immunother* 31, no. 6 (2008): 591–598.

102. Bachleitner-Hofmann et al., "Pilot Trial of Autologous Dendritic Cells." Palmer et al., "A Phase II Study." A. Van Driessche, A. L. Van de Velde, G. Nijs, T. Braeckman, B. Stein, J. M. De Vries, Z. N. Berneman, and V. F. Van Tendeloo, "Clinical-Grade Manufacturing of Autologous Mature mRNA-Electroporated Dendritic Cells and Safety Testing in Acute Myeloid Leukemia Patients in a Phase I Dose-Escalation Clinical Trial," *Cytotherapy* 11, no. 5 (2009): 653–68. J.

H. Kim, Y. Lee, Y. S. Bae, W. S. Kim, K. Kim, H. Y. Im, W. K. Kang, K. Park, H. Y. Choi, H. M. Lee, S. Y. Baek, H. Lee, H. Doh, B. M. Kim, C. Y. Kim, C. Jeon, and C. W. Jung, "Phase I/II Study of Immunotherapy Using Autologous Tumor Lysate-Pulsed Dendritic Cells in Patients with Metastatic Renal Cell Carcinoma," *Clin Immunol* 125, no. 3 (2007): 257–67.

103. Kimura et al., "Prospective Phase II Study."

104. A. M. Dohnal, V. Witt, H. Hügel, W. Holter, H. Gadner, T. Felzmann, "Phase I Study of Tumor Ag-Loaded IL-12 Secreting Semi-Mature DC for the Treatment of Pediatric Cancer," *Cytotherapy* 9, no. 8 (2007): 755–70. S. De Vleeschouwer, S. Fieuws, S. Rutkowski, F. Van Calenbergh, J. Van Loon, J. Goffin, R. Sciot, G. Wilms, P. Demaerel, M. Warmuth-Metz, N. Soerensen, J. E. Wolff, S. Wagner, E. Kaempgen, and S. W. Van Gool, "Postoperative Adjuvant Dendritic Cell-Based Immunotherapy in Patients with Relapsed Glioblastoma Multiforme," *Clin Cancer Res* 14, no. 10 (2008): 3098–104.

105. Ibid.

106. B. G. Molenkamp, B. J. Sluijter, P. A. van Leeuwen, S. J. Santegoets, S. Meijer, P. G. Wijnands, J. B. Haanen, A. J. van den Eertwegh, R. J. Scheper, and T. D. de Gruijl, "Local Administration of PF-3512676 CpG-B Instigates Tumor-Specific CD8+ T-Cell Reactivity in Melanoma Patients," *Clin Cancer Res* 14, no. 14 (2008): 4532–42.

107. Mashino et al., "Effective Strategy of Dendritic Cell-Based Immunotherapy."

108. Ibid. Tanaka et al., "Potential Role of Dendritic Cell Vaccination." Molenkamp et al., "Local Administration of PF-3512676 CpG-B." D. V. Kouiavskaia, C. A. Berard, E. Datena, A. Hussain, N. Dawson, E. N. Klyushnenkova, and R. B. Alexander, "Vaccination with Agonist Peptide PSA: 154-163 (155L) Derived from Prostate Specific Antigen Induced CD8 T-Cell Response to the Native Peptide PSA: A Phase 2 Study in Patients with Recurrent Prostate Cancer," *J Immunother* 32, no. 6 (2009): 655–66. C. Ménard, J. Y. Blay, C. Borg, S. Michiels, F. Ghiringhelli, C. Robert, C. Nonn, N. Chaput, J. Taïeb, N. F. Delahaye, C. Flament, J. F. Emile, A. Le Cesne, and L. Zitvogel, "Natural Killer Cell IFN-Gamma Levels Predict Long-Term Survival with Imatinib Mesylate Therapy in Gastrointestinal Stromal Tumor-Bearing Patients," *Cancer Res* 69, no. 8 (2009): 3563–9. M. N. López, C. Pereda, G. Segal, L. Muñoz, R. Aguilera, F. E. González, A. Escobar, A. Ginesta, D. Reyes, R. González, A. Mendoza-Naranjo, M. Larrondo, A. Compán, C. Ferrada, and F. Salazar-Onfray, "Prolonged Survival of Dendritic Cell-Vaccinated Melanoma Patients Correlates with Tumor-Specific Delayed Type

IV Hypersensitivity Response and Reduction of Tumor Growth Factor Beta-Expressing T Cells," *J Clin Oncol* 27, no. 6 (2009): 945–52. A. Berntsen, R. Trepiakas, L. Wenandy, P. F. Geertsen, P. thor Straten, M. H. Andersen, A. E. Pedersen, M. H. Claesson, T. Lorentzen, J. S. Johansen, and I. M. Svane, "Therapeutic Dendritic Cell Vaccination of Patients with Metastatic Renal Cell Carcinoma: A Clinical Phase 1/2 Trial," *J Immunother* 31, no. 8 (2008): 771–80. I. M. Svane, A. E. Pedersen, K. Nikolajsen, and M. B. Zocca, "Alterations in p53-Specific T Cells and Other Lymphocyte Subsets in Breast Cancer Patients during Vaccination with p53-Peptide Loaded Dendritic Cells and Low-Dose Interleukin-2," *Vaccine* 26, no. 36 (2008): 4716–24.

109. R. Fontana, M. Bregni, A. Cipponi, L. Raccosta, C. Rainelli, D. Maggioni, F. Lunghi, F. Ciceri, S. Mukenge, C. Doglioni, P. Colau, P. G. Coulie, C. Bordignon, C. Traversari, and V. Russo, "Peripheral Blood Lymphocytes Genetically Modified to Express the Self/Tumor Antigen MAGE-A3 Induce Antitumor Immune Responses in Cancer Patients," *Blood* 113, no. 8 (2009): 1651–60.

110. Van Driessche et al., "Clinical-Grade Manufacturing." O. Y. Leplina, V. V. Stupak, Y. P. Kozlov, I. V. Pendyurin, S. D. Nikonov, M. A. Tikhonova, N. V. Sycheva, A. A. Ostanin, and E. R. Chernykh, "Use of Interferon-Alpha-Induced Dendritic Cells in the Therapy of Patients with Malignant Brain Gliomas," *Bull Exp Biol Med* 143, no. 4 (2007): 528–34.

111. Van Driessche et al., "Clinical-Grade Manufacturing." I. Hus, M. Schmitt, J. Tabarkiewicz, S. Radej, K. Wojas, A. Bojarska-Junak, A. Schmitt, K. Giannopoulos, A. Dmoszyfska, and J. Rolifski, ?Vaccination of B-CLL Patients with Autologous Dendritic Cells Can Change the Frequency of Leukemia Antigen-Specific CD8+ T Cells as well as CD4+CD25+FoxP3+ Regulatory T Cells toward an Antileukemia Response," *Leukemia* 22, no. 5 (2008): 1007–17.

112. Molenkamp et al., "Local Administration of PF-3512676 CpG-B." M. Di Nicola, R. Zappasodi, C. Carlo-Stella, R. Mortarini, S. M. Pupa, M. Magni, L. Devizzi, P. Matteucci, P. Baldassari, F. Ravagnani, A. Cabras, A. Anichini, and A. M. Gianni, "Vaccination with Autologous Tumor-Loaded Dendritic Cells Induces Clinical and Immunologic Responses in Indolent B-Cell Lymphoma Patients with Relapsed and Measurable Disease: A Pilot Study," *Blood* 113, no. 1 (2009): 18–27.

113. Tanaka et al., "Potential Role of Dendritic Cell Vaccination." Molenkamp et al., "Local Administration of PF-3512676 CpG-B."

114. Svane et al., "Alterations in p53-Specific T Cells."

115. Tanaka et al., "Potential Role of Dendritic Cell Vaccination." Molenkamp et al., "Local Administration of PF-3512676 CpG-B."

116. Palmer et al., "A phase II Study of Adoptive Immunotherapy."

117. Kimura et al., "Prospective Phase II Study of Post-Surgical Adjuvant Chemo-Immunotherapy."

118. Y. Hirooka, A. Itoh, H. Kawashima, K. Hara, K. Nonogaki, T. Kasugai, E. Ohno, T. Ishikawa, H. Matsubara, M. Ishigami, Y. Katano, N. Ohmiya, Y. Niwa, K. Yamamoto, T. Kaneko, M. Nieda, K. Yokokawa, and H. Goto, "A Combination Therapy of Gemcitabine with Immunotherapy for Patients with Inoperable Locally Advanced Pancreatic Cancer," *Pancreas* 38, no. 3 (2009): 69–74.

119. Mashino et al., "Effective Strategy of Dendritic Cell-Based Immunotherapy." Berntsen et al., "Therapeutic Dendritic Cell Vaccination." D. E. Avigan, B. Vasir, D. J. George, W. K. Oh, M. B. Atkins, D. F. McDermott, P. W. Kantoff, R. A. Figlin, M. J. Vasconcelles, Y. Xu, D. Kufe, and R. M. Bukowski, "Phase I/II Study of Vaccination with Electrofused Allogeneic Dendritic Cells/Autologous Tumor-Derived Cells in Patients with Stage IV Renal Cell Carcinoma," *J Immunother* 30, no. 7 (2007): 749–61.

120. Bachleitner-Hofmann et al., "Pilot Trial of Autologous Dendritic Cells."

121. Kouiavskaia et al., "Vaccination with Agonist Peptide PSA: 154-163 (155L)."

122. "FDA Approves New Prostate Cancer Therapy," retrieved from www.fda.gov/ForConsumers/ConsumerUpdates/ucm210620.htm. "FDA Approves a Cellular Immunotherapy for Men with Advanced Prostate Cancer," retrieved from www.fda.gov/NewsEvents/Newsroom/PressAnnouncements/ucm210174.htm.

123. Bachleitner-Hofmann et al., "Pilot Trial of Autologous Dendritic Cells

124. C. Papewalis, B. Jacobs, M. Wuttke, E. Ullrich, T. Baehring, R. Fenk, H. S. Willenberg, S. Schinner, M. Cohnen, J. Seissler, K. Zacharowski, W. A. Scherbaum, and M. Schott, "IFN-Alpha Skews Monocytes into CD56+-Expressing Dendritic Cells with Potent Functional Activities In Vitro and In Vivo," *J Immunol* 180, no. 3 (2008): 1462–70.

125. Hus et al., "Vaccination of B-CLL Patients

126. Kim et al., "Phase I/II Study of Immunotherapy."

127. Di Nicola et al., "Vaccination with Autologous Tumor-Loaded Dendritic Cells."

128. Kimura et al., "Prospective Phase II Study."

129. Ménard et al., "Natural Killer Cell IFN-Gamma Levels."

130. López et al., "Prolonged Survival of Dendritic Cell-Vaccinated Melanoma Patients."

131. Svane et al., "Alterations in p53-Specific T Cells."

132. Palmer et al., "A Phase II Study of Adoptive Immunotherapy."

133. Tanaka et al., "Potential Role of Dendritic Cell Vaccination."

134. R. Gorter, unpublished data, Medical Center Cologne (Cologne, Germany), 2010.

135. Mashino et al., "Effective Strategy of Dendritic Cell-Based Immunotherapy."

136. Kouiavskaia et al., "Vaccination with Agonist Peptide PSA: 154-163 (155L)."

Chapter 8

137. R. Grossarth-Maticek and R. Ziegler, "Randomized and Non-randomized Prospective Controlled Cohort Studies in Matched Pair Design for the Long-Term Therapy of Corpus Uteri Cancer Patients with a Mistletoe Preparation (Iscador)," *Eur J Med Res* 13, no. 3 (2008): 107–20.

138. J. Beuth, B. Schneider, and J. M. Schierholz, "Impact of Complementary Treatment of Breast Cancer Patients with Standardized Mistletoe Extract during Aftercare: A Controlled Multicenter Comparative Epidemiological Cohort Study," *Anticancer Res* 28, no. 1B (2008): 523–7.

139. A. Loewe-Mesch, J. J. Kuehn, K. Borho, U. Abel, C. Bauer, I. Gerhard, A. Schneeweiss, C. Sohn, T. Strowitzki, and C. v. Hagens, "Adjuvant Simultaneous Mistletoe Chemotherapy in Breast Cancer—Influence on Immunological Parameters, Quality of Life and Tolerability [article in German]," *Forsch Komplementmed* 15, no. 1 (2008): 22–30. V. F. Semiglazov, V. V. Stepula, A. Dudov, J. Schnitker, and U. Mengs, "Quality of Life Is Improved in Breast Cancer Patients by Standardised Mistletoe Extract PS76A2 during Chemotherapy and Follow-Up: A Randomised, Placebo-Controlled, Double-Blind, Multicentre Clinical Trial," *Anticancer Res* 26, no. 2B (2006): 1519–29.

140. U. Elsässer-Beile, C. Leiber, U. Wetterauer, P. Bühler, P. Wolf, M. Lucht, and U. Mengs, "Adjuvant Intravesical Treatment with a Standardized Mistletoe Extract to Prevent Recurrence of Superficial Urinary Bladder Cancer," *Anticancer Res* 25, no. 6C (2005): 4733–6.

141. M. Mabed, L. El-Helw, and S. Shamaa, "Phase II Study of Viscum Fraxini-2 in Patients with Advanced Hepatocellular Carcinoma," *Br J Cancer* 90, no. 1 (2004): 65–69.

142. R. W. Gorter , M. van Wely, M. Reif, and M. Stoss, "Tolerability of an Extract of European Mistletoe among Immunocompromised and Healthy Individuals," *Altern Ther Health Med* 5, no. 6 (1999): 37–44, 47–48.

143. Beuth et al., Impact of Complementary Treatment."

144. R. Grossarth-Maticek and R. Ziegler, "Randomised and Non-randomised Prospective Controlled Cohort Studies in Matched-Pair Design for the Long-Term Therapy of Breast Cancer Patients with a Mistletoe Preparation (Iscador): A Re-analysis," *Eur J Med Res* 11, no. 11 (2006): 485–95.

145. R. Grossarth-Maticek and R. Ziegler, "Prospective Controlled Cohort Studies on Long-Term Therapy of Ovarian Cancer Patients with Mistletoe *(Viscum album L.)* Extracts Iscador," *Arzneimittelforschung* 57, no. 10 (2007): 665–78.

146. R. Grossarth-Maticek and R. Ziegler, "Randomized and Non-randomized Prospective Controlled Cohort Studies in Matched Pair Design for the Long-Term Therapy of Corpus Uteri Cancer Patients with a Mistletoe Preparation (Iscador)," *Eur J Med Res* 13, no. 3 (2008): 107–20.

147. R. Grossarth-Maticek and R. Ziegler, "Prospective Controlled Cohort Studies on Long-Term Therapy of Cervical Cancer Patients with a Mistletoe Preparation (Iscador)," *Forsch Komplementmed* 14, no. 3 (2007): 140–7.

148. R. Huber, M. Rostock, R. Goedl, R. Lüdtke, K. Urech, and R. Klein, "Immunologic Effects of Mistletoe Lectins: A Placebo-Controlled Study in Healthy Subjects," *J Soc Integr Oncol* 4, no. 1 (2006): 3–7.

149. W. Dohmen, M. Breier, and U. Mengs, "Cellular Immunomodulation and Safety of Standardized Aqueous Mistletoe Extract PS76A2 in Tumor Patients Treated for 48 Weeks," *Anticancer Res* 24, no. 2C (2004): 1231–7. M. Schink, W. Tröger, A. Dabidian, A. Goyert, H. Scheuerecker, J. Meyer, I. U. Fischer, and F. Glaser, "Mistletoe Extract Reduces the Surgical Suppression of Natural Killer Cell Activity in Cancer Patients: A Randomized Phase III Trial," *Forsch Komplementmed* 14, no. 1 (2007): 9–17.

150. L. Heinzerling, V. von Baehr, C. Liebenthal, R. von Baehr, and H. D. Volk, "Immunologic Effector Mechanisms of a Standardized Mistletoe Extract on the Function of Human Monocytes and Lymphocytes In Vitro, Ex Vivo, and In Vivo," *J Clin Immunol* 26, no. 4 (2006): 347–59. J. Beuth, B. Stoffel, H. L. Ko, G. Buss, L. Tunggal, and G. Pulverer, "Immunoactive Effects of Various Mistletoe Lectin-1 Dosages in Mammary Carcinoma Patients [article in German]," *Arzneimittelforschung* 45, no. 4 (1995): 505–7.

151. Huber et al., "Immunologic Effects of Mistletoe Lectins." Heinzerling

et al., "Immunologic Effector Mechanisms." P. Schöffski, S. Riggert, P. Fumoleau, M. Campone, O. Bolte, S. Marreaud, D. Lacombe, B. Baron, M. Herold, H. Zwierzina, K. Wilhelm-Ogunbiyi, H. Lentzen, and C. Twelves, "Phase I Trial of Intravenous Aviscumine (rViscumin) in Patients with Solid Tumors: A Study of the European Organization for Research and Treatment of Cancer New Drug Development Group," *Ann Oncol* 15, no. 12 (2004): 1816–24.

152. Schöffski et al., "Phase I Trial of Intravenous Aviscumine (rViscumin)." R. Klein, K. Classen, P. A. Berg, R. Lüdtke, M. Werner, and R. Huber, "In Vivo-Induction of Antibodies to Mistletoe Lectin-1 and Viscotoxin by Exposure to Aqueous Mistletoe Extracts: A Randomised Double-Blinded Placebo Controlled Phase I Study in Healthy Individuals," *Eur J Med Res* 7, no. 4 (2002): 155–63.

153. E. Kovacs, T. Hajto, and K. Hostanska, "Improvement of DNA Repair in Lymphocytes of Breast Cancer Patients Treated with Viscum Album Extract (Iscador)," *Eur J Cancer* 27, no. 12 (1991): 1672–6. E. Kovacs, "The In Vitro Effect of Viscum Album (VA) Extract on DNA Repair of Peripheral Blood Mononuclear Cells (PBMC) in Cancer Patients," *Phytother Res* 16, no. 2 (2002): 143–7.

154. H. S. Riordan, J. J. Casciari, M. J. González, N. H. Riordan, J. R. Miranda-Massari, P. Taylor, and J. A. Jackson, "A Pilot Clinical Study of Continuous Intravenous Ascorbate in Terminal Cancer Patients," *P R Health Sci J* 24, no. 4 (2005): 269–76.

155. A. J. Waring, I. M. Drake, C. J. Schorah, K. L. White, D. A. Lynch, A. T. Axon, and M. F. Dixon, "Ascorbic Acid and Total Vitamin C Concentrations in Plasma, Gastric Juice, and Gastrointestinal Mucosa: Effects of Gastritis and Oral Supplementation," *Gut* 38, no. 2 (1996): 171–6.

156. Riordan et al., "A Pilot Clinical Study."

157. A. Pakdaman, "Symptomatic Treatment of Brain Tumor Patients with Sodium Selenite, Oxygen, and Other Supportive Measures," *Biol Trace Elem Res* 62, no. 1–2 (1998): 1–6.

158. L. Kiremidjian-Schumacher, M. Roy, R. Glickman, K. Schneider, S. Rothstein, J. Cooper, H. Hochster, M. Kim, and R. Newman, "Selenium and Immunocompetence in Patients with Head and Neck Cancer," *Biol Trace Elem Res* 73, no. 2 (2000): 97–111.

159. S. S. Khanna and F. R. Karjodkar, "Circulating Immune Complexes and Trace Elements (Copper, Iron and Selenium) as Markers in Oral Precancer and Cancer: A Randomised, Controlled Clinical Trial," *Head Face Med* 2 (2006): 33.

160. Kiremidjian-Schumacher et al., "Selenium and Immunocompetence."

161. S. J. Padayatty, H. Sun, Y. Wang, H. D. Riordan, S. M. Hewitt, A. Katz, R. A. Wesley, and M. Levine, "Vitamin C Pharmacokinetics: Implications for Oral and Intravenous Use," *Ann Intern Med* 140, no. 7 (2004): 533–7.

162. L. J. Hoffer, M. Levine, S. Assouline, D. Melnychuk, S. J. Padayatty, K. Rosadiuk, C. Rousseau, L. Robitaille, and W. H. Miller Jr., "Phase I Clinical Trial of I.V. Ascorbic Acid in Advanced Malignancy," *Ann Oncol* 19, no. 11 (2008): 1969–74.

163. S. Sasazuki, T. Hayashi, K. Nakachi, S. Sasaki, Y. Tsubono, S. Okubo, M. Hayashi, and S. Tsugane, "Protective Effect of Vitamin C on Oxidative Stress: A Randomized Controlled Trial," *Int J Vitam Nutr Res* 78, no. 3 (2008): 121–8.

164. Riordan et al., "A Pilot Clinical Study."

165. Padayatty et al., "Vitamin C Pharmacokinetics."

166. H. Sakagami, K. Satoh, Y. Hakeda, and M. Kumegawa, "Apoptosis-Inducing Activity of Vitamin C and Vitamin K," *Cell Mol Biol* 46, no. 1 (2000): 129–43.

167. J. J. Casciari, N. H. Riordan, T. L. Schmidt, X. L. Meng, J. A. Jackson, and H. D. Riordan, "Cytotoxicity of Ascorbate, Lipoic Acid, and Other Antioxidants in Hollow Fibre In Vitro Tumours," *Br J Cancer* 84, no. 11 (2001): 1544–50.

168. Hoffer et al., "Phase I Clinical Trial."

169. S. J. Padayatty and M. Levine, "Reevaluation of Ascorbate in Cancer Treatment: Emerging Evidence, Open Minds and Serendipity," *J Am Coll Nutr* 19, no. 4 (2000): 423–5.

170. Padayatty et al., "Vitamin C Pharmacokinetics."

171. K. Margolin, M. Atkins, J. Sparano, J. Sosman, G. Weiss, M. Lotze, J. Doroshow, J. Mier, K. O'Boyle, R. Fisher, E. Campbell, J. Rubin, D. Federighi, and S. Bursten, "Prospective Randomized Trial of Lisofylline for the Prevention of Toxicities of High-Dose Interleukin 2 Therapy in Advanced Renal Cancer and Malignant Melanoma," *Clin Cancer Res* 3, no. 4 (1997): 565–72.

172. H. D. Riordan, N. H. Riordan, J. A. Jackson, J. J. Casciari, R. Hunninghake, M. J. Gonzalez, E. M. Mora, J. R. Miranda-Massari, N. Rosario, and A. Rivera, "Intravenous Vitamin C as a Chemotherapy Agent: A Report on Clinical Cases," *P R Health Sci J* 23, no. 2 (2004): 115–8.

173. M. J. González, E. M. Mora, J. R. Miranda-Massari, J. Matta, H. D. Riordan, and N. H. Riordan, "Inhibition of Human Breast Carcinoma Cell Proliferation by Ascorbate and Copper," *P R Health Sci J* 21, no. 1 (2002): 21–3.

174. Q. Chen, M. G. Espey, A. Y. Sun, C. Pooput, K. L. Kirk, M. C. Krishna, D. B. Khosh, J. Drisko, and M. Levine, "Pharmacologic Doses of Ascorbate Act as a Prooxidant and Decrease Growth of Aggressive Tumor Xenografts in Mice," *Proc Natl Acad Sci USA* 105, no. 32 (2008): 11105–9.

175. Sakagami et al., "Apoptosis-Inducing Activity."

176. C. H. Park, B. F. Kimler, S. Y. Yi, S. H. Park, K. Kim, C. W. Jung, S. H. Kim, E. R. Lee, M. Rha, S. Kim, M. H. Park, S. J. Lee, H. K. Park, M. H. Lee , S. S. Yoon, Y. H. Min, B. S. Kim, J. A. Kim, and W. S. Kim, "Depletion of L-Ascorbic Acid Alternating with Its Supplementation in the Treatment of Patients with Acute Myeloid Leukemia or Myelodysplastic Syndromes," *Eur J Haematol* 83, no. 2 (2009): 108–18.

177. Hoffer et al., "Phase I Clinical Trial."

178. Riordan et al., "A Pilot Clinical Study."

179. Ibid.

180. R. Gorter, unpublished clinical data, Medical Center Cologne (Cologne, Germany), 2010.

181. O. Micke, F. Bruns, R. Mücke, U. Schäfer, M. Glatzel, A. F. DeVries, K. Schönekaes, K. Kisters, and J. Büntzel, "Selenium in the Treatment of Radiation-Associated Secondary Lymphedema," *Int J Radiat Oncol Biol Phys* 56, no. 1 (2003): 40–9.

182. J. Büntzel, "Experiences with Sodium Selenite in Treatment of Acute and Late Adverse Effects of Radiochemotherapy of Head-Neck Carcinomas: Cytoprotection Working Group in AK Supportive Measures in Oncology within the Scope of MASCC and DKG [article in German]," *Med Klin* (Munich) 94, suppl. 3 (1999): 49–53.

183. A. Pakdaman, "Symptomatic Treatment of Brain Tumor Patients with Sodium Selenite, Oxygen, and Other Supportive Measures," *Biol Trace Elem Res* 62, no. 1–2 (1998): 1–6.

184. I. A. Asfour, S. El Shazly, M. H. Fayek, H. M. Hegab, S. Raouf, and M. A. Moussa, "Effect of High-Dose Sodium Selenite Therapy on Polymorphonuclear Leukocyte Apoptosis in Non-Hodgkin's Lymphoma Patients," *Biol Trace Elem Res* 110, no. 1 (2006): 19–32.

185. Ibid.

186. Ibid.

187. Büntzel, "Experiences with Sodium Selenite."

188. Asfour et al., "Effect of High-Dose Sodium Selenite."

189. Micke et al., "Selenium in the Treatment of Radiation-Associated Secondary Lymphedema."

190. Büntzel, "Experiences with Sodium Selenite."

191. Pakdaman, "Symptomatic Treatment of Brain Tumor Patients."

192. R. Kasseroller, "Sodium Selenite as Prophylaxis against Erysipelas in Secondary Lymphedema," *Anticancer Res* 18, no. 3C (1998): 2227–30. T. Zimmermann, H. Leonhardt, S. Kersting, S. Albrecht, U. Range, and U. Eckelt, "Reduction of Postoperative Lymphedema after Oral Tumor Surgery with Sodium Selenite," *Biol Trace Elem Res* 106, no. 3 (2005): 193–203.

193. W. Li, Y. Zhu, X. Yan, Q. Zhang, X. Li, Z. Ni, Z. Shen, H. Yao, J. Zhu, "The Prevention of Primary Liver Cancer by Selenium in High Risk Populations [article in Chinese]," *Zhonghua Yu Fang Yi Xue Za Zhi* 34, no. 6 (2000): 336–8.

194. O. H. Al-Taie, J. Seufert, S. Karvar, C. Adolph, H. Mörk, M. Scheurlen, J. Köhrle, and F. Jakob, "Selenium Supplementation Enhances Low Selenium Levels and Stimulates Glutathione Peroxidase Activity in Peripheral Blood and Distal Colon Mucosa in Past and Present Carriers of Colon Adenomas," *Nutr Cancer* 46, no. 2 (2003): 125–30.

195. C. H. Bunker, A. C. McDonald, R. W. Evans, N. de la Rosa, J. M. Boumosleh, and A. L. Patrick, "A Randomized Trial of Lycopene Supplementation in Tobago Men with High Prostate Cancer Risk," *Nutr Cancer* 57, no. 2 (2007): 130–7.

196. M. E. Wright, J. Virtamo, A. M. Hartman, P. Pietinen, B. K. Edwards, P. R. Taylor, J. K. Huttunen, and D. Albanes, "Effects of Alpha-Tocopherol and Beta-Carotene Supplementation on Upper Aerodigestive Tract Cancers in a Large, Randomized Controlled Trial," *Cancer* 109, no. 5 (2007): 891–8.

197. S. Sasazuki, S. Sasaki, Y. Tsubono, S. Okubo, M. Hayashi, T. Kakizoe, and S. Tsugane, "The Effect of 5-Year Vitamin C Supplementation on Serum Pepsinogen Level and Helicobacter Pylori Infection," *Cancer Sci* 94, no. 4 (2003): 378–82.

198. Chen et al., "Pharmacologic Doses of Ascorbate."

199. B. Tareen, J. L. Summers, J. M. Jamison, D. R. Neal, K. McGuire, L. Gerson, and A. Diokno, "A 12 Week, Open Label, Phase I/IIa Study Using Apatone for the Treatment of Prostate Cancer Patients Who Have Failed Standard Therapy," *Int J Med Sci* 5, no. 2 (2008): 62–7.

200. J. R. Berenson, O. Yellin, D. Woytowitz, M. S. Flam, A. Cartmell, R. Patel, H. Duvivier, Y. Nassir, B. Eades, C. D. Abaya, J. Hilger, R. A. Swift, "Borte-

zomib, Ascorbic Acid and Melphalan (BAM) Therapy For Patients with Newly Diagnosed Multiple Myeloma: An Effective and Well-Tolerated Frontline Regimen," *Eur J Haematol* 82, no. 6 (2009): 433–9.

201. Additional references on the Newcastle disease virus follow: R. M. Lorence, M. S. Roberts, W. S. Groene, and H. Rabin, "Replication-Competent, Oncolytic Newcastle Disease Virus for Cancer Therapy," in *Replication-Competent Viruses for Cancer Therapy: Monographs in Virology*, vol. 22, eds. P. H. Driever and S. D. Rabkin (Doerr, HW: Karger, 2001), 160–182. J. Szeberenyi, Z. Fabian, B. Torocsik, K. Kiss, and L. K. Csatary, "Newcastle Disease Virus-Induced Apoptosis in PC 12 Pheochromocytoma Cells," *Am J Therap* 10, no. 4 (2003): 282–288. K. W. Reichard, R. M. Lorence, and C. J. Cascino, "Selective Replication of Newcastle Disease Virus (NDV) in Cancer Cells Is Associated with Virus-Induced Cell Fusion," *Proc Am Assoc Cancer Res* 33 (1992): 521. K. W. Reichard, R. M. Lorence, C. J. Cascino, M. E. Peeples, R. J. Walter, M. B. Fernando, H. M. Reyes, and J. A. Greager, "Newcastle Disease Virus Selectively Kills Human Tumor Cells," *J Surg Res* 52 (1992): 448–53. J. Fazakerley and T. E. Allsopp, "Programmed Cell Death in Virus Infections of the Nervous System," in *The Mechanisms of Neuronal Damage in Virus Infections of the Nervous System*, ed. G. Gosztonyi, *CTMI* 253 (2001): 95–119. Z. Fabian, B. Torocsik, L. K. Csatary, K. Kiss, and J. Szeberenyi, "Induction of Apoptosis by a Newcastle Disease Virus Vaccine (MTH-68/H) in PC12 Rat Phaeochromocytoma Cells," *Anti-cancer Res* 21 (2001): 125–136. K. W. Reichard, R. M. Lorence, B. B. Katubig, M. E. Peeples, and H. M. Reyes, "Retinoic Acid Enhances Killing of Neuroblastoma Cells by Newcastle Disease Virus," *J Pediatr Surg* 28 (1993): 1221–1225. K. M. Lam, A. C. Vasconcelos, and A. A. Bickford, "Apoptosis as a Cause of Death in Chicken Embryos Inoculated with Newcastle Disease Virus," *Microb Pathol* 19 (1995): 169–174. K. W. Reichard, R. M. Lorence, and C. J. Cascino, "Selective Replication of Newcastle Disease Virus (NDV) in Cancer Cells Is Associated with Virus-Induced Cell Fusion," *Proc Am Assoc Cancer Res* 33 (1992): 521. H. E. Webb and C. E. Gordon Smith, "Viruses in the Treatment of Cancer," *Lancet* 1 (1970): 1206–1208. P. H. Driever and S. D. Rabkin, eds., *Replication-Competent Viruses for Cancer Therapy: Monographs in Virology*, vol. 22 (Basel: Karger, 2001). J. Nemunaitis, "Live Viruses in Cancer Treatment," *Oncology* 16 (2002): 1483–1492. N. J. Nelson, "Viruses and Cancer," *J Natl Cancer Inst* 91 (1999): 1709. L. K. Csatary, "Viruses in the Treatment of Cancer," *Lancet* 2 (1971): 825. L. K. Csatary, R. W. Moss, I. Beuth, B. Torocsik, J. Szeberenyi, and T. Bakacs, "Beneficial Treatment of Patients with

Advanced Cancer Using a Newcastle Disease Virus Vaccine (MTH-68/H)." L. K. Csatary, S. Eckhardt, I. Bukosza, F. Czegledi, C. Fenyvesi, P. Gergely, B. Bodey, and C. M. Csatary, "Attenuated Veterinary Virus Vaccine for the Treatment of Cancer," *Cancer Detect Prev* 17 (1993): 619–627. L. Pollak, R. Gur, N. Walach, R. Reif, L. Tamir, J. Schiffer, "Clinical Determinants of Long-Term Survival in Patients with Glioblastoma Multiforme," *Turnori* 83 (1997): 613–617. M. Salvati, L. Cervoni, M. Artico, R. Caruso, and F. M. Gagliardi, "Long-Term Survival in Patents with Supratentorial Glioblastoma," *J Neuro-Oncol* 36 (1998): 61–64. T. Yoshida, N. Kawano, H. Oka, K. Fujii, and Y. Nakazato, "Clinical Cure of Glioblastoma: Two Case Reports," *Neurol Med Chir* (Tokyo) 40 (2000): 224–229. R. Klein, G. Molenkamp, N. Sorensen, and W. Roggendorf, "Favorable Outcome of Giant Cell Glioblastoma in a Child: Report of an 11-Year Survival Period," *Childs Nerv Syst* 14 (1998): 288–291. B. Meyer-Puttlitz, Y. Hayashi, A. Wahaa, B. Rollbrocker, J. Bostrom, O. D. Wiestler, D. N. Louis, G. Reifenberger, and A. von Deimling, "Molecular Genetic Analysis of Giant Cell Glioblastomas," *Am J Pathol* 151 (1997): 853–857. R. Alemany, C. Gomez-Manzano, C. Balague, W. K. Yung, D. T. Curiel, A. P. Kyritsis, and J. Fueyo, "Gene Therapy for Glioblas Tomas: Molecular Targets, Adenoviral Vectors, and Oncolytic Adenoviruses," *Exp Cell Res* 252 (1999): 1–12. J. M. Markert, G. Y. Gillespie, R R. Weichselbaum, B. Roizman, and R. J. Whitley, "Genetically Engineered HSV in the Treatment of Glioma: A Review," *Rev Med Virol* 10 (2000): 17–30. P. Tunici, D. Gianni, and G. Finocchiaro, "Gene Therapy of Glioblas Tomas: From Suicide to Homicide," *Prog Brain Res* 132 (2001): 711–719. G. Karpati, H. Li, and J. Nalbantoglu, "Molecular Therapy for Glioblastoma," *Curr Opin Mol Ther* 1 (1999): 545–552. E. Pennisi, "Training Viruses to Attack Cancers," *Science* 282 (1998): 1244–1246. N. J. Nelson, "Scientific Interest in Newcastle Disease Virus Is Reviving: Viruses and Cancer," *J Natl Cancer Inst* 91 (1999): 1708–1710. J. Fueyo, R. Alemany, C. Gomez-Marzano, G. N. Fuller, A. Khan, C. A. Conrad, T. J. Liu, H. Jiang, M. G. Lemoine, K. Suzuki, R. Sawaya, D. T. Curiel, W. K. Alfred Yung, and F. F. Lang, "Preclinical Characterization of the Antiglioma Activity of a Tropism-Enhanced Adenovirus Targeted to the Retinoblastoma Pathway," *J Ntl Cancer Inst* 95 (2003): 652–660. L. J. Xue, N. Y. Jin, W. Gong, H. W. Wang, D. H. Sun, Q. F. Luo, T. Ge, and P. Li, "The Effect of Newcastle Disease Virus on the Biological Behavior of Tumor Cells," *Xi Bao Yu Fen Zi Mian Yi Xue Za Zhi* 19, no. 1 (2003): 29–31. L. K. Csatary, G. Gosztonyi, J. Szeberenyi, Z. Fabian, V. Liszka, B. Bodey, and C. M. Csatary, "MTH-68/H Oncolytic Viral Treatment in Human High-Grade Gliomas," *J Neu-*

rooncol 67, no. 1–2 (2004): 83–93. V. Zaitsev, M. von Itzstein, D. Groves, M. Kiefel, T. Takimoto, A. Portner, and G. Taylor, "Second Sialic Acid Binding Site in Newcastle Disease Virus Hemagglutinin-Neuraminidase: Implications for Fusion," *J Virol* 78, no. 7 (2004): 3733–41. V. Dolganiuc, L. McGinnes, E. J. Luna, and T. G. Morrison, "Role of the Cytoplasmic Domain of the Newcastle Disease Virus Fusion Protein in Association with Lipid Rafts," *J Virol* 77, no. 24 (2003): 12968–7. N. Bar-Eli, H. Giloh, M. Schlesinger, and Z. Zakay-Rones, "Preferential Cytotoxic Effect of Newcastle Disease Virus on Lymphoma Cells," *J Cancer Res Clin Oncol* 122, no. 7 (1996): 409–15. Z. Huang, A. Panda, S. Elankumaran, D. Govindarajan, D. D. Rockemann, and S. K. Samal, "The Hemagglutinin-Neuraminidase Protein of Newcastle Disease Virus Determines Tropism and Virulence," *J Virol* 78, no. 8 (2004): 4176–84.

202. Z. Fabian, B. Torocsik, L. K. Csatary, K. Kiss, and J. Szeberenyi, "Induction of Apoptosis by a Newcastle Disease Virus Vaccine (MTH-68/H) in PC12 Rat Phaeochromocytoma Cells," *Anti-cancer Res* 21 (2001): 125–136. K. M. Lam, A. C. Vasconcelos, and A. A. Bickford, "Apoptosis as a Cause of Death in Chicken Embryos Inoculated with Newcastle Disease Virus," *Microb Pathol* 19 (1995): 169–174. H. E. Webb and C. E. Gordon Smith, "Viruses in the Treatment of Cancer," *Lancet* 1 (1970): 1206–1208. P. H. Driever and S. D. Rabkin, eds., *Replication-Competent Viruses for Cancer Therapy: Monographs in Virology,* vol. 22 (Basel: Karger, 2001). J. Nemunaitis, "Live Viruses in Cancer Treatment," *Oncology* 16 (2002): 1483–1492. N. J. Nelson, "Viruses and Cancer," *J Natl Cancer Inst* 91 (1999): 1709.

203. H. E. Webb and C. E. Gordon Smith, "Viruses in the Treatment of Cancer," *Lancet* 1 (1970): 1206–1208.

204. W. A. Cassell and R. E. Garrett, "Newcastle Disease Virus as an Antineoplastic Agent," *Cancer* 18 (1965): 863–868.

205. L. K. Csatary, S. Eckhardt, I. Bukosza, F. Czegledi, C. Fenyvesi, P. Gergely, B. Bodey, and C. M. Csatary, "Attenuated Veterinary Virus Vaccine for the Treatment of Cancer," *Cancer Detect Prev* 17, no. 6 (1993): 619–27. P. Schlag, M. Manasterski, T. Gerneth, P. Hohenberger, M. Dueck, C. Herfarth, W. Liebrich, and V. Schirrmacher, "Active Specific Immunotherapy with Newcastle-Disease-Virus-Modified Autologous Tumor Cells Following Resection of Liver Metastases in Colorectal Cancer: First Evaluation of Clinical Response of a Phase II-Trial," *Cancer Immunol Immunother* 35, no. 5 (1992): 325–30.

206. A. I. Freeman, Z. Zakay-Rones, J. M. Gomori, E. Linetsky, L. Rasooly, E. Greenbaum, S. Rozenman-Yair, A. Panet, E. Libson, C. S. Irving, E. Galun,

T. Siegal, "Phase I/II Trial of Intravenous NDV-HUJ Oncolytic Virus in Recurrent Glioblastoma Multiforme," *Mol Ther* 13, no. 1 (2006): 221–8.

207. E. Hagmüller, N. Beck, D. Ockert, V. Schirrmacher, "Adjuvant Therapy of Liver Metastases: Active Specific Immunotherapy [article in German]," *Zentralbl Chir* 120, no. 10 (1995): 780–5.

208. A. L. Pecora, N. Rizvi, G. I. Cohen, N. J. Meropol, D. Sterman, J. L. Marshall, S. Goldberg, P. Gross, J. D. O'Neil, W. S. Groene, M. S. Roberts, H. Rabin, M. K. Bamat, R. M. Lorence, "Phase I Trial of Intravenous Administration of PV701, an Oncolytic Virus, in Patients with Advanced Solid Cancers," *J Clin Oncol* 20, no. 9 (2002): 2251–66.

209. H. H. Kirchner, P. Anton, and J. Atzpodien, "Adjuvant Treatment of Locally Advanced Renal Cancer with Autologous Virus-Modified Tumor Vaccines," *World J Urol* 13, no. 3 (1995): 171–3.

210. Ibid.

211. P. T. Emmerson, *Newcastle Disease Virus (Paramyxoviridae): Virology and Microbiology* (Newcastle, UK: University of Newcastle Upon Tyne Academic Press, 1999).

212. L. K. Csatary, E. Csatary, and R. W. Moss, "Scientific Interest in Newcastle Disease Virus Is Reviving," *J Natl Cancer Inst* 92 (2000): 493–494.

213. C. Pfirschke and V. Schirrmacher, "Cross-Infection of Tumor Cells by Contact with T Lymphocytes Loaded with Newcastle Disease Virus," *Int J Oncol* 34, no. 4 (2009): 951–52.

214. M. Jarahian, C. Watzl, P. Fournier, A. Arnold, D. Djandji, S. Zahedi, A. Cerwenka, A. Paschen, V. Schirrmacher, and F. Momburg, "Activation of Natural Killer Cells by Newcastle Disease Virus Hemagglutinin-Neuraminidase," *J Virol* 83, no. 16 (2009): 8108–21.

215. V. Schirrmacher and P. Fournier, "Newcastle Disease Virus: A Promising Vector for Viral Therapy, Immune Therapy, and Gene Therapy of Cancer," *Methods Mol Biol* 542 (2009): 565–605.

216. W. A. Cassel and D. R. Murray, "A Ten-Year Follow-Up on Stage II Malignant Melanoma Patients Treated Postsurgically with Newcastle Disease Virus Oncolysate," *Med Oncol Tumor Pharmacother* 9, no. 4 (1992): 169–71.

217. F. M. Batliwalla, B. A. Bateman, D. Serrano, D. Murray, S. Macphail, V. C. Maino, J. C. Ansel, P. K. Gregersen, and C. A. Armstrong, "A 15-Year Follow-Up of AJCC Stage III Malignant Melanoma Patients Treated Postsurgically with Newcastle Disease Virus (NDV) Oncolysate and Determination of Alterations in the CD8 T Cell Repertoire," *Mol Med* 4, no. 12 (1998): 783–94.

218. T. Schneider, R. Gerhards, E. Kirches, and R. Firsching, "Preliminary Results of Active Specific Immunization with Modified Tumor Cell Vaccine in Glioblastoma Multiforme," *J Neurooncol* 53, no. 1 (2001): 39–46.

219. H. H. Kirchner, P. Anton, and J. Atzpodien, "Adjuvant Treatment of Locally Advanced Renal Cancer with Autologous Virus-Modified Tumor Vaccines," *World J Urol* 13, no. 3 (1995): 171–3.

220. Schlag et al., "Active Specific Immunotherapy."

221. Ibid.

222. Csatary et al., "Attenuated Veterinary Virus Vaccine."

Chapter 9

223. Adapted from R. Sapolsky, *Why Zebras Don't Get Ulcers* (New York: Owl Books, 2004).

224. Even though support is very helpful, paradoxically, it can sometimes backfire and be unhelpful. We recommend that patients do not be afraid to ask for what they need and also to ignore what they don't need. For example, people have an uncanny knack for telling newly diagnosed cancer patients graphic stories about family or friends who have suffered miserably and died. Remember that at the time of diagnosis, patients are highly suggestible and thus susceptible to these traumatizing messages. The messages need to be supportive and nurturing.

225. Be open to explore or use any approach that has not been proven harmful. Remember that the absence of proof does not mean it does not work; it means that the research has not yet been performed. Most cancer research has been funded by pharmaceutical companies, especially if the new treatments can be patented. At the present time, developing a single new medication and performing the appropriate clinical trials leading to FDA approval may cost $900 million or more.

226. M. Pollan, *In Defense of Food: An Eater's Manifesto* (New York: Penguin Press, 2009).

227. For the revised international table see www.mendosa.com/ gilists.htm.

228. F. S. Atkinson, K. F. Foster-Powell, and J. C. Brand-Miller, "International Tables of Glycemic Index and Glycemic Load Values: 2008," *Diabetes Care* 31, no. 12 (2008): 2281–2283.

229. T. C. Campbell and T. M. Campbell, *The China Study* (Dallas, TX: Benbella Books, 2006).

230. D. Ornish, G. Weidner, W. R. Fair, et al., "Intensive Lifestyle Changes

May Affect the Progression of Prostate Cancer," *Journal of Urology* 174, no. 3 (2005): 165–69.

231. The President's Cancer Panel, *Reducing Environmental Cancer Risk: What We Can Do Now,* National Cancer Institute, National Institutes of Health, U.S. Department of Health and Human Services, April 2010.

232. National Cancer Institute (NCI) and the National Institute of Environmental Health Sciences (NIEHS), *Cancer and the Environment: What You Need to Know What You Can Do,* NIH Publication No. 03–2039, 2003. U.S. Department of Health and Human Services, Public Health Service, National Toxicology Program, *Report on Carcinogens* (11th ed.).

233. R. O'Neill, "Burying the Evidence," *Hazards Magazine* 92 (2005), available at www.hazards.org/cancer/buryinghthevidence.pdf. S. Steingraber, *Living Downstream: An Ecologist's Personal Investigation of Cancer and the Environment,* 2nd ed. (New York: Da Capo, 2010).

234. J. D. Brown and J. M. Siegel, "Exercise as a Buffer of Life Stress: A Prospective Study of Adolescent Health," *Health Psychology* 7, no. 4 (1988): 341–353.

235. Therapeutic eurhythmy or curative eurhythmy is an art expression that synthesizes movement, music, and speech. In this art form the body is an instrument for physical, emotional, and spiritual expression. It is the medical form of eurhythmy, the terpsichorean mode of anthroposophy, and can be applied therapeutically to support the healing efforts of the body. The design of eurhythmy is a direct expression of a rhythm that pervades Nature. Eurhythmy is described as a visual form of speech and music. Curative eurhythmy causes the inward conveyance of a harmonizing process that influences diseased organs and their life processes. For more information see www.eana.org/.

236. M. Fleshner, "Physical Activity and Stress Resistance: Sympathetic Nervous System Adaptations Prevent Stress-Induced Immunosuppression," *Exercise and Sport Sciences Reviews* 33, no. 3 (2005): 120–126.

237. J. Blumenthal, M. A. Babyak, K. Moore, E. Craighead, S. Herman, P. Khatri, R. Waugh, M. A. Napolitana, L. M. Forman, M. Appelbaum, M. Doraiswamy, and K. R. Krishnan, "Effects of Exercise Training on Older Patients with Major Depression," *Archives of Internal Medicine* 159 (1999): 2349–2356.

238. L. Cohen, C. Warneke, R. T. Fouladi, M. A. Rodriguez, and A. Chaoul-Reich, "Psychological Adjustment and Sleep Quality in a Randomized Trial of the Effects of a Tibetan Yoga Intervention in Patients with Lymphoma," *Cancer* 100, no. 10 (2004): 2253–60.

239. S. C. Danhauer, S. L. Mihalko, G. B. Russell, C. R. Campbell, L. Felder, K. Daley, and E. A. Levine, "Restorative Yoga for Women with Breast Cancer: Findings from a Randomized Pilot Study," *Psychooncology* 18, no. 4 (2009): 360–8.

240. A. B. Moadel, C. Shah, J. Wylie-Rosett, M. S. Harris, S. R. Patel, C. B. Hall, and J. A. Sparano, "Randomized Controlled Trial of Yoga among a Multiethnic Sample of Breast Cancer Patients: Effects on Quality of Life," *J Clin Oncol* 25, no. 28 (2007): 4387–95.

241. J. W. Carson, K. M. Carson, L. S. Porter, F. J. Keefe, H. Shaw, and J. M. Miller, "Yoga for Women with Metastatic Breast Cancer: Results from a Pilot Study," *J Pain Symptom Manage* 33, no. 3 (2007): 331–41.

242. L. E. Carlson, M. Speca, K. D. Patel, and E. Goodey, "Mindfulness-Based Stress Reduction in Relation to Quality of Life, Mood, Symptoms of Stress and Levels of Cortisol, Dehydroepiandrosterone Sulfate (DHEAS) and Melatonin in Breast and Prostate Cancer Outpatients," *Psychoneuroendocrinology* 29, no. 4 (2004): 448–74.

243. L. E. Carlson, M. Speca, P. Faris, and K. D. Patel, "One Year Pre-Post Intervention Follow-Up of Psychological, Immune, Endocrine and Blood Pressure Outcomes of Mindfulness-Based Stress Reduction (MBSR) in Breast and Prostate Cancer Outpatients," *Brain Behav Immun* 21, no. 8 (2007): 1038–49.

244. R. M. Raghavendra, R. Nagarathna, H. R. Nagendra, K. S. Gopinath, B. S. Srinath, B. D. Ravi, S. Patil, B. S. Ramesh, and R. Nalini, "Effects of an Integrated Yoga Programme on Chemotherapy-Induced Nausea and Emesis in Breast Cancer Patients," *Eur J Cancer Care* (Engl) 16, no. 6 (2007): 462–74.

245. S. N. Culos-Reed, L. E. Carlson, L. M. Daroux, S. Hately-Aldous, "A Pilot Study of Yoga for Breast Cancer Survivors: Physical and Psychological Benefits," *Psychooncology* 15, no. 10 (2006): 891–7.

246. B. Banerjee, H. S. Vadiraj, A. Ram, R. Rao, M. Jayapal, K. S. Gopinath, B. S. Ramesh, N. Rao, A. Kumar, N. Raghuram, S. Hegde, H. R. Nagendra, and M. Prakash Hande, "Effects of an Integrated Yoga Program in Modulating Psychological Stress and Radiation-Induced Genotoxic Stress in Breast Cancer Patients Undergoing Radiotherapy," *Integr Cancer Ther* 6, no. 3 (2007): 242–50.

247. M. R. Rao, N. Raghuram, H. R. Nagendra, K. S. Gopinath, B. S. Srinath, R. B. Diwakar, S. Patil, S. R. Bilimagga, N. Rao, and S. Varambally, "Anxiolytic Effects of a Yoga Program in Early Breast Cancer Patients Undergoing Conventional Treatment: A Randomized Controlled Trial," *Complement Ther Med* 17, no.

1 (2009): 1–8. H. S. Vadiraja, R. M. Raghavendra, R. Nagarathna, H. R. Nagendra, M. Rekha, V. Vanitha, K. S. Gopinath, B. S. Srinath, M. S. Vishweshwara, Y. S. Madhavi, B. S. Ajaikumar, B. S. Ramesh, R. Nalini, and V. Kumar, "Effects of a Yoga Program on Cortisol Rhythm and Mood States in Early Breast Cancer Patients Undergoing Adjuvant Radiotherapy: A Randomized Controlled Trial," *Integr Cancer Ther* 8, no. 1 (2009): 37–46.

248. J. R. Satin, W. Linden, and M. J. Phillips, "Depression as a Predictor of Disease Progression and Mortality in Cancer Patients: A Meta-Analysis," *Cancer* 115, no. 22 (2010): 5349–5361. R. Van Overbruggen, *Healing Psyche* (Charleston, SC: BookSurge, 2006).

249. B. L. Andersen, Y. Hae-Chung, W. B. Farrar, D. M. Golden-Kreutz, et al., "Psychologic Intervention Improves Survival for Breast Cancer Patients: A Randomized Clinical Trial," *Cancer* 113 (2008): 3450–3458.

250. J. S. de Vendômois, F. Roullier, D. Cellier, and G. E. Séralini, "A Comparison of the Effects of Three GM Corn Varieties on Mammalian Health," *Int J Biol Sci* 5 (2009): 706–726.

Chapter 10

251. V. Klinkenborg, "Our Vanishing Night," *National Geographic,* November 2008, 102–123.

252. H. G. Bastian, A. Kornmann, R. Hafen, and M. Koch, *Musik(erziehung) und ihre Wirkung* (Mainz, Germany: Schott Musik International, 2000).

253. R. G. Foster and L. Kreitzman, *Rhythms of Life: The Biological Clocks That Control the Daily Lives of Every Living Thing* (New Haven: Yale University Press, 2005).

254. J. O'Donnell, "Insomnia in Cancer Patients," *Clinical Cornerstone* 6, no. 1 (2004): S6–S14. J. Savard and C. M. Morin, "Insomnia in the Context of Cancer: A Review of a Neglected Problem," *Journal of Clinical Oncology* 19, no. 3 (2001): 895–908.

255. J. F. Duffy, D. J. Dijk, E. B. Klerman, and C. A. Czeisler, "Altered Circadian Phase of Awakening in Older People," *Am J Physiol Regulatory Integrative Comp Physiol* 275 (1998): 1478–1487.

256. M. Moser, D. v. Bonin, et al., *Diagnostik Rhythmus trägt Leben* (Weiz, Austria: Joanneum Research Instittue für Nichtinvasive Diagnostik, 2003). R. E. Kleiger, J. P. Miller, J. T. Bigger, et al., and the Multicenter Post Infarction Research Group, "Decreased Heart Rate Variability and Its Association with Increased Mortality after Acute Myocardial Infarction," *American Journal of Cardiology* 59 (1987): 256–262.

257. D. F. Kripke, L. Garfinkel, D. L. Wingard, M. R. Klauber, and M. R. Marler, "Mortality Associated with Sleep Duration and Insomnia," *Arch Gen Psychiatry* 59, no. 2 (2002): 131–6. G. Belleville, "Mortality Hazard Associated with Anxiolytic and Hypnotic Drug Use in the National Population Health Survey," *Canadian Journal of Psychiatry* 55, no. 9 (2010): 558–567

258. J. Kabat-Zinn, *Full Catastrophe Living* (New York: Delacorte Press, 1990). D. D. Burns, *Feeling Good: The New Mood Therapy—Revised and Updated* (New York: Harper, 1999).

259. N. Cousins, *Anatomy of an Illness as Perceived by the Patient* (New York: W.W. Norton, 2005).

260. To stroke the legs, you need to sit up and bend down toward your legs since it is impossible to do while lying flat on your back. Alternatively, roll to the side and bring your knees up as you stroke down your legs.

261. R. Pollycove and N. Faass, *The Pocket Idiot's Guide to Bioidentical Hormones* (New York: Alpha/Penguin, 2010).

262. H. Bettermann, D. von Bonin, M. Frühwirth, and M. Moser, "Effects of Speech Therapy with Poetry on Heart Rate Rhythmicity and Cardiorespiratory Coordination," *International Journal of Cardiology* 84 (2002): 77–88. D. Campbell, *Die Heilkraft der Musik: Klänge für Körper und Seele* (Munich: Droemersche Verlagsanstalt, 1998). D. Cysarz, D. von Bonin, H. Lackner, P. Heusser, M. Moser, and H. Bettermann, "Oscillations of Heart Rate and Respiration Synchronize during Poetry Recitation," *Am J Physiol Heart Circ Physiol* 287 (2004): H579–87. G. Hildebrandt, M. Moser, and M. Lehofer, *Chronobiologie und Chronomedizin: Kurzgefaßtes Lehr- und Arbeitsbuch* (Hippokrates Verlag, 1998). Joanneumresearch, available at www.joanneum.at/ind. H. R. Maturana and F. J. Varela, 1980, "Autopoiesis and Cognition: The Realization of the Living," *Boston Studies in the Philosophy of Science* 42 (1980). M. Moser, 1999, "Zwischen Chaos und Ordnung: Überlegungen zur Entstehung von Gestalt und Form" in *Chaostheorie und Medizin: Selbstorganisation im komplexen System Mensch,* ed. Karl Toifl. M. Moser, D. v. Bonin, M. Frühwirth, J. Herfert, H. Lackner, F. Muhry, and C. Puelacher, "Luftkunst: Von der Fähigkeit, mit dem Atem das Herz und den Körper zum Klingen zu bringen," in *Luft: Elemente des Naturhaushalts, 4, Kunst- und Ausstellungshalle der BRD,* ed. S. Forum, 2003. M. Moser, M. Frühwirth, D. von Bonin, D. Cysarz, R. Penter, C. Heckmann, and G. Hildebrandt, *Das autonome (autochrone) Bild als Methode zur Darstellung der Rhythmen des menschlichen Herzschlags: Hygiogenese* (Bern: Peter Heusser, 1999).

M. Moser, M. Lehofer, G. Hildebrandt, M. Voica, S. Egner, and T. Kenner, "Phase- and Frequency Coordination of Cardiac and Respiratory Function," *Biological Rhythm Research* 26, no. 1 (1994): 100–111. M. Moser, M. Lehofer, A. Sedminek, M. Lux, H. G. Zapotoczky, T. Kenner, and A. Noordergraaf, "Heart Rate Variability as a Prognostic Tool in Cardiology," *Circulation* 90 (1994): 1078–1082. J. Newman, J. H. Rosenbach, K. L. Burns, B. C. Latimer, H. R. Matocha, and E. R. Vogt, "An Experimental Test of 'the Mozart effect': Does Listening to His Music Improve Spatial Ability?" *Percept Mot Skills* 81 (1995): 1379–87. Novalis, *Die Enzyklopädie: Die Philosophischen Wissenschaften*, 1798/1799. F. Raschke, *Die Kopplung zwischen Herzschlag und Atmung beim Menschen* (Phillips-Universität Marburg/Lahn, 1981). F. H. Rauscher and G. L. Shaw, "Key Components of the Mozart Effect," *Percept Mot Skills* 86 (1998): 835–41. F. H. Rauscher, G. L. Shaw, and K. N. Ky, "Listening to Mozart Enhances Spatial-Temporal Reasoning: Towards a Neurophysiological Basis," *Neurosci Lett* 185 (1995): 44–7. A. Schulenburg, M. Frühwirth, and M. Moser, unpusblished observations, 1999. S. Strogatz, *Synchron: Vom rätselhaften Rhythmus der Natur* (Berlin: Berlin Verlag, 2004).

Chapter 11

263. E. Easwaran, *Dialogue with Death* (Tomales, CA: Nilgiri Press, 1981).

264. L. LeShan, *Cancer as a Turning Point* (New York: Plume, 1999).

265. E. Green, A. Green, and D. Walters, "Voluntary Control of Internal States: Psychological and Physiological," *Journal of Transpersonal Psychology* 1 (1970): 1–26. See also E. Green and A. Green, *Beyond Biofeedback* (New York: Knoll, 1989).

266. S. Folkman and J. T. Moskowitz, "Stress, Positive Emotion, and Coping," *Current Directions in Psychological Science* 9 (2000): 115–118. J. T. Moskowitz, "Positive Affect Predicts Lower Risk of AIDS Mortality," *Psychosomatic Medicine* 65 (2003): 620–626.

267. R. Daniel, *The Cancer Directory* (London: HarperCollins, 2005). C. Hirschberg and M. Barasch, *Remarkable Recovery: What Extraordinary Healings Tell Us about Getting Well and Staying Well* (Darby, PA: Diane Publishing Company, 1999).

268. N. Cousins, *Anatomy of an Illness as Perceived by the Patient* (New York: W.W. Norton, 2005).

269. D. C. McClelland and C. Kirshnit, "The Effect of Motivational Arousal through Films on Salivary Immunoglobulin A," *Psychology and Health* 1, no. 2 (1988): 31–52.

270. V. E. Wilson and E. Peper, "The Effects of Upright and Slumped Postures on the Generation of Positive and Negative Thoughts," *Applied Psychophysiology and Biofeedback* 29, no. 3 (2004): 189–195.

271. R. Thayer, *The Origin of Everyday Moods* (New York: Oxford University Press, 1966).

272. One of the best resources on how to talk to yourself is the wonderful little book that launched this entire concept: D. D. Burns, *Feeling Good: The New Mood Therapy* (New York: Harper, 1999).

273. Adapted from the teaching of therapeutic touch by Dora Kunz. Some of her wisdom is published in D. Kunz, *Spiritual Aspects of the Healing Arts* (Wheaton, IL: Quest Books, 1985).

274. Adapted from a lecture by Martin Seligman, PhD, presented at TED, February 2004, available at www.ted.com/index.php/talks/martin_seligman_on_the_state_of_psychology.html.

275. R. J. Davidson, J. Kabat-Zinn, J. Schumacher, M. Rosenkranz, D. Muller, S. F. Santorelli, F. Urbanowski, A. Harrington, K. Bonus, and J. F. Sheridan, "Alterations in Brain and Immune Function Produced by Mindfulness Meditation," *Psychosomatic Medicine* 65, no. 4 (2003): 564–570.

276. S. James, "Steven James' Totally Subjective, Non-Scientific Guide to Illness and Health: Ten Step Programs," in *Surviving and Thriving with Aids: Hints for the Newly Diagnosed,* ed. M. Callen (1987). See also M. Callen, *Surviving AIDS* (New York: Perennial, 1991).

Chapter 12

277. E. Peper and M. MacHose, "Symptom Prescription: Inducing Anxiety by 70% Exhalation," *Biofeedback and Self-Regulation* 18, no. 3 (1993): 133–139.

278. J. K. Kiecolt-Glaser, P. T. Marucha, A. M. Mercado, W. B. Malarkey, and R. Glaser, "Slowing of Wound Healing by Psychological Stress," *Lancet* 346, no. 8984 (1995): 1194–1196. L. Vileikyte, "Stress and Wound Healing," *Clinics in Dermatology* 25, no. 1 (2009): 49–55.

279. E. Peper, V. E. Wilson, J. Gunkelman, M. Kawakami, M. Sata, W. Barton, and J. Johnston, "Tongue Piercing by a Yogi: QEEG Observations," *Applied Psychophysiology and Biofeedback* 34, no. 4 (2006): 331–338.

Chapter 13

280. In many cases our moods improve when we do some physical movement. See R. E. Thayer, *The Origin of Everyday Moods* (New York: Oxford University Press, 1996).

281. Adapted from practice taught by V. E. Wilson.

282. Adapted from the practices described in E. Peper, K. H. Gibney, and C. Holt, *Make Health Happen: Training Yourself to Create Wellness* (Dubuque, IA: Kendall-Hunt, 2002).

Chapter 14

283. Many patients after treatment will automatically avoid the location and any associations to the place where they received treatment. Almost any cue associated with the cancer, the diagnostic procedures, or the cancer treatment tends to evoke worry and fear. Patients have been conditioned that any thought, association, or symbol associated with the treatment will tend to trigger panic. Just thinking I have to go there for a follow-up will trigger fear and anxiety. This occurs even though the treatment has been beneficial. The trauma induced by cancer treatment can be debilitating, as between 4 and 19 percent of all cancer patients develop post traumatic stress as a result of the experience of the horrendous treatment; L. J. Kwekeboom and S. J. Seng, "Recognizing and Responding to Post-Traumatic Stress Disorder in People with Cancer," *Oncology Nursing Forum* 29, no. 4 (2002): 643–649. J. K. Kiecolt-Glaser, P. T. Marucha, A. M. Mercado, W. B. Malarkey, and R. Glaser, "Slowing of Wound Healing by Psychological Stress," *Lancet* 346, no. 8984 (1995): 1194–1196. National Cancer Institute, US National Institutes of Health, Post-traumatic Stress Disorder (PDQ®), www.cancer.gov/cancertopics/pdq/support-ivecare/post-traumatic-stress/Patient/page2. M. Y. Smith, W. H. Redd, C. Peyser, and D. Vogl, "Post-traumatic Stress Disorder in Cancer: A Review," *Psycho-Oncology* 8, no. 6 (1999): 521–537.

284. O. C. Simonton, S. Matthews-Simonton, and J. L. Creighton, *Getting Well Again* (New York: Bantam Books, 1992 [1978]). J. Achterberg and G. F. Lawlis, *Imagery of Cancer* (Champaign, IL: Institute for Personality and Ability Testing, 1978).

Chapter 15

285. P. Enck, F. Benedetti, and M. Schedlowski, "New Insights into the Placebo and Nocebo Responses," *Neuron* 59, no. 2 (2009): 195–206. H. A. Guess, A. Kleinman, J. W. Kusek, and L. W. Engel, eds., *The Science of the Placebo: Toward an Interdisciplinary Research Agenda* (London: BMJ Books, 2002). D. E. Moerman and W. B. Jonas, "Deconstructing the Placebo Effect and Finding the Meaning Response," *Annals of Internal Medicine* 136, no. 6 (2002): 471–476.

286. Available at www.washingtonpost.com/ac2/wp-dyn/A2709-2002Apr29.

287. F. Benedetti, "The Placebo and Nocebo Effect: How the Therapist's Words Act on the Patient's Brain," *Karger Gazette* 69 (2007): 7–9.

288. E. M. Sternberg, *Healing Spaces: The Science of Place and Well-Being* (Cambridge, MA: Harvard University Press, 2009).

289. J. Groopman, *The Anatomy of Hope* (New York: Random House, 2004), xiv–xvii.

290. N. Cousins, *Head First: The Biology of Hope* (New York: E.P. Dutton, 1989).

291. R. van Overbruggen, *Healing Psyche* (Charleston, SC: BookSurge, 2006).

292. P. Norris and G. Porter, *I Choose Life* (Walpole, NH: Stillpoint Publishing, 1985).

Appendix A

293. One of the best books describing the challenges in making choices and the broad range of legitimate treatment options available is M. Lerner, *Choices in Healing* (Cambridge: MIT Press, 1994). See also www.commonweal .org/pubs/ choices-healing.html.

294. This process can be equally effective when you talk through it or discuss it with a compassionate friend or family member who is open to explore options.

Index

About the Authors

ROBERT GORTER earned his medical degree at the University of Amsterdam Medical School in the Netherlands in 1973. The same year he completed specialty training in anthroposophical medicine, with an emphasis on oncology, in Switzerland. From 1974–1982, he was in private practice in Amsterdam and from 1983–1986 he received post-doctoral training at the University of California San Francisco (UCSF) Medical School. Dr. Gorter was a full UCSF faculty member from 1986 to 2008. He earned a PhD from the University of Witten/Herdecke in Germany, where from 1992–1993 he was Vice Dean and where he continues to serve as a faculty member. In the 1980s he was a physician and researcher on AIDS at San Francisco General Hospital in the world-renowned Ward 86. Subsequently, for four years, Dr. Gorter was medical director of the Department of AIDS Epidemiology and Biostatistics at UCSF. In 1993 he founded the European Institute for Oncological and Immunological Research in Berlin, which he oversaw until 2000. In 2000 he founded the Medical Center Cologne, dedicated to the treatment of cancer using dendritic cell vaccinations and adult mesenchymal stem cells in combination with immune supportive therapies and hyperthermia, and has been its director since then. Dr. Gorter has written numerous articles and abstracts, contributed to many books, and been featured on ABC, CNN, and numerous television programs in the EU and in the Middle East.

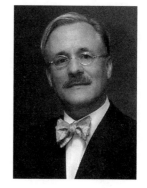

ERIK PEPER is an internationally known expert on holistic health, stress management, and biofeedback. He received his BA from Harvard University in 1968 and his PhD in psychology from Union Graduate Institute in 1975. Since 1976 he has taught at San Francisco State University (SFSU), where he was instrumental in establishing the Institute for Holistic Health Studies, the first holistic health program at a public university in the U.S. Dr. Peper is president of the Biofeedback Foundation of Europe, former president of the Association for Applied Psychophysiology and Biofeedback and of the Biofeedback Society of California, and was the sports psychologist for the U.S. Olympic Gymnastic Team for four years. He received a State of California Governor's Employee Safety Award in 2004 for his contributions to improving workplace health for computer users. Dr. Peper lectures and teaches frequently all over the world and runs a biofeedback practice at BiofeedbackHealth in Berkeley, California. A recognized expert on stress management and workplace health and the author of numerous books and articles, he has been the editor of *Psychophysiology Today* since 2004 and has been featured on ABCNews.com and in *GQ, Glamour, Men's Health, Reader's Digest,* the *San Francisco Chronicle, Shape,* and *Women's Health.*

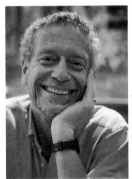

Photo by Jana Asenbrennerova